ORTHOPEDIC PHYSICAL ASSESSMENT ATLAS AND VIDEO

SELECTED SPECIAL TESTS AND MOVEMENTS

ORTHOPEDIC PHYSICAL ASSESSMENT ATLAS AND VIDEO

SELECTED SPECIAL TESTS AND MOVEMENTS

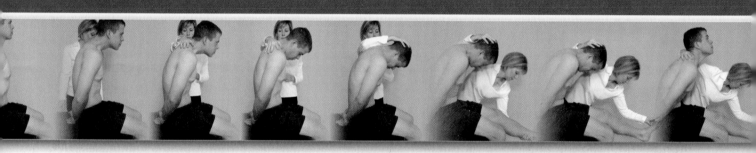

David J. Magee, PhD, BPT

Professor and Associate Dean
Department of Physical Therapy
Faculty of Rehabilitation Medicine
University of Alberta
Edmonton, Alberta, Canada

Derrick Sueki, DPT, GCPT, OCS

Adjunct Orthopedic Faculty
Mount St. Mary's College
Los Angeles, California
Owner and President
Knight Physical Therapy Inc
Garden Grove, California

Video narration by **Judy Chepeha, BScPT, MScPT,** Assistant Professor, Department of Physical Therapy, University of Alberta, Edmonton, Alberta, Canada

ELSEVIER
SAUNDERS

3251 Riverport Lane
St. Louis, Missouri 63043

Notices

Knowledge and best practice in this field are constantly changing. As new research and experience broaden our understanding, changes in research methods, professional practices, or medical treatment may become necessary.

Practitioners and researchers must always rely on their own experience and knowledge in evaluating and using any information, methods, compounds, or experiments described herein. In using such information or methods they should be mindful of their own safety and the safety of others, including parties for whom they have a professional responsibility.

With respect to any drug or pharmaceutical products identified, readers are advised to check the most current information provided (i) on procedures featured or (ii) by the manufacturer of each product to be administered, to verify the recommended dose or formula, the method and duration of administration, and contraindications. It is the responsibility of practitioners, relying on their own experience and knowledge of their patients, to make diagnoses, to determine dosages and the best treatment for each individual patient, and to take all appropriate safety precautions.

To the fullest extent of the law, neither the Publisher nor the authors, contributors, or editors, assume any liability for any injury and/or damage to persons or property as a matter of products liability, negligence or otherwise, or from any use or operation of any methods, products, instructions, or ideas contained in the material herein.

Acquisitions Editor: Kathy Falk
Developmental Editor: Bev Evjen
Publishing Services Manager: Julie Eddy
Project Manager: Rich Barber
Design Direction: Amy Buxton

Printed in the United States of America

Last digit is the print number: 9 8 7 6 5 4 3 2 1

PREFACE

Orthopedic Physical Assessment Atlas and Video: Selected Special Tests and Movements was developed to provide students and clinicians with a means of seeing the movements and tests most commonly used in an orthopedic examination. With a still picture, specific motions and details of an assessment technique often may be overlooked or missed. Building on the content in *Orthopedic Physical Assessment*, this text provides succinct step-by-step guidance for evaluating movements and performing the most common special tests in musculoskeletal assessment. Full-color clinical photographs and illustrations in the atlas are supplemented by detailed video demonstrations of tests and procedures. A quick reference table of contents for the video clips helps match the video clips to the atlas content.

The reader should note that this atlas and video are not meant to replace the text, *Orthopedic Physical Assessment*, but instead they are meant to serve as an adjunct to the text. The atlas and video are not intended to cover all aspects of a musculoskeletal assessment. Key elements, such as the History, Observation, and other parts of the orthopedic examination detailed in *Orthopedic Physical Assessment* are not included in the atlas. In addition, some regions of the body are also not covered.

This manual is the culmination of the work of several individuals. In particular, we would like to thank:

Bev Evjen, our irreplaceable developmental editor, friend, and "security blanket"
Judy Chepeha and Carolyn Crowell, the models for the video
Don Spence, director, producer, and video editor
Richard Gustavsen, cameraman
Randy Tomiuk, camerman
Judy Sara, our secretary
Kathy Falk, Christie Hart, Rich Barber, and the production people at Elsevier

David Magee
Derrick Sueki

Atlas Contents

DVD Contents

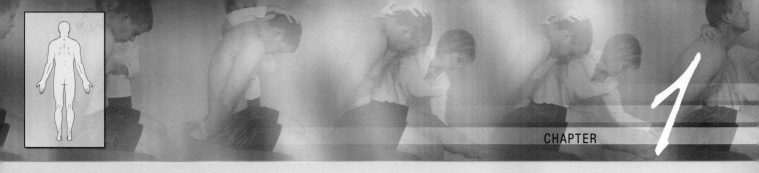

GENERAL PRINCIPLES AND CONCEPTS OF SELECTED MOVEMENTS AND SPECIAL TESTS

Principles of Movement Examination

- Before beginning the physical examination, the examiner should have a working hypothesis on which to base the assessment. If you cannot make a preliminary diagnosis from the history, supplemented by observation, before you begin the examination, either you have not asked enough questions or you have not asked the right questions.
- Communication and rapport are essential to gaining a patient's trust. The patient has the right to be informed about all aspects of the examination process. Be sure to tell the patient what you are doing and to explain clearly what you want the patient to do and why it is necessary.
- Unless bilateral movement is required, you should test the normal (uninvolved) side first. Testing the normal side first allows the examiner to establish a baseline for normal movement of the joint being tested. It also demonstrates to the patient what to expect, which increases the patient's confidence and eases the patient's apprehension when the injured side is tested.
- In comparing the normal and injured limbs, you must use the same testing methods for both limbs. This means using the same initial starting position and applying the same amount of gentle force at the same point or throughout the range. You should note the position at which any changes occur.
- The patient performs active movements before you perform passive movements. Passive movements are followed by resisted isometric movements. This approach gives the examiner a better idea of what the patient thinks he or she can do before the structures are fully tested.
- You should perform any movements that are painful last, if possible, to prevent an overflow of painful symptoms to the next movement, which actually may be symptom free.

- During active movements, if the range of motion (ROM) is full, you may apply overpressure carefully to determine the end feel of the joint. This often negates the need to do passive movements.
- If active ROM is not full, you may apply overpressure but only with extreme care to prevent an exacerbation of symptoms.
- You may repeat each active, passive, or resisted isometric movement several times or hold (sustain) the contraction for a certain amount of time to see whether:
  - Symptoms increase or decrease
  - A different pattern of movement results
  - Weakness increases or indications of possible vascular insufficiency are noted
- This repetitive or sustained activity is especially important if the patient has complained that repetitive movement or sustained postures alter symptoms.
- You should do resisted isometric movements with the joint *in a neutral or resting position* so that stress on the inert tissues is minimal. Any symptoms produced by the movement then are more likely to be caused by problems with contractile tissue.
- For passive ROM or ligament testing, it is important that you determine not only the *degree* (i.e., amount) of movement, but also the *quality* (i.e., end feel) of the movement.
- When you are testing the ligaments, apply the appropriate stress gently and repeat this several times. The stress is increased up to but not beyond the point of pain, thereby demonstrating maximum instability without causing muscle spasm.
- When testing myotomes (i.e., groups of muscles supplied by a single nerve root), you should hold each contraction for a minimum of 5 seconds to see whether weakness becomes evident. Myotomal weakness takes time to develop,

1

because the muscles are supplied by more than one nerve root.

- A thorough examination often involves stressing and aggravating different tissues. At the completion of an assessment, you must warn the patient that symptoms may be exacerbated as a result of the assessment. This prevents the patient from thinking that any initial treatment may have made the condition worse, which in turn might make the patient hesitant to return for further treatment.
- Clinical decision making is a continuous process of communication, hypothesis generation, assessment, and hypothesis revision. During the examination, you will look for subjective signs and symptoms (i.e., what the patient feels) and objective signs and symptoms (i.e., what you deduce from the various tests the patient performs) and then use this information to shape your hypothesis and subsequent decisions.
- A quick scanning examination is not meant to rule in or out a particular pathologic condition. Rather, it is performed to determine whether a more thorough examination of a region is needed. A scanning examination is used in the following circumstances:
  - To rule out signs and symptoms referred distally from the spine, spinal cord, or nerve roots to other parts of the body (e.g., sciatica)
  - To help rule out problems in the spine that may be causing signs and symptoms elsewhere
  - To determine the level of the spine that is affected
  - When signs and symptoms are felt in a peripheral joint or one of the limbs but the patient has no history of injury in that area
  - When radicular signs are present
  - When the patient has no history of injury or overuse
  - When trauma with radicular signs is present
  - When altered sensation in a limb is present
  - When spinal cord ("long track") signs are present
  - When abnormal signs and symptoms are present
  - When psychological overlay is suspected
- When testing movement, you must determine whether pain or restriction is the predominant problem.

Active Movements

Active movements combine tests of joint range, motor control, muscle power, and the patient's willingness to perform the movement. During active movements, the examiner should compare the two sides and watch for:
- When and where pain occurs during each movement
- Whether movement changes the intensity and quality of the pain
- The patient's reaction to pain
- The pattern of movement:
  - Does there appear to be neural control?
  - Are the proper muscles recruited and in the proper sequence?
  - Does the movement occur at the correct speed?
  - Are the movement sequences synchronized appropriately?
  - Are the muscle force-couples functioning correctly?
- The rhythm and quality of movement
- The amount of observable restriction (i.e., freedom of movement)
- The movement of associated joints
- The patient's willingness to move

Passive Movements

Passive movements are used to determine how much ROM actually exists in a joint, as well as the "feel" at the end of the joint ROM (i.e., end feel). During passive movements, you should compare the two sides and watch for:
- When and where pain occurs during each movement
- Whether the movement changes the intensity or quality of the pain
- The pattern of limitation of movement
- The end feel of movement
- The movement of associated joints
- The ROM available:
  - What is the normal ROM for that joint and that individual?
  - Is the joint normal, hypomobile, or hypermobile?
  - Are adjacent joints compensating?
  - Which joint (or joints) is painful?

Resisted Isometric Movements

Resisted isometric movements are designed primarily to test contractile tissue (i.e., muscles, tendons, and their attachments). During resisted isometric movements, you should compare the two sides to determine:
- Whether the contraction is painful
- The strength of the contraction
- The type of contraction that causes symptoms (e.g., concentric, eccentric)
- The patient's ability to control movement (i.e., the ability to do the movement correctly)
- The way the muscle is functioning (e.g., as an agonist or a synergist)
- Whether the muscle is *weak* and long (phasic) or *tight* and strong (weak and long muscles are often considered phasic and strong; and shortened muscles are considered postural/tonic)
- Whether any muscle imbalance is present
- Whether the muscle is acting as a stabilizer or mobilizer

Special Diagnostic Tests

Special diagnostic tests are designed to confirm a diagnosis. As such, they may:
- Test specific structures (e.g., stability tests)
- Stress specific tissues

- Differentiate between tissues (e.g., for thoracic outlet syndrome)
- Provoke symptoms (e.g., provocative or neurodynamic tests)
- Relieve symptoms (e.g., distraction tests)

Points to remember about special diagnostic tests include the following:

- They depend on (1) the examiner's ability to perform the test, (2) the examiner's skill in doing the test; and (3) the patient's ability to relax.
- They should **never** be used alone or in isolation. As an examiner, you will use these tests in conjunction with other testing *to confirm a diagnosis.*
- They are most accurate (1) immediately after an injury (because of tissue shock); (2) when the patient is under anesthesia; and (3) in chronic conditions.

Special tests should be used *with caution* in the presence of:

- Severe pain
- Acute and irritable joint conditions
- Instability
- Osteoporosis
- Pathological bone diseases
- Acute active disease
- Unusual signs and symptoms
- Major neurological signs
- Patient apprehension
- Inability of the patient to understand verbal cueing, explanations, and/or instructions

Joint Play Movements

Joint play movements are accessory movements that are not under a patient's control. Normal joint play is necessary for full, painless functioning and full ROM of a joint. Joint dysfunction signifies a loss of joint play movement. When doing joint play movements, you should compare the two sides ensuring that:

- The patient is relaxed and fully supported
- You are relaxed and using a firm but comfortable grasp
- You examine one joint at a time
- You examine one movement at a time

CERVICAL SPINE

Précis of the Cervical Spine Assessment*

History (sitting)
Observation (sitting or standing)
Examination
   Active movements
      Flexion
      Extension
      Side flexion (right and left)
      Rotation (right and left)
      Combined movements (if necessary)
      Repetitive movements (if necessary)
      Sustained positions (if necessary)
   Passive movements
      Flexion (tissue stretch)†
      Extension (tissue stretch)
      Side flexion (tissue stretch)
      Rotation (tissue stretch)
   Resisted isometric movements (as in active movements but in the resting position of the joint)
   Scanning examination
      Peripheral joint scan:
         Temporomandibular joints (open mouth and closed mouth)
         Shoulder girdle (elevation through abduction, elevation through forward flexion, elevation through plane of the scapula, medial and lateral rotation with arm at side; medial and lateral rotation at 90° abduction)
         Elbow (flexion, extension, supination, pronation)
         Wrist (flexion, extension, radial and ulnar deviation)
         Fingers and thumb (flexion, extension, abduction, adduction)
      Myotomes:
         Neck flexion (C1, C2)
         Neck side flexion (C3)
         Shoulder elevation (C4)
         Shoulder abduction (C5)
         Elbow flexion (C6) and/or extension (C7)
         Wrist flexion (C7) and/or extension (C6)
         Thumb extension (C8) and/or ulnar deviation (C8)
         Hand intrinsics (abduction or adduction) (T1)
      Sensory scanning examination
   Special tests
      Foraminal compression test (Spurling's test)
      Distraction test
      Shoulder abduction test
      Vertebral artery tests
   Reflexes and cutaneous distribution
      Biceps (C5-C6)
      Triceps (C7-C8)
      Hoffmann's sign (or Babinski's test)

Examination, supine
   Passive movements
      Flexion
      Extension
      Side flexion
      Rotation
   Special tests
      Upper limb tension test
      Vertebral artery tests
   Note 1: The following tests should be performed if the examiner anticipates treating the patient by mobilization or manipulation. In this case, they are called clearing tests for treatment:
      Vertebral artery tests (supine or sitting)
      Sharp-Purser test (sitting)
      Pettman's distraction test (supine)
      Anterior shear test (supine)
      Transverse ligament stress test (supine)
      Lateral shear test (supine)
      Lateral flexion alar ligament stress test (supine)
   Note 2: If any of the previous tests are positive, mobilization or manipulation should be performed only with extreme care, and the level exhibiting the positive signs should be stabilized during the treatment.
   Joint play movements
      Side glide of cervical spine‡
      Anterior glide of cervical spine‡
      Posterior glide of cervical spine‡
      Traction glide of cervical spine‡
      Rotation of occiput on C1§
   Palpation
Examination, prone
   Joint play movements
      Posteroanterior central vertebral pressure§
      Posteroanterior unilateral vertebral pressure§
      Transverse vertebral pressure§
   Palpation
Diagnostic imaging

---

*The précis is shown in an order that limits the amount of moving the patient must do but ensures that all necessary structures are tested. After any examination, the patient should be warned that symptoms may be exacerbated as a result of the assessment.
† (end feel)
‡ Movements involve the whole cervical spine (general techniques)
§ Movements involve individual segments of the cervical spine (specific techniques)

SELECTED MOVEMENTS

ACTIVE MOVEMENTS[1-9]   DVD

GENERAL INFORMATION	While the patient performs the active movements, the examiner looks for limitation of movement and possible reasons for pain, spasm, stiffness, or blocking, and also the pattern of movement. The movements should be done in a particular order so that the most painful movements are done last; this ensures that no residual pain is carried over from the previous movement. With a very acute condition of the cervical spine, only some movements—those that give the most information—are done to prevent undue exacerbation of symptoms. As the patient reaches the full range of active movement, passive overpressure may be applied very carefully, but only if the movement appears to be full and not too painful (see discussion of passive movement later in the chapter). The overpressure helps the examiner to determine the end feel of the movement and to differentiate between physiological (active) end range and anatomical (passive) end range. The examiner must be careful when applying overpressure during rotation or any combination of rotation, side flexion, and extension. In these positions, the vertebral artery often is compressed, which can lead to a reduction in the blood supply to the brain; also, the movements can cause narrowing of the spinal and intervertebral canals.
PATIENT POSITION	The patient is sitting.
EXAMINER POSITION	The examiner is positioned directly in front of the patient so that he or she can instruct the patient, observe motion, and apply overpressure as needed.

Flexion—Upper Cervical Spine

TEST PROCEDURE	To test flexion movement in the upper cervical spine (*A*), the patient is asked to nod forward or to place the chin on the Adam's apple.
INDICATIONS OF A POSITIVE TEST	Normally, this movement is pain free. Positive test results (e.g., tingling in the feet, an electrical shock sensation down the neck [Lhermitte's sign], severe pain, nausea, and cord signs) all indicate a severe pathological condition (e.g., meningitis, tumor, dens fracture).
CLINICAL NOTES/CAUTIONS	• As the patient flexes (nods) the head, the examiner can palpate the relative movement between the mastoid and transverse process of C1 on each side, comparing the two sides for hypomobility or hypermobility between C0 and C1. The examiner also can palpate the posterior arch of C1 and the lamina of C2 during the nodding movement to compare the relative movement.
	• As the patient forward-flexes, the examiner should look for a posterior bulging of the spinous process of the axis (C2). This bulging may result from forward subluxation of the atlas, which allows the spinous process of the axis to become more prominent. If this sign appears, the examiner should exercise extreme caution during the remainder of the cervical assessment. To verify the subluxation, the Sharp-Purser test may be performed (see that test under Special Tests for Cervical Instability); however, it must be done with extreme care.
	• The mastoid process moves away from the C1 transverse process on flexion and extension.

Continued

ACTIVE MOVEMENTS[1-9]—*cont'd*

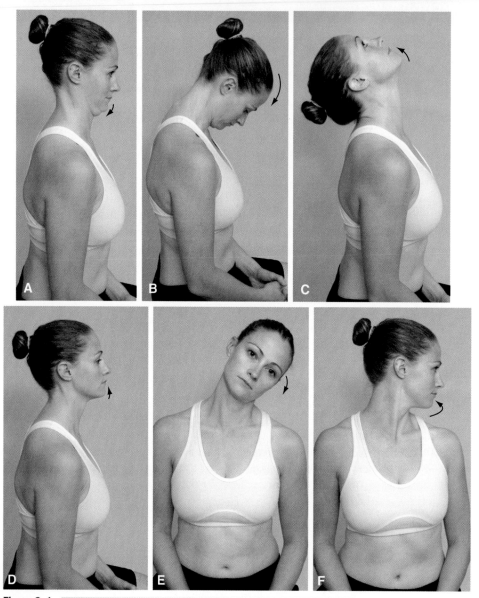

Figure 2–1
Active movements of the cervical spine. **A,** Anterior nodding (upper cervical spine). **B,** Flexion.
C, Extension. **D,** Posterior nodding (upper cervical spine). **E,** Side flexion. **F,** Rotation.

Extension—Upper Cervical Spine

TEST PROCEDURE	To test extension in the upper cervical spine, the patient is asked to nod backward or to lift the chin up without moving the neck (*D*).
INDICATIONS OF A POSITIVE TEST	Positive test results include the occurrence of pain, limited range of motion (ROM), tingling in the arms or feet, loss of balance, and drop attacks (collapsing for no apparent reason).
CLINICAL NOTE/CAUTION	• Manifestation of serious symptoms (e.g., tingling in the feet, loss of balance, drop attack) suggests spinal cord compression or vertebrobasilar dysfunction.

ACTIVE MOVEMENTS[1-9]—*cont'd*

Side Flexion/Side Bend—Upper Cervical Spine

CLINICAL NOTE	• Very little side bend occurs at the upper cervical region. Therefore, this movement is not typically part of the active movement assessment.

Rotation (Testing Rotation of C1 or C2)—Upper Cervical Spine

TEST PROCEDURE	The patient is asked to nod or to bring the chin to the Adam's apple. From this position, the patient is instructed to rotate the head left and/or right (*F*).
INDICATIONS OF A POSITIVE TEST	Normal rotation for the upper cervical spine is 45° right and left. Positive test results include the occurrence of pain, limited ROM, tingling in the arms, and loss of balance.
CLINICAL NOTE/CAUTION	• Most of the cervical rotation occurs between C1 and C2. If the patient can rotate 40° to 50°, it is unlikely that the C1-C2 articulation is at fault. However, if side flexion occurs early in the movement to allow full motion, C1-C2 probably is involved.

Flexion—Lower Cervical Spine

TEST PROCEDURE	To test flexion movement in the lower cervical spine, the patient is asked to bring the chin to the chest (*B*).
INDICATIONS OF A POSITIVE TEST	For flexion, or forward bending, of the lower cervical spine, the maximum range of motion (ROM) is 80° to 90°. The extreme of ROM normally is found if the chin is able to reach the chest with the mouth closed; however, a space of up to two finger widths between chin and chest is considered normal.
CLINICAL NOTES	• If the deep neck flexors are weak, the sternocleidomastoid muscles will initiate the flexion movement; this causes the jaw, rather than the nose, to lead the movement, because the sternocleidomastoid muscles cause the chin to elevate before flexion occurs. • In flexion, the intervertebral disc widens posteriorly and narrows anteriorly. • The intervertebral foramen is 20% to 30% larger on flexion than on extension. • The vertebrae shift forward in flexion and backward in extension.

Extension—Lower Cervical Spine

TEST PROCEDURE	To test extension in the lower cervical spine, the patient is asked to look upward as far as possible (*C*).
INDICATIONS OF A POSITIVE TEST	Extension, or backward bending, of the cervical spine usually is limited to 70°. Normally, extension is sufficient to allow the plane of the nose and forehead to be nearly horizontal.
CLINICAL NOTES/CAUTIONS	• Because no anatomical block prevents extension from going past the normal limit position, problems often result from whiplash or cervical strain. • When the head is held in extension, the atlas tilts upward, resulting in posterior compression between the atlas and occiput.

Continued

ACTIVE MOVEMENTS[1-9]—cont'd

Side Flexion/Side Bend—Lower Cervical Spine

TEST PROCEDURE	The patient is instructed to bring the ear toward the shoulder (*E*).
INDICATIONS OF A POSITIVE TEST	Side or lateral flexion is approximately 20° to 45° to the right and left.
CLINICAL NOTES	• As the patient does the movement, the examiner can palpate adjacent transverse processes on the convex side to determine relative movement at each level. • When the patient does the movement, the examiner should make sure the ear moves toward the shoulder and not the shoulder toward the ear. • As with rotation, the examiner should look for compensations that occur with the side flexion motion. The most common deviations are flexion and rotation. These compensations should be corrected and the motion retested. The end of motion is the point where these compensations begin to occur.

Rotation—Lower Cervical Spine

TEST PROCEDURE	The patient is instructed to rotate the head left or right, starting on the pain-free side (*F*).
INDICATIONS OF A POSITIVE TEST	Normally, rotation is 70° to 90° right and left, and the chin does not quite reach the plane of the shoulder.
CLINICAL NOTES	• Rotation and side flexion always occur together (coupled movement) but not necessarily in the same direction. This combined movement, which may or may not be visible in a given patient, occurs because of the coronally oblique shape of the articular surfaces of the facet joints. • As the patient rotates the head, the examiner should note when the person begins to physically side-bend the head instead of rotate it. Although rotation and side flexion are coupled movements, visually to the examiner patients should be able to do both movements individually. This is a normal compensation for lack of rotation. The patient should be instructed not to side-bend the head, and the motion should be retested. The end of the motion is the point where the compensation begins to occur.

PASSIVE MOVEMENTS[4,5,10-13]

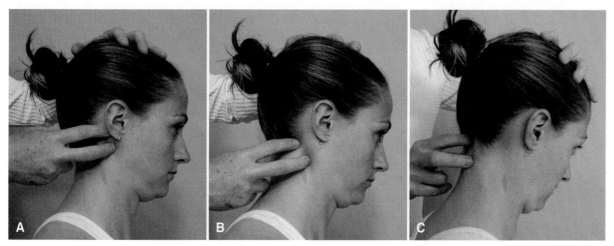

Figure 2–2
Testing passive movement in the cervical spine. **A,** Position testing for the occipitoatlantal joint.
B, Position testing for the atlantoaxial joint. **C,** Flexion testing of C2-T1.

GENERAL INFORMATION   Passive movements are performed to determine the end feel of each movement. This may give the examiner an idea of the pathological condition involved. The normal end feels of the cervical spine motions are tissue stretch for all four movements. As with active movements, the most painful movements are done last. The examiner should also note whether a capsular pattern is present (i.e., side flexion and rotation equally limited; extension less limited). Overpressure may be used to test the entire spine by testing it at the end of the ROM, or proper positioning may be used to test different parts of the cervical spine.

PATIENT POSITION   The patient is sitting or supine.

EXAMINER POSITION   The examiner generally is seated at the top of the patient's head or standing directly in front of the patient.

Flexion—Upper Cervical Spine

TEST PROCEDURE   The examiner places the pad of the index or middle finger between the mastoid process and the transverse process for movement between C0 and C1, and between the arch of C1 and the spinous process of C2 for movement between C1 and C2, to palpate between adjacent vertebrae to feel the relative amount of movement on each side. The examiner then passively flexes the patient's head and upper cervical region several times to determine the amount of movement.

INDICATIONS OF A POSITIVE TEST   A positive test result is indicated if movement occurs sooner (hypomobile) or later (hypermobile) than normal at the caudal spinal segment than in patients without a pathological condition.

CLINICAL NOTES   • The test can be performed unilaterally.
• To flex the upper cervical spine, the examiner can focus on bringing the patient's chin to the Adam's apple. A common mistake is to flex the patient's chin to the chest; this, however, tests the lower cervical region.

Continued

PASSIVE MOVEMENTS[4,5,10-13]—cont'd

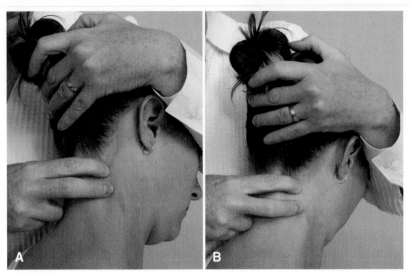

Figure 2–3
Testing passive movement in the cervical spine. **A,** Side flexion. **B,** Rotation.

Extension—Upper Cervical Spine

TEST PROCEDURE The examiner places the pad of the index or middle finger between the mastoid process and the transverse process for movement between C0 and C1, and between the arch of C1 and the spinous process of C2 for movement between C1 and C2, to palpate between adjacent vertebrae to feel the relative amount of movement on each side. The examiner then passively extends the patient's head and upper cervical region.

INDICATIONS OF A POSITIVE TEST A positive test result is indicated if movement occurs sooner (hypomobile) or later (hypermobile) at the caudal spinal segment than in a patient without a pathological condition.

CLINICAL NOTE • The test can be performed unilaterally.

Side Flexion/Side Bend—Upper Cervical Spine

TEST PROCEDURE The examiner palpates the transverse processes of C1. First the examiner must find the mastoid process on each side and then move the fingers inferiorly and anteriorly until a hard bump (i.e., the transverse process of C1) is palpated on each side (usually below the earlobe and just behind the jaw). The examiner palpates between the occiput and C1 to feel the relative amount of movement on each side. After C0-C1 motion has been tested, the fingers are moved caudally to the transverse process of C2 to test C1-C2 motion. To test side bend between the occiput (C0) and C1, the examiner holds the patient's head in position and then side-bends the head in the desired direction. Care must be taken to side-bend only at the upper cervical region. A common mistake is to side-bend the entire cervical region. The examiner side-bends the patient's head until movement is felt at the C1 transverse process. This procedure is repeated for testing of C1-C2 motion.

PASSIVE MOVEMENTS[4,5,10-13]—*cont'd*

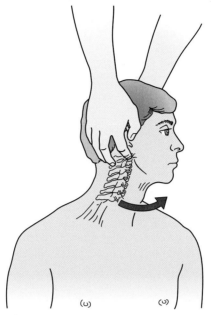

Figure 2–4
Left rotation of the occiput on C1. Note the index finger palpating the right transverse process of C1.

INDICATIONS OF A POSITIVE TEST   A positive test result is indicated by excessive or restricted motion of the head before motion occurs at the C1 (or C2) transverse process. Motion is compared to the contralateral side. If both sides are symptomatic or have motion abnormalities, the clinician must use prior clinical experience as a guide for normality.

CLINICAL NOTES   • Very little side bend occurs in the upper cervical region.
• If excessive motion occurs with this test, the examiner should suspect a pathological condition or laxity in the upper cervical region. Examiner error also may be a factor if the examiner is side-bending through the middle and lower cervical regions.

Rotation—Upper Cervical Spine

TEST PROCEDURE   The examiner palpates the transverse processes of C1. First the examiner must find the mastoid process on each side and then move the fingers inferiorly and anteriorly until a hard bump (i.e., the transverse process of C1) is palpated on each side (usually below the earlobe and just behind the jaw). The examiner palpates between the occiput (C0) and C1 to feel the relative amount of movement on each side. After C0-C1 motion has been tested, the fingers are moved caudally to the transverse process of C2 to test C1-C2 motion. To test rotation between C0 and C1, the examiner holds the patient's head in position and then rotates the head while palpating the transverse processes. Normally, the transverse process on the side to which the head is rotated seems to disappear (bottom one), whereas the transverse process on the other side (top one) seems to be accentuated. This procedure is repeated for testing of C1-C2 motion.

INDICATIONS OF A POSITIVE TEST   If the disappearance/accentuation of C1 does not occur, restriction of movement is present between C0 and C1 (or C1 and C2) on that side. Very little rotation occurs at C0-C1. In comparison, 50% of the entire cervical rotational motion occurs at C1-C2.

PASSIVE MOVEMENTS[4,5,10-13]—*cont'd*

| CLINICAL NOTES/CAUTIONS | • Movement at each segment during side flexion and rotation may be felt by palpating the adjacent transverse processes on each side while doing the movement.
• Palpation in the area of the C1 transverse process generally is painful, so care must be taken during this technique.
• With all of these movements, the end feel should be tissue stretch. |

Flexion—Lower Cervical Spine

| TEST PROCEDURE | The examiner places the pad of the index or middle finger between the spinous processes of two adjacent spinal segments (e.g., the finger is placed between the spinous processes of C3 and C4 to feel the relative movement between C3 and C4). The examiner passively flexes the patient's head and cervical region. The examiner palpates between adjacent vertebrae to feel the relative amount of movement between each spinal segment. |

| INDICATIONS OF A POSITIVE TEST | A positive test result is indicated if movement occurs sooner (hypomobile) or later (hypermobile) than in a patient without a pathological condition or relative to adjacent vertebrae. |

| CLINICAL NOTES | • The test can be performed unilaterally by placing the pads of the fingers between the transverse processes of adjacent spinal segments.
• The examiner will find that as he or she works down the spine from C2 to C7, more flexion is required to feel the movement. |

Extension—Lower Cervical Spine

| TEST PROCEDURE | The examiner places the pad of the index or middle finger between the spinous processes of two adjacent spinal segments (e.g., a finger is placed between the spinous processes of C3 and C4 to feel the relative movement between C3 and C4). The examiner passively extends the patient's head and cervical region. The examiner palpates between adjacent vertebrae to feel the relative amount of movement between each spinal segment. |

| INDICATIONS OF A POSITIVE TEST | A positive test result is indicated if movement occurs sooner (hypomobile) or later (hypermobile) than in a patient without a pathological condition or relative to adjacent vertebrae. |

| CLINICAL NOTES | • The test can be performed unilaterally by placing the pads of the fingers between the transverse processes of adjacent spinal segments.
• The examiner will find that as he or she works down the spine from C2 to C7, more extension will be required to feel the movement. |

Side Flexion/Side Bend—Lower Cervical Spine

| TEST PROCEDURE | The examiner places the pad of the index or middle finger between the transverse processes of two adjacent spinal segments (e.g., a finger is placed between the transverse processes of C3 and C4 to feel the relative movement between C3 and C4). To test side bend, the examiner holds the patient's head in position and then side-bends the patient in the desired direction. Care must be taken to side-bend only at the desired spinal level. A common mistake is to side-bend the entire cervical region. The examiner side-bends the patient's head, feeling the relative movement between the transverse processes. |

PASSIVE MOVEMENTS[4,5,10-13]—*cont'd*

INDICATIONS OF A POSITIVE TEST A comparison is made between the two sides or between other adjoining spinal segments on the same side. A positive test result is indicated if movement occurs sooner (hypomobile) or later (hypermobile) than one would normally expect or relative to adjacent vertebrae. If the joint moves sooner than anticipated, this is an indication of hypomobility. If the joint moves later than anticipated, it is an indication of hypermobility of the joint.

CLINICAL NOTE • Dysfunction is indicated if differences are noted between the two sides or between adjoining spinal segments on the same side.

Rotation—Lower Cervical Spine

TEST PROCEDURE The examiner places the pad of the index or middle finger between the transverse processes of two adjacent spinal segments (i.e., a finger is placed between the transverse processes of C3 and C4 to feel the relative movement between C3 and C4). To test rotation, the examiner holds the patient's head in position and then rotates the head while palpating the transverse processes.

INDICATIONS OF A POSITIVE TEST A comparison is made between the two sides or between other adjoining spinal segments on the same side. A positive test result is indicated if movement occurs sooner (hypomobile) or later (hypermobile) than one would normally expect or relative to adjacent vertebrae. If the joint moves sooner than anticipated, this is an indication of hypomobility. If the joint moves later than anticipated, it is an indication of hypermobility of the joint.

CLINICAL NOTES • Movement at each segment during side flexion and rotation may be felt by palpating the adjacent transverse processes on each side while doing the movement.
• With all of these movements, the end feel should be a solid tissue stretch.

RESISTED ISOMETRIC MOVEMENTS

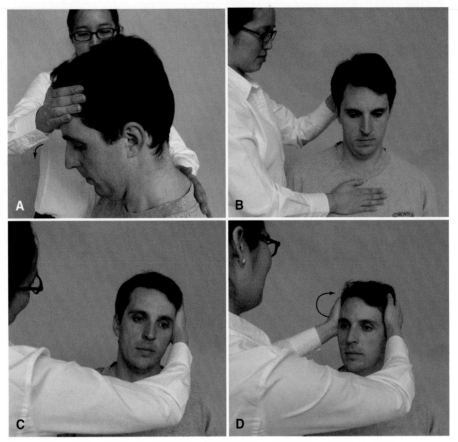

Figure 2–5
Positioning for resisted isometric movement. **A,** Flexion. Note the slight flexion of the neck before giving resistance. **B,** Extension. Note the slight flexion of the neck before giving resistance. **C,** Side flexion (left side flexion is shown). **D,** Rotation (left rotation is shown).

PURPOSE	To assess the strength of the cervical musculature.
PATIENT POSITION	The patient may be sitting or supine. The patient's head is placed in a neutral posture (i.e., no rotation, side bend, flexion, or extension with a slight nod).
EXAMINER POSITION	If the patient is sitting, the examiner is positioned directly in front of the patient. If the patient is supine, the examiner is positioned directly superior to the patient's head.
TEST PROCEDURE (SITTING)	**Flexion.** The examiner places the palm of the hand on the patient's forehead and the other hand on the patient's upper back for stabilization (*A*). **Extension.** The examiner places the palm of the hand on the patient's occipital region and the other hand on the sternum for stabilization (*B*). **Side flexion.** The examiner places the palm of the hand on the patient's temporal region and the other hand on the contralateral shoulder for stabilization (*C*). **Rotation.** The examiner places both hands on the patient's temples (*D*).

RESISTED ISOMETRIC MOVEMENTS—*cont'd*

The examiner tests resisted isometric strength by applying force to the head through the palm of the hand. The patient should be instructed, "Don't let me move you," rather than, "Contract the muscle as hard as possible." In this way, the examiner makes sure the movement is as isometric as possible and that minimal movement occurs while at the same time gauging the strength of the movement.

INDICATIONS OF A POSITIVE TEST   Weakness or pain (or both) in the cervical spine when the muscles are tested.

CLINICAL NOTES
- If the patient's history includes a complaint that certain loaded or combined movements (i.e., movements that give resistance other than gravity) are painful, the examiner should not hesitate to carefully test these movements isometrically to better determine the problem.
- The examiner should make sure these movements are done with the cervical spine in the neutral position and that painful movements are done last. Resistance to the head should be built up slowly.

PERIPHERAL JOINT SCANNING EXAMINATION

PERIPHERAL JOINT SCAN[14]

PURPOSE   The peripheral joint scan is used to rule out other, associated (peripheral) joints as a source of or a contributor to the patient's pain or dysfunction and also to note areas that may need more detailed examination. With all of the following screening tests, overpressure at the end ROM may be added to the test if active motions are pain free. Overpressure to the joint helps to further clear it of association with the patient's complaint.

SUSPECTED INJURY   Possible injury to a peripheral joint, its inert tissue support, or the muscles that move the joint; or, referral of symptoms to the joint.

PATIENT POSITION   The patient is sitting or standing.

EXAMINER POSITION   The examiner is positioned directly in front of the patient so as to instruct the patient, observe motion, and apply overpressure as needed.

Temporomandibular Joints (TMJs)

TEST PROCEDURE   The examiner first explains to the patient that he or she will place the index or little fingers in the patient's ears to feel TMJ movement. The examiner places the fingers in the patient's ears with the pulp aspect of the finger facing forward so as to feel for equality of movement of the condyles of the temporomandibular joints and for clicking or grinding in the joints. The patient is then asked to open and close the mouth.

INDICATIONS OF A POSITIVE TEST   Pain or tenderness, especially on closing the mandible, usually indicates posterior capsulitis. As the patient opens the mouth, the condyle normally moves forward. To open the mouth fully, the condyle must rotate and translate equally bilaterally. If this does not occur, mouth opening will be limited and/or deviation of the mandible will occur, indicating positive test results.

Continued

PERIPHERAL JOINT SCAN[14]—*cont'd*

CLINICAL NOTES	• The examiner should observe the patient as the person opens and closes the mouth and should watch for any deviation during the movement. • The examiner will be able to see the mandibular condyle move anteriorly (visually, it appears to move laterally) on the side of dysfunction as the patient opens the mouth.

Shoulder Girdle

TEST PROCEDURE	The examiner quickly scans this complex of joints (glenohumeral, acromioclavicular, sternoclavicular and "scapulothoracic" joints) by asking the patient to actively elevate each arm through abduction, followed by active elevation through forward flexion and elevation through the plane of the scapula (scaption). In addition, the examiner quickly tests medial and lateral rotation of each shoulder with the arm at the side and with the arm abducted to 90°.
INDICATIONS OF A POSITIVE TEST	Any pattern of restriction (movement deviations or pain production) or abnormal movement should be noted as positive test results.
CLINICAL NOTE	• If the patient is able to reach full abduction without difficulty or pain, this usually is an indication that there is no problem with the shoulder complex.

Elbow Joints

TEST PROCEDURE	The patient is asked to actively move the elbow joints through flexion, extension, supination, and pronation.
INDICATIONS OF A POSITIVE TEST	Any restriction or abnormality of movement, or abnormal signs and symptoms should be noted, because they may indicate a pathological condition and a positive test result.
CLINICAL NOTE	• The examiner also can have the patient repeat elbow flexion and extension motions while the forearm is in the fully pronated and supinated positions.

Wrist and Hand

TEST PROCEDURE	The patient actively performs flexion, extension, and radial and ulnar deviation of the wrist. Active movements (flexion, extension, abduction, adduction, and opposition) are performed for the fingers and thumb. These actions of the fingers and thumb can be accomplished by having the patient make a fist and then spread the fingers and thumb wide.
INDICATIONS OF A POSITIVE TEST	Any restriction or abnormality of movement, or abnormal signs and symptoms should be noted, because they may indicate a pathological condition and a positive test result.

MYOTOME TESTING

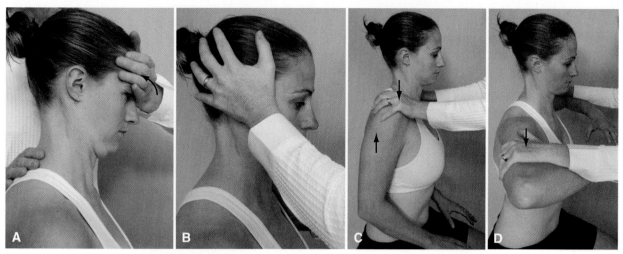

Figure 2–6

Positioning for myotome testing. **A,** Neck flexion (C1, C2). **B,** Neck side flexion to the left (C3). **C,** Shoulder elevation (C4). **D,** Shoulder abduction (C5).

Continued

PURPOSE	To assess the integrity of the cervical spine nerve roots supplying the muscles of the upper limb.
SUSPECTED INJURY	Pathological condition of the spinal nerve root.
PATIENT POSITION	The patient is sitting.
EXAMINER POSITION	The examiner is positioned directly in front of or to the side of the patient's upper extremity.
TEST PROCEDURE	Myotomes are tested by resisted *isometric* contractions with the joint at or near the resting position. As with the resisted isometric movements previously mentioned, the examiner should position the joint being tested and instruct the patient, "Don't let me move you," so that an isometric contraction is obtained. The contraction should be held *at least 5 seconds,* because myotome weakness commonly takes time to develop.

C1-C2 myotome (neck flexion). The patient's head should be slightly flexed (a nod). The examiner applies pressure to the patient's forehead while stabilizing the patient's trunk with a hand between the scapulae (*A*). The examiner should make sure the patient's neck does not extend when pressure is applied to the forehead.

C3 myotome and cranial nerve XI (neck side flexion). The examiner places one hand above the patient's ear and applies a side-flexion force to the head while stabilizing the patient's trunk with the other hand on the opposite shoulder (*B*). Both right and left side flexion must be tested.

C4 myotome and cranial nerve XI (shoulder elevation). The examiner asks the patient to elevate the shoulders to about half of full elevation. The examiner applies a downward force on both of the patient's shoulders while the patient attempts to hold them in position (*C*). The examiner should make sure the patient is not "bracing" the arms against the thighs if testing is done with the patient sitting.

Continued

MYOTOME TESTING—*cont'd*

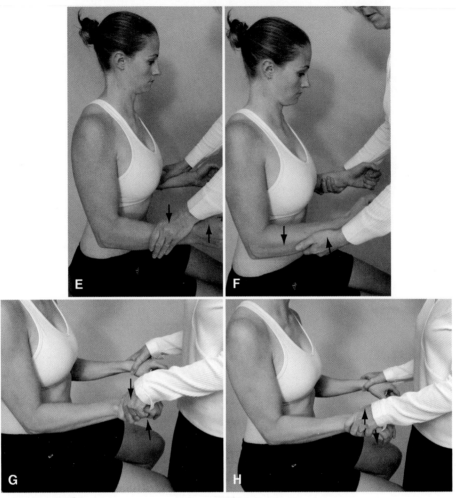

Figure 2–6 cont'd
E, Elbow flexion (C6). **F,** Elbow extension (C7). **G,** Wrist extension (C6). **H,** Wrist flexion (C7).

Continued

C5 myotome (shoulder abduction). The examiner asks the patient to elevate the arms to about 75° to 80° in the scapular plane with the elbows flexed to 90° and the forearms pronated or in neutral. The examiner applies a downward force on the humeral shaft while the patient attempts to hold the arms in position (*D*). To prevent rotation, the examiner places his or her forearms over the patient's forearms while applying pressure to the humerus.

C6 and C7 (elbow flexion and extension). The examiner asks the patient to put the arms by the sides with the elbows flexed to 90° and the forearms in neutral. The examiner applies a downward isometric force to the forearms to test the elbow flexors (C6 myotome) (*E*) and an upward isometric force to test the elbow extensors (C7 myotome) (*F*). For testing of wrist movements (extension, flexion, and ulnar deviation), the patient has the arms by the side, the elbows at 90°, the forearms pronated, and the wrists, hands, and fingers in neutral. The examiner applies a downward force to the hands to test wrist extension (C6 myotome) (*G*) and an upward force to test wrist flexion (C7 myotome) (*H*).

MYOTOME TESTING—*cont'd*

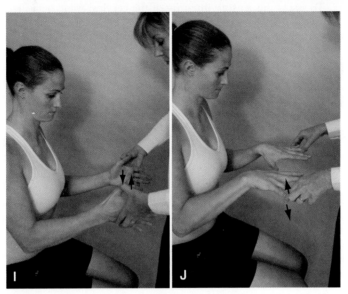

Figure 2–6 cont'd
I, Thumb extension (C8). **J,** Finger abduction (T1).

C8 myotome (thumb extension). The patient extends the thumb just short of full ROM. The examiner applies an isometric force to bring the thumb into flexion (*I*). A lateral force (radial deviation) to test ulnar deviation may also be performed to test the C8 myotome. The clinician stabilizes the patient's forearm with one hand and applies a radial deviation force to the side of the hand.

T1 myotome (finger abduction/adduction). To test hand intrinsics (T1 myotome), the examiner may have the patient squeeze a piece of paper between the fingers (usually the fourth and fifth fingers) while the examiner tries to pull it away. Alternatively, the patient may squeeze the examiner's fingers, or the patient may abduct the fingers slightly with the examiner isometrically adducting the fingers (*J*).

INDICATIONS OF A POSITIVE TEST	Delayed muscle weakness during myotome testing.
CLINICAL NOTES/CAUTIONS	• Where applicable, the two sides are tested at the same time to allow comparison. • If possible, the examiner must avoid applying pressure over the joints, because this may mask symptoms if the joints are tender.
RELIABILITY/SPECIFICITY/ SENSITIVITY	Unknown

SENSORY SCANNING EXAMINATION

PURPOSE

To assess the sensory integrity of the cervical spine nerve roots.

SUSPECTED INJURY

Pathological condition of a spinal nerve root or peripheral nerve.

PATIENT POSITION

The patient is supine or sitting with the eyes closed.

EXAMINER POSITION

The examiner is positioned directly in front of the patient.

TEST PROCEDURE

The examiner tests an area of intact sensation (e.g., the cheek) to give the patient a reference point for normal sensation. The examiner instructs the patient to compare the sensation on the cheek (or area of normal sensation) with the area that is tested. The examiner then uses very light pressure of the hands to test the patient's sensation systematically. To perform the "sensory scan," the examiner runs relaxed hands over the patient's head (sides and back); down over the shoulders, upper chest and back; and down the arms, making sure to cover all aspects of the arm.

INDICATIONS OF A POSITIVE TEST

Alterations in sensation from side to side or area to area are considered a positive test result. The examiner must be able to differentiate between the sensory areas of a nerve root (dermatome) and a peripheral nerve.

CLINICAL NOTE/CAUTION

- The examiner may use a pinwheel, pin, cotton batting, or brush (or a combination of these) to map out the exact area of sensory difference and to determine whether any sensory difference is due to a nerve root, peripheral nerve, or some other neurological deficit.

RELIABILITY/SPECIFICITY/ SENSITIVITY

Unknown

SPECIAL TESTS FOR NEUROLOGICAL SIGNS AND SYMPTOMS

Relevant Special Tests

Foraminal compression test (Spurling's test)
Maximum cervical compression test
Jackson's compression test
Distraction test
Upper limb tension tests (ULTTs) (brachial plexus tension
  or Elvey test)
Shoulder abduction (relief) test (Bakody's sign)

Definition

Nerves are sensitized structures designed to propagate electrical impulses along their axons. The axon of the nerve also functions to transmit nutrients and chemicals down its lumen. Any pathological condition that prevents the nerve from completing these activities produces varying degrees of neurological symptoms. Cervical tests for neurological symptoms fall into two categories: those designed to identify patients who have cervical radiculopathy and those designed to identify patients who have limits in the mobility of the upper extremity nerves.

Suspected Injury

With cervical radiculopathy tests, test positions are designed to narrow or open the intervertebral foramen so that an increase or a decrease in symptoms may indicate conditions such as stenosis; cervical spondylosis; osteophytes; trophic, arthritic, or inflamed facet joint pathology; a herniated disc, which also narrows the foramen; or even vertebral fractures.

The upper limb tension tests (ULTTs) and the shoulder abduction test identify patients who have limited nerve or nerve root mobility. Any pathological condition that limits the mobility of the upper extremity nerves could be a source of symptoms.

Epidemiology and Demographics

Radicular and neurological symptoms cannot be diagnosed solely on the basis of demographics or epidemiology. The neurological symptoms are a reflection of another pathological condition (that is, the nerve is damaged or irritated, but the source of the damage or irritation is another structure or a part of the injury healing process); therefore, the symptoms take on the demographics of that particular pathological condition. According to a study by Wainner et al.,[15] the prevalence of radicular symptoms was 23% in a sample of patients who underwent a standardized electrophysiological examination.

Relevant History

Patients often have a progressive history of cervical and/or arm symptoms. Each episode may manifest progressively worse symptoms and require a longer recovery time for return to the previous status. The initial mechanism of injury may be a traumatic event, such as a motor vehicle accident or a fall, often combined with degenerative changes. Repetitive activities may also be a precursor to neurological symptoms. Patients commonly complain of pain or weakness (or both) into the shoulder (anterior and posterior) or arm, especially when standing or with neck movements.

Relevant Signs and Symptoms

A common pattern for this pathological condition may or may not include the following:
- Pain in the neck, intrascapular region, or upper extremity
- Radiation of symptoms into the shoulder, elbow, or distal component of the dorsal and/or palmar aspect of the hand, depending on whether a nerve root (dorsal and palmar) or peripheral nerve (dorsal and/or palmar) is involved
- Pain, tingling, and/or numbness into the shoulder (anterior or posterior) and/or arm
- Aggravation of symptoms by neck movement or different postures
- Symptoms of short or long duration
- A history of trauma
- A patient over 40 years of age
- Limited ROM as a result of muscle spasm
- Muscle wasting/atrophy
- Joint instability
- Loss of reflexes
- Weakness (atrophy may or may not be present, depending on the amount and duration of pressure on the nerve)
- Pain associated with limited ROM of the cervical spine (usually as a result of muscle spasm)
- Sensation changes along the dermatome pattern of the suspected radiculopathy or peripheral nerve lesion

Mechanism of Injury

Trauma to the neck (e.g., a whiplash-associated disorder [WAD] type of injury, a herniated disc, or degenerative osteoarthritis [spondylosis]) can produce neurological symptoms. Trauma or degeneration leads to muscle spasm, which, combined with inflammation, can result in narrowing of the intervertebral foramen; this, in turn, leads to increased pressure on the nerve root.

Because a wide variety of pathological conditions ultimately can result in radicular or neurological symptoms, the mechanism of injury is highly variable. Injury or trauma related to extension of the cervical spine or any form of axial compression or loading may be the mechanism of injury in patients with an acute onset of symptoms. An insidious onset of symptoms may arise from a gradual buildup of symptoms involving the neck and arm over a certain period. Cervical radiculopathy is characterized by spinal nerve root dysfunction. Commonly, this is due to degenerative changes within the spine; these changes can create either a foraminal impingement on an associated cervical nerve root or an inflammatory condition around the nerve root itself. Pathological conditions such as cervical disc herniation or spondylosis also are common sources of this disorder.

RELIABILITY/SPECIFICITY/SENSITIVITY COMPARISON[15-20]

	Interrater Reliability	Intrarater Reliability	Specificity	Sensitivity
Foraminal Compression Test	Unknown	Unknown	92%	77%
Maximum Cervical Compression Test	Unknown	Unknown	Unknown	Unknown
Jackson's Compression Test	Unknown	Unknown	Unknown	Unknown
Distraction Test	0.88	Unknown	100%	43%
Upper Limb Tension Test 1	0.76	Unknown	22%	97%
Shoulder Abduction Test	Unknown	Unknown	100% neurological 80% radicular	36% neurological 31% radicular

FORAMINAL COMPRESSION TEST (SPURLING'S TEST)[15-17,21,22]

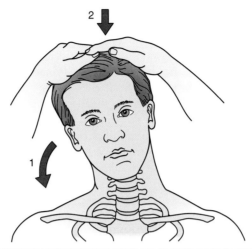

Figure 2–7

Foraminal compression test. The patient flexes the head to one side *(1)*, and the examiner presses straight down on the head *(2)*.

PURPOSE	The foraminal compression test is performed if the patient history includes a complaint of nerve root symptoms, but these symptoms are diminished or absent at the time of examination. The test is designed to provoke symptoms. It is especially useful if the patient has complained of radicular symptoms on neck movement, especially side flexion.
SUSPECTED INJURY	Cervical radiculopathy
PATIENT POSITION	The patient is sitting.
EXAMINER POSITION	The examiner stands slightly behind the patient.
TEST PROCEDURE	The patient bends or side-flexes the head to the unaffected side first and then to the affected side. The examiner places both hands on the top of the patient's head. The examiner then carefully presses straight down on the head, noting any manifestation of or change in signs and symptoms.
INDICATIONS OF A POSITIVE TEST	A positive test result is indicated if pain radiates into the arm (dermatome) during compression to the side to which the head is side flexed. The pain indicates pressure on a nerve root (cervical radiculitis). Neck pain with no radiation into the shoulder or arm does not constitute a positive test result.

Continued

FORAMINAL COMPRESSION TEST (SPURLING'S TEST)[15-17,21,22]—cont'd

CLINICAL NOTES/CAUTIONS

- Bradley et al.[22] advocated doing this test in three stages, each of which is increasingly provocative; if symptoms are produced, the examiner does not proceed to the next stage. The first stage involves compression with the head in neutral. The second stage involves compression with the head in extension. The final stage involves compression with the head in extension and rotation to the unaffected side. If this is negative, compression with the head in extension and rotation to the affected side is tested.
- Radiculitis implies pain in the dermatomal distribution of the affected nerve root.
- If pain is felt in the side opposite that to which the head is taken, this is called a reverse Spurling's sign. It indicates muscle spasm in conditions such as tension myalgia.
- Bilateral symptoms may indicate a myelopathy.
- A common clinical mistake is to pull the head into further rotation and extension when loading the spine. Instead, the force should be compressive with no further rotation or extension occurring.

RELIABILITY/SPECIFICITY/ SENSITIVITY[16,17]

Reliability range: k = 0.60-0.62
Specificity range: 50% to 74%
Sensitivity range: 50% to 56%

MAXIMUM CERVICAL COMPRESSION TEST[23,24]

DVD

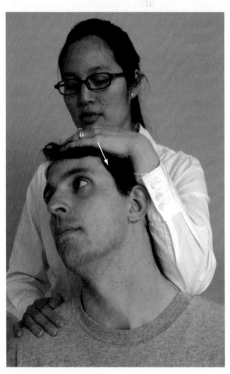

Figure 2–8
Maximum cervical compression test.

MAXIMUM CERVICAL COMPRESSION TEST[23,24]—*cont'd*

PURPOSE

The maximum cervical compression test is performed if the patient history includes a complaint of nerve root symptoms, but these symptoms are diminished or absent at the time of examination. The test is designed to provoke symptoms. This test is especially useful if the patient has complained of radicular symptoms, especially on rotation, side flexion, and/or rotation neck movements or when these movements are combined.

SUSPECTED INJURY

Cervical radiculopathy

PATIENT POSITION

The patient is sitting.

EXAMINER POSITION

The examiner stands slightly behind the patient.

TEST PROCEDURE

The side without symptoms is addressed first. The patient side-flexes the head and then rotates it to the same side. The examiner places one hand on the contralateral shoulder to stabilize the trunk and the other hand on top of the patient's head; a downward force is then applied to the head. The test is repeated on the affected side. If the head then is taken into extension (as well as side flexion and rotation) and compression is applied, the intervertebral foramen is closed maximally to the side of movement and symptoms will be accentuated.

INDICATIONS OF A POSITIVE TEST

A positive test result is pain that radiates into the arm toward which the head is side flexed during compression; this indicates pressure on a nerve root (cervical radiculitis). Pain on side towards which the neck is bent indicates a pathological condition of a nerve root if pain is felt into the dermatome. Localized cervical pain on the side towards which the head is turned may be the result of facet joint pathology. Pain experienced on the contralateral side may be indicative of a muscle strain.

CLINICAL NOTES/CAUTIONS

- The second position (side flexion, rotation, and extension) may also compress the vertebral artery. If the vertebral artery is being tested, the position should be held for 20 to 30 seconds to elicit symptoms (e.g., dizziness, nystagmus, feeling faint, nausea) that would indicate compression of the vertebral artery rather than a neurological problem.
- Neck pain with no radiation into the shoulder or arm does not constitute a positive test result.

RELIABILITY/SPECIFICITY/ SENSITIVITY

Unknown but probably similar to those for the foraminal compression test.

JACKSON'S COMPRESSION TEST[25]

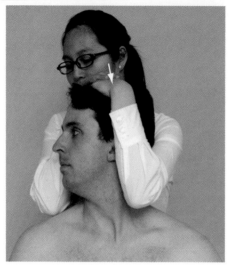

Figure 2–9
Jackson's compression test.

PURPOSE	Jackson's compression test is performed if the patient history includes a complaint of nerve root symptoms, but these symptoms are diminished or absent at the time of examination. This test is designed to provoke symptoms and is especially useful if the patient has complained of radicular symptoms with neck rotation movements.
SUSPECTED INJURY	Cervical radiculopathy
PATIENT POSITION	The patient is sitting.
EXAMINER POSITION	The examiner stands slightly behind the patient.
TEST PROCEDURE	The patient rotates the head to the uninvolved side first. The examiner then places both hands on top of the patient's head and carefully presses straight down on the head. The test is repeated with the head rotated to the involved side.
INDICATIONS OF A POSITIVE TEST	The test result is positive if pain radiates into the arm, indicating pressure on a nerve root. The pain distribution (dermatome) can give some indication of which nerve root is affected.
CLINICAL NOTE	• This test is a modification of the foraminal compression test (Spurling's test).
RELIABILITY/SPECIFICITY/ SENSITIVITY	Unknown but probably similar to those for the foraminal compression test.

DISTRACTION TEST[4,15,16]

DVD

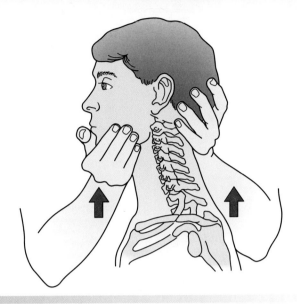

Figure 2–10
Distraction test.

PURPOSE	The distraction test is used to assess for cervical involvement in patients whose history includes a complaint of radicular symptoms and who demonstrate radicular signs (e.g., pain into a dermatome, a weak myotome) during the examination. It also may be used to help differentiate nerve root pain (cervical spine) and shoulder pain.
SUSPECTED INJURY	Cervical radiculopathy
PATIENT POSITION	The patient is sitting.
EXAMINER POSITION	The examiner stands immediately adjacent to the patient.
TEST PROCEDURE	The examiner places one hand under the patient's chin and the other hand under the occiput. The examiner then slowly lifts the patient's head, in effect applying traction to the cervical spine.
INDICATIONS OF A POSITIVE TEST	The test result is classified as positive if the pain is relieved or diminished when the head is lifted; this indicates that the pressure on nerve roots has been relieved.
CLINICAL NOTES/CAUTIONS	• If the patient abducts the arms while traction is applied, the symptoms in the shoulder often are further relieved or lessened, especially if the C4 or C5 nerve roots are involved. Nevertheless, the test findings still indicate nerve root pressure in the cervical spine, not a pathological condition of the shoulder. • Increased pain on distraction may be the result of muscle spasm, ligament sprain, muscle strain, dural irritability, or disc herniation. • It may take a few minutes for the neurological symptoms to change.
RELIABILITY/SPECIFICITY/ SENSITIVITY[15,16]	Reliability: k = 0.88 Specificity: 100% Sensitivity range: 26% to 43%

UPPER LIMB TENSION TESTS (ULTTs) (Brachial Plexus Tension or Elvey Test)[12,15,17-20,24,26,27]

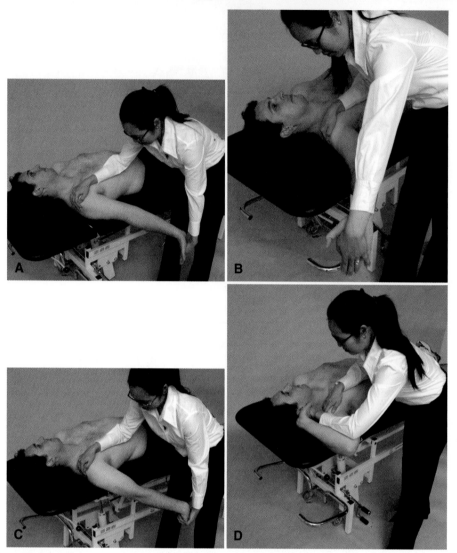

Figure 2–11
Upper limb tension tests (ULTTs) (Elvey tests). **A,** ULTT1. **B,** ULTT2. **C,** ULTT3. **D,** ULTT4.

PURPOSE   The upper limb tension tests (ULTTs) are designed to put stress or tension on the neurological structures of the upper limb, although stress actually is put on all the tissues of the upper limb. With these tests, the examiner looks for exacerbation of the patient's symptoms. The neurological tissue is differentiated by what is defined as *sensitizing* tests (e.g., neck side flexion test). This process, first described by Elvey, since has been divided into four tests to stress different peripheral nerves and the nerve roots. Modification of the position of the shoulder, elbow, forearm, wrist, and fingers places greater stress on specific nerves (nerve bias).

SUSPECTED INJURY   Limitations in upper extremity nerve mobility may occur because of trauma or degeneration anywhere along the course of the spinal cord, nerve roots, or peripheral nerves. Bilateral symptoms indicate a *myelopathy* (upper motor neuron lesion), whereas unilateral symptoms indicate *radiculopathy* (lower motor neuron lesion).

UPPER LIMB TENSION TESTS (ULTTs) (Brachial Plexus Tension or Elvey Test)[12,15,17-20,24,26,27]—cont'd

PATIENT POSITION   The patient lies supine on the treatment table. The head should be placed in a neutral position with no pillow beneath the head or knees. The legs should not be allowed to cross.

EXAMINER POSITION   The examiner is positioned directly adjacent to the shoulder being tested.

TEST PROCEDURE   The examiner decides which of the four tests would be relevant based on the patient's symptoms (Table 2-1). In each test, the unaffected side is tested first. The examiner positions the shoulder first, followed by the forearm, wrist, fingers, and, last, because of its large ROM, the elbow. This allows easier measurement of the available ROM, which can change as the condition improves or worsens. Each phase is added until neurological symptoms are produced. Once symptoms have been produced, the location of the symptoms is noted and the test is stopped. To further "sensitize" the test, side flexion of the cervical spine may be performed to further increase symptoms.

When the shoulder is positioned, it is essential to maintain shoulder depression throughout the test so that the shoulder girdle remains depressed even with abduction. If the shoulder is not held depressed, the test is less likely be effective. While the shoulder girdle is depressed, the glenohumeral joint is taken to the appropriate abduction position (110° or 10°, depending on the test), and the forearm, wrist, and fingers are taken to their appropriate end-of-range position. For example, for most of the upper limb tension tests, the fingers are extended and the wrist is in full extension, the forearm is supinated, and the elbow is extended. If symptoms are minimal or no symptoms appear, the head and cervical spine are taken into contralateral side flexion (sensitizing tests).

INDICATIONS OF A POSITIVE TEST   A positive test result is indicated by neurological symptoms along the course of the affected nerve. Because numerous structures are stressed by the test, the result should be considered positive only if (1) the patient's symptoms are reproduced; (2) a difference is noted between the unaffected side and the symptom side; or (3) the symptoms are altered by the sensitizing test (i.e., neck movements).

Table 2-1

Upper Limb Tension Tests (ULTT) Showing Order of Joint Positioning and Nerve Bias

	ULTT1	ULTT2	ULTT3	ULTT4
Shoulder	Depression and abduction (110°)	Depression and abduction (10°)	Depression and abduction (10°)	Depression and abduction (10° to 90°), hand to ear
Elbow	Extension	Extension	Extension	Flexion
Forearm	Supination	Supination	Pronation	Supination
Wrist	Extension	Extension	Flexion and ulnar deviation	Extension and radial deviation
Fingers and thumb	Extension	Extension	Flexion	Extension
Shoulder	—	Lateral rotation	Medial rotation	Lateral rotation
Cervical spine	Contralateral side flexion	Contralateral side flexion	Contralateral side flexion	Contralateral side flexion
Nerve bias	Median nerve, anterior interosseous nerve, C5, C6, C7	Median nerve, musculocutaneous nerve, axillary nerve	Radial nerve	Ulnar nerve, C8 and T1 nerve roots

Continued

UPPER LIMB TENSION TESTS (ULTTs) (Brachial Plexus Tension or Elvey Test)[12,15,17-20,24,26,27]—cont'd

CLINICAL NOTES/CAUTIONS	• These stress tests are contraindicated if the neurological signs are worsening or in the acute phase when the patient history is taken. • During tension testing, symptoms are more easily aggravated with upper limb testing than with lower limb testing. • The elbow position often is not performed until last, because the large elbow ROM is easiest to measure if the available range is being recorded to show change in the condition over time. • The tests are designed to stress tissues. In addition to the neurological tissues, they stress some contractile and inert tissues. Differentiation among the types of tissues depends on the signs and symptoms manifested.
RELIABILITY/SPECIFICITY/ SENSITIVITY[17-20]	Reliability range: k = 0.76-0.83 Specificity range: 22% to 33% Sensitivity range: 72% to 97%

SHOULDER ABDUCTION (RELIEF) TEST (BAKODY'S SIGN)[16,25,28-30]

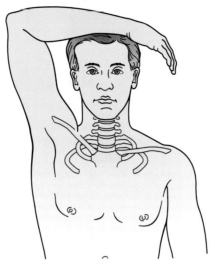

Figure 2–12
Shoulder abduction test (Bakody's sign).

PURPOSE	To test for radicular symptoms, especially those involving the C4 or C5 nerve roots. This test is especially useful if the patient has indicated in the history that putting the arm or hand on the head relieves the symptoms.
SUSPECTED INJURY	Cervical radiculopathy
PATIENT POSITION	The patient is sitting. (The patient may be tested in the supine position, but sitting appears to be more effective.)
EXAMINER POSITION	The examiner is positioned either in front of or behind the patient to allow observation of the patient abducting the arm.
TEST PROCEDURE	The examiner passively (or the patient actively) elevates the arm through abduction so that the hand or forearm rests on top of the patient's head.
INDICATIONS OF A POSITIVE TEST	A decrease in or relief of neurological symptoms indicates a cervical extradural compression problem, such as a herniated disc, epidural vein compression, or nerve root compression, usually in the C4-C5 or C5-C6 area. An increase in pain with the positioning of the arm implies that pressure is increasing in the interscalene triangle.
CLINICAL NOTES	• Differentiation is done by the dermatome (and possibly myotome) distribution of the symptoms. • Abduction of the arm reduces the length of the neurological pathway and decreases the pressure on the lower nerve roots. • It may take a few minutes for the neurological symptoms to change.
RELIABILITY/SPECIFICITY/ SENSITIVITY[16]	Specificity range: 80% to 100% Sensitivity range: 31% to 43%

SPECIAL TEST FOR VASCULAR SIGNS AND SYMPTOMS[31-33]

Relevant Special Test

Vertebral artery (cervical quadrant) test

Definition

Damage to or pressure on the vertebral artery in the neck, especially as it winds around C1 and enters the skull, can result in the loss of the artery's ability to supply blood to the brain and brain stem. Because the primary distribution of the basilar artery (formed from the vertebral arteries) is the posterior aspect of the brain, loss of blood supply affects activities controlled by the pons, medulla, thalamus, cerebellum, midbrain, and occipital region of the cortex.

Suspected Injury

Vertebrobasilar ischemia
Vertebral artery insufficiency
Vertebrobasilar circulatory disorders

Epidemiology and Demographics

In the United States, 25% of strokes occur in a vertebrobasilar distribution. Age is a factor in that the incidence of vertebrobasilar insufficiency (VBI) increases with age. The incidence is highest in individuals 60 to 70 years old. Men are more prone to VBI then women, and African Americans have a greater prevalence then Caucasians.[34-36]

Relevant History

The patient may have a history of head trauma, whiplash, a motor vehicle accident, manipulation of the upper cervical spine, or other trauma to the region. Risk factors include hypertension, diabetes, and smoking.

Relevant Signs and Symptoms (5*D*s, 3*N*s and an *A*)

- Dizziness (vertigo, giddiness, lightheadedness)
- Drop attacks (collapsing for no apparent reason)
- Diplopia
- Dysarthria (speech difficulties)
- Dysphagia (plus hoarseness/hiccups)
- Nausea
- Numbness (unilateral)
- Nystagmus
- Ataxia

Mechanism of Injury

Occlusion of the vertebral or basilar arteries can occur as a result of cervical rotation or rotation coupled with extension. Therefore, activities such as painting, yoga, backing up a car, and getting the hair washed all can lead to symptoms of vertebrobasilar insufficiency.

Dissections or acute trauma to the vessels can be the result of motor vehicle accidents, whiplash, and cervical manipulations. Head and neck positions appear to alter vertebral artery vascular flow. It has been speculated that end-range rotational activities could alter this vascular flow. The current research on cervical motion and circulation to the brain is mixed. Cadaveric studies have implicated rotation as the single movement most likely to alter blood flow. With rotation, the contralateral artery was compromised more often; however, when extension was coupled with rotation, the ipsilateral vertebral artery was involved as frequently as the contralateral vessel.

Licht et al.[37,38] conducted two studies that addressed the effect of cervical position on blood flow. They found no significant decrease in contralateral blood flow volume despite decreases in blood flow velocity. Yi-Kai et al.[39] found that vertebral artery flow decreased with extension and rotation in both the contralateral and ipsilateral vertebral arteries, with the most significant decrease occurring in the contralateral artery.

After an extensive review of studies on vertebral artery blood flow, Terrett[40] concluded that rotation with or without extension applies the most stress to the vertebral arteries, with the greatest stress to the vertebral artery occurring between the atlas and axis transverse foramina. Lateral flexion of the neck appeared to have little effect on vertebral artery blood flow.

Reliability/Specificity/Sensitivity Comparison

Unknown

VERTEBRAL ARTERY (CERVICAL QUADRANT) TEST[41-54]

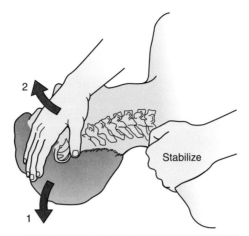

Figure 2–13
Vertebral artery (cervical quadrant) test. The examiner passively moves the patient's head and neck into extension and side flexion *(1)* and then rotation *(2)*, holding for 30 seconds.

PURPOSE	To determine the ability of the vertebral arteries to provide adequate blood flow to cortical regions of the brain when placed in certain cervical positions.
SUSPECTED INJURY	Vertebrobasilar insufficiency
PATIENT POSITION	The patient is supine.
EXAMINER POSITION	The examiner is positioned at the head of the table.
TEST PROCEDURE	If the patient history includes a complaint of arterial symptoms, the movements that are least likely to cause the symptoms are tested first. The examiner passively takes the patient's head and neck into extension and side flexion. After this movement has been achieved, the examiner rotates the patient's neck to the same side and holds it for approximately 30 seconds unless symptoms occur. Most commonly the test is done before mobilizing the cervical spine. In this case, the examiner positions the patient in the position to be mobilized, holding the end range for up to 30 seconds.
INDICATIONS OF A POSITIVE TEST	With a positive test result, referring symptoms (see Relevant Signs and Symptoms in the preceding section) are provoked if the opposite artery is affected. This test must be done with care. If dizziness or nystagmus occurs, the test is stopped immediately, because this is an indication that the vertebral arteries are being compressed and compromised.
CLINICAL NOTES/CAUTIONS	• The DeKleyn-Nieuwenhuyse test performs a similar function but involves extension and rotation rather than extension and side flexion. Both tests may be used to assess nerve root compression in the lower cervical spine, but the symptoms will be different. • To test the upper cervical spine, the examiner "pokes" the patient's chin and follows with extension, side flexion, and rotation of the cervical spine and holds the position for 30 seconds or until symptoms appear. • The vertebral artery (cervical quadrant) test is similar to Spurling's test for nerve root compression. The chief difference is that no compressive force is placed through the spine when the examiner is assessing blood flow.
RELIABILITY/SPECIFICITY/ SENSITIVITY[45]	Reliability (interrater): k = 0.90

SPECIAL TESTS FOR CERVICAL INSTABILITY

Relevant Special Tests

Sharp-Purser test
Aspinall's transverse ligament test
Transverse ligament stress test
Anterior shear or sagittal stress test
Atlantoaxial lateral (transverse) shear test
Lateral flexion alar ligament stress test
Rotational alar ligament stress test

Definition

Cervical instability is a generalized term used to define a loss of structural or muscular support or cohesiveness within the cervical region. Instability may be present in any of the cervical segments, but most special tests focus on the upper cervical region. Upper cervical instability is most commonly the result of injury or a pathological condition of the alar ligament, the transverse ligament, or the odontoid process of the upper cervical spine. The function of these structures is to stabilize the head on the neck. Injury or damage to these structures can result in instability and can risk compromise of the brain stem and spinal cord. The ligaments and their supporting musculature allow head motions while protecting the brain stem and the spinal cord as it runs through the region.

Suspected Injury

Cervical instability
Odontoid process (dens) fracture
Transverse ligament tear
Alar ligament tear
Odontoid dysplasia

Epidemiology and Demographics

In adults, 15% of all fractures of the cervical spine involve the odontoid process; in children under age 7 years, 75% of these fractures involve the odontoid.[55-57] Cervical spine subluxations are seen in 43% to 86% of patients with rheumatoid arthritis. They occur more frequently in men, even though women have a greater propensity for rheumatoid arthritis. Atlantoaxial subluxation occurs in 11% to 39% of patients with rheumatoid arthritis.[58-60] Cervical instability should be highly suspected if the patient history includes a complaint of a feeling of instability, a lump in the throat, lip paresthesia, severe headache (especially with movement), muscle spasm, nausea, or vomiting.[4]

Relevant History

In the case of trauma, no past history need be present. However, in the case of nontraumatic instability, the patient may have a history of diseases that affect ligaments or bone, such as Down's syndrome, rheumatoid arthritis, osteoporosis, or Cushing's disease.

Relevant Signs and Symptoms

The examiner may find the patient reluctant to do forward flexion if the transverse ligament or odontoid process has been damaged. The patient commonly is very hesitant to move the head or neck in any direction. When the head and neck are moved, the patient may experience the following symptoms:
• Diplopia (double vision)
• Dysarthria (difficulty speaking)
• Dysphasia (difficulty swallowing)
• Dizziness
• Drop attacks (collapsing for no apparent reason)
• Tinnitus (ringing in the ears)
• Headaches
• Blurry vision
• Nausea
• Lump in the throat
• Difficulty concentrating
• Bilateral paresthesia in the hands and feet

Mechanism of Injury

Common means of injury include motor vehicle accidents and falls that involve head trauma. Biomechanically, if the transverse ligament or odontoid process is damaged, C1 translates forward (subluxes) on C2 during upper cervical flexion. This results in spinal cord or brain stem symptoms as the posterior aspect of C1 encroaches on the spinal cord. Some have hypothesized that odontoid fractures occur as a result of trauma that involves a combination of flexion, extension, and rotation.[55,56] Although the mechanism of injury typically is trauma, some disease processes (e.g., rheumatoid arthritis, Cushing's disease, and Down's syndrome) can weaken the bone and ligaments to the point of failure or increased laxity.

Clinical Note/Caution

• The examiner should use caution when testing for upper cervical instability. Generally, these patients have significant muscle guarding in the upper cervical region, and if spinal segments truly are injured or lax, care must be taken not to injure the involved structures further. Slow, gentle motions should be used for the test.

SHARP-PURSER TEST[61]

DVD

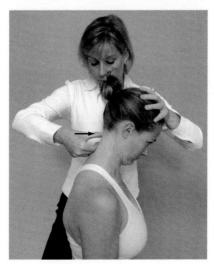

Figure 2–14
Sharp-Purser test for subluxation of the atlas on the axis.

PURPOSE	To detect subluxation of the atlas on the axis.
SUSPECTED INJURY	Cervical instability Odontoid process (dens) fracture Transverse ligament tear
PATIENT POSITION	The patient is seated.
EXAMINER POSITION	The examiner stands to the side of the patient.
TEST PROCEDURE	The examiner places one hand over the patient's forehead and then places the thumb of the other hand over the spinous process of the axis (C2) to stabilize it. The patient is asked to flex the head slowly (if instability is present, the head will slide forward on the neck). The examiner then presses backward with the palm on the patient's forehead.
INDICATIONS OF A POSITIVE TEST	A positive test result is obtained if the examiner feels the head slide backward during the flexion movement when the head is pushed backward. The slide backward indicates that the subluxation of the atlas has been reduced (indicating that the transverse ligament has been disrupted); the slide may be accompanied by a "clunk" as the odontoid process contacts the posterior aspect of the anterior part of the atlas (C1). Symptoms such as difficulty swallowing, a fullness in the throat, dizziness, difficulty speaking, and double vision all may occur when the head is flexed. These symptoms diminish when the head is pushed posteriorly.
CLINICAL NOTES/CAUTIONS	• If the odontoid process is intact, the patient may be reluctant to forward flex the head, because if the transverse ligament has been torn, the odontoid process could press against the spinal cord. • Caution should be used in testing for upper cervical instability. Generally, these patients have significant muscle guarding in the upper cervical region, and if spinal segments are truly injured or lax, care must be taken not to injure the involved structures further. Slow, gentle motions should be used for the test.
RELIABILITY/SPECIFICITY/ SENSITIVITY[61]	Specificity: 96% Sensitivity: 69%

ASPINALL'S TRANSVERSE LIGAMENT TEST[62]

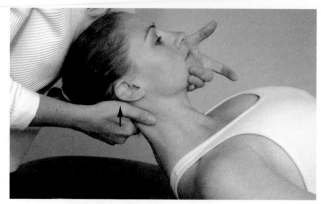

Figure 2–15
Aspinall's transverse ligament test.

PURPOSE	To detect subluxation of the atlas on the axis.
SUSPECTED INJURY	Cervical instability Odontoid process (dens) fracture Transverse ligament tear
PATIENT POSITION	The patient is supine.
EXAMINER POSITION	The examiner is positioned at the head of the table
TEST PROCEDURE	The examiner places one hand centrally on the posterior aspect of the atlas (C1). The other hand is placed over the patient's chin and is used to control cervical flexion. The examiner stabilizes the occiput on the atlas in flexion and holds the occiput in this flexed position. An anteriorly directed force then is applied to the posterior aspect of the atlas, moving the atlas (C1) forward on the axis (C2).
INDICATIONS OF A POSITIVE TEST	Normally, the patient does not perceive any movement or symptoms. A positive test result is indicated if the patient feels a lump in the throat as the atlas moves toward the esophagus; this indicates hypermobility at the atlantoaxial articulation.
CLINICAL NOTE	• Aspinall[62] advocated use of this additional test if the Sharp-Purser test produced a negative result.
RELIABILITY/SPECIFICITY/ SENSITIVITY	Unknown

TRANSVERSE LIGAMENT STRESS TEST[63,64]   DVD

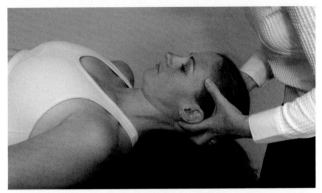

Figure 2–16
Testing the transverse ligament of C1. The examiner's hands support the head and C1.

PURPOSE	To detect subluxation of the atlas on the axis. The test detects hypermobility at the atlantoaxial articulation.
SUSPECTED INJURY	Cervical instability Odontoid process (dens) fracture Transverse ligament tear
PATIENT POSITION	The patient is supine.
EXAMINER POSITION	The examiner is positioned at the head of the table.
TEST PROCEDURE	The examiner supports the occiput (C0) with the palms and the third, fourth, and fifth fingers. The index fingers are placed in the space between the occiput and the C2 spinous process such that the index fingertips are overlying the neural arch of C1. The examiner then carefully lifts the head and C1 anteriorly together, allowing no flexion or extension. This anterior shear is normally resisted by the transverse ligament. The position is held for 10 to 20 seconds to see whether symptoms occur, indicating a positive test result.
INDICATIONS OF A POSITIVE TEST	Positive test results include a soft end feel; muscle spasm; dizziness; nausea; paresthesia of the lip, face, or limb; nystagmus; or a lump sensation in the throat
RELIABILITY/SPECIFICITY/ SENSITIVITY	Unknown

ANTERIOR SHEAR OR SAGITTAL STRESS TEST[64,65]   DVD

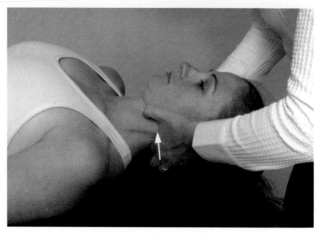

Figure 2–17
Anterior sagittal stress test.

PURPOSE	To test the integrity of the supporting ligamentous and capsular tissues of the cervical spine.
SUSPECTED INJURY	Cervical instability Cervical myelopathy Cervical spondylolisthesis
PATIENT POSITION	The patient is supine with the head in neutral position resting on the table.
EXAMINER POSITION	The examiner is positioned at the head of the table.
TEST PROCEDURE	The examiner places either the tips of the index fingers or the radial side of the second metacarpophalangeal (MCP) joint of each hand on the posterior arch or spinous process of the vertebra to be tested. Each segment may be tested individually. An anteriorly directed force then is applied through the posterior arch of C1 or the spinous processes of C2 to T1 or bilaterally through the lamina of each vertebral body. In each case, the normal end feel is tissue stretch with an abrupt stop. This procedure tests the superior segment's motion on the inferior spinal segment (e.g., posteroanterior [PA] pressure is placed on C1 to test the translation of C1 on C2).
INDICATIONS OF A POSITIVE TEST	Positive test results, especially when the upper cervical spine is tested, include nystagmus, pupillary changes, dizziness, a soft end feel, nausea, facial or lip paresthesia, and a lump sensation in the throat.
CLINICAL NOTES/CAUTIONS	• This test is designed to move an unstable superior segment anteriorly on a stable caudal segment in the cervical spine. If enough instability exists, the anterior motion results in compression of the spinal cord or the inferior portion of the brain stem. In either case, care should be taken not to injure these two structures. • Motions should be slow and controlled. Excessive force or motion is not required to produce symptoms if instability exists.
RELIABILITY/SPECIFICITY/ SENSITIVITY	Unknown

ATLANTOAXIAL LATERAL (TRANSVERSE) SHEAR TEST[63,64]

DVD

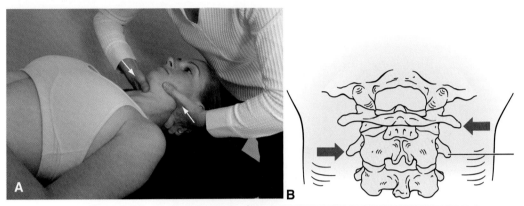

Figure 2–18

A, Atlantoaxial lateral shear test. **B,** The metacarpophalangeal joints against the transverse processes.

PURPOSE	To detect instability of the atlantoaxial articulation.
SUSPECTED INJURY	Cervical instability Odontoid process (dens) fracture Transverse ligament tear Odontoid dysplasia
PATIENT POSITION	The patient is supine with the head supported.
EXAMINER POSITION	The examiner is positioned at the head of the table.
TEST PROCEDURE	The examiner places the radial side of the second MCP joint of one hand against the transverse process of the atlas (C1) and the second MCP joint of the other hand against the opposite transverse process of the axis (C2). The examiner then carefully pushes the hands together (in a medial direction), causing a shear of one vertebra on the other (i.e., the vertebra above shears on the vertebra below). Each vertebral level can be tested in a similar fashion.
INDICATIONS OF A POSITIVE TEST	Normally, minimal motion and no symptoms (cord or vascular) are produced, although the patient may feel pain because of the pressure of the MCP joints against the transverse processes. Positive test results, especially when the upper cervical spine is tested, include nystagmus, pupillary changes, dizziness, a soft end feel, nausea, facial or lip paresthesia, and a lump sensation in the throat.
CLINICAL NOTES/CAUTIONS	• The patient should be warned before the test is performed that pain is a normal sensation, because soft tissues are compressed against bone. • This technique also can be used to test other levels of the cervical spine (e.g., C2 to C7). • Caution should be used in testing for upper cervical instability. Generally, these patients have significant muscle guarding in the upper cervical region, and if spinal segments truly are injured and lax, care must be taken not to injure the involved structures further. Slow, gentle motions should be used for the test.
RELIABILITY/SPECIFICITY/ SENSITIVITY	Unknown

LATERAL FLEXION ALAR LIGAMENT STRESS TEST[63,64,66]

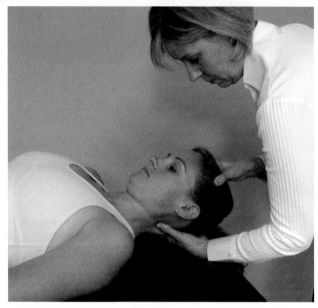

Figure 2–19
Lateral flexion alar ligament stress test. The examiner attempts to side-flex the patient's head while stabilizing the axis.

PURPOSE	To detect instability of the atlantoaxial articulation and to test the integrity of the alar ligament.
SUSPECTED INJURY	Cervical instability Odontoid process (dens) fracture Alar ligament tear Odontoid dysplasia
PATIENT POSITION	The patient is supine with the head in the physiological neutral position.
EXAMINER POSITION	The examiner is positioned at the head of the table.
TEST PROCEDURE	The examiner uses one hand to stabilize the axis (C2) with a wide pinch grip around the spinous process and lamina of C2 (this region generally is tender in a patient with instability; therefore, a firm but gentle grip is necessary). The other hand is placed on the patient's head and used to move the head on the patient's neck. The examiner attempts to side-flex the head and atlas (C1) while maintaining the axis (C2) as fixed as possible.
INDICATIONS OF A POSITIVE TEST	Normally, if the ligament is intact, minimal side flexion occurs, and the examiner notes a strong capsular end feel and solid stop. Excessive movement or reproduction of the patient's symptoms indicate a positive test result.
CLINICAL NOTES/CAUTIONS	• Caution should be used in testing for upper cervical instability. Slow, gentle motions should be used for the test. • This technique was first designed to test for upper cervical instability in patients with rheumatoid arthritis.
RELIABILITY/SPECIFICITY/ SENSITIVITY	Unknown

ROTATIONAL ALAR LIGAMENT STRESS TEST[64]

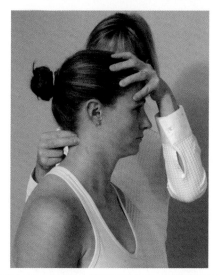

Figure 2–20

Rotational alar ligament stress test. The examiner grips the lamina of C2 with one hand and then uses the other hand to rotate the patient's head left and right.

PURPOSE	To detect instability of the atlantoaxial articulation.
SUSPECTED INJURY	Cervical instability Odontoid process (dens) fracture Alar ligament tear Odontoid dysplasia
PATIENT POSITION	The patient is sitting.
EXAMINER POSITION	The examiner stands to the side of the patient.
TEST PROCEDURE	The examiner firmly but gently grips the lamina and spinous process of C2 between the finger and thumb of one hand. The other hand is placed on top of the patient's head. While stabilizing C2, the examiner passively rotates the patient's head left or right, moving to the symptom-free side first.
INDICATIONS OF A POSITIVE TEST	More than 20° to 30° of rotation without movement of C2 indicates injury to the contralateral alar ligament, especially if the lateral flexion alar stress test result is positive in the same direction. If the excessive motion is in the opposite direction for both tests, the instability is due to an increase in the neutral zone in the joint.
CLINICAL NOTES/CAUTIONS	• Caution should be used in testing for upper cervical instability. Slow, gentle motions should be used for the test. • This technique was first designed to test for upper cervical instability in patients with rheumatoid arthritis.
RELIABILITY/SPECIFICITY/ SENSITIVITY	Unknown

SPECIAL TEST FOR MUSCLE STRENGTH

Relevant Special Test

Craniocervical flexion test

Definition

The craniocervical flexion test is done to detect a reduction in muscle strength due directly to injury to the muscles of the cervical spine, especially the deep neck flexors. Reduction of muscle strength may also be due indirectly to compensation for injury in associated areas.

Suspected Injury

Any pathological condition of the neck could result in alterations in the strength of the deep neck flexors. Muscles are designed to move joints, but they also play a protective role. A change in muscle strength is normal in patients with a cervical spine injury; however, it also may be present as compensation for a pathological condition in other regions. Injury to the muscle itself is defined as a *cervical strain.*

Epidemiology and Demographics

Neck pain affects 10% of the population in the United States at any given time. It is more common in women then in men.[67] Although the exact number of patients with altered muscle recruitment patterns is not known, it seems logical to hypothesize that many, if not all, individuals with neck pain also have altered muscle strength and endurance in the cervical deep neck flexors.

Relevant History

Most patients present with acute or chronic pain in the cervical spine or in regions associated with the cervical spine. Injury or trauma may or may not be associated with the onset of muscle symptoms. Patients also may have a history of or occupations that require repetitive motion of the neck or sustained positions (e.g., using a computer all day) that result in repetitive stress on the structures of the cervical region. Poor posture and positioning also have been suggested as contributors to neck pain and altered cervical strength.

Relevant Signs and Symptoms

- Local or generalized cervical pain
- Decreased range of cervical motion (muscle spasm)
- Upper thoracic and/or midscapular pain (possible in severe cases)
- Occipital headaches
- Symptoms that sometimes may radiate into the upper extremity, especially the scapular region

Mechanism of Injury

Injury affects muscle recruitment. This effect is seen throughout the body; inflammation, pain, and muscle guarding can change the body's neuromuscular activity. Local inflammation reduces the body's ability to voluntarily recruit a muscle. As inflammation spreads from local regions to adjacent areas, the muscles in these new areas are affected. Therefore, local muscles, such as the deep neck flexors, become weakened and have poor endurance. Because of the changes in local muscle control, a pattern emerges of weakened local stabilizer musculature and overactive global stabilizer/mobilizer muscles. The global muscles increase their activity to compensate for the lack of local muscle control. Weak or easily fatigued deep flexor muscles are commonplace in patients with a pathological condition of the neck or associated areas.

CRANIOCERVICAL FLEXION TEST[68-70]

DVD

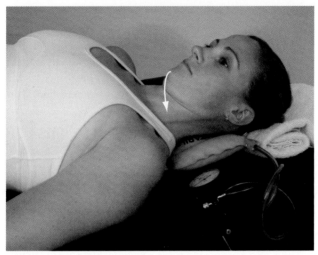

Figure 2–21
Craniocervical flexion test.

PURPOSE	To assess the strength and endurance of the deep neck flexors.
SUSPECTED INJURY	Any pathological condition of the neck may result in changes in the strength of the deep neck flexors.
PATIENT POSITION	The patient is supine in crook-lying position so that the forehead and chin are parallel to the bed (horizontal). The head should be positioned so that the craniocervical and cervical spine are in the neutral position.
EXAMINER POSITION	No patient contact is required for this test, so the examiner should be positioned where the pressure sensor can be viewed along with the patient's facial expressions.
TEST PROCEDURE	The patient's head is supported on a folded towel, and an inflatable pressure sensor is positioned behind the neck and below the occiput. The bladder is inflated just enough to fill the space between the bed and the neck, with no pressure being felt on the neck. The patient then is asked to slowly nod the chin toward the sternum and to maintain the end-range hold for 10 seconds.
INDICATIONS OF A POSITIVE TEST	The movement should increase the pressure reading by at least 10 mm Hg. Inability to do the test or to increase the pressure indicates weakness of the deep cervical flexors.
CLINICAL NOTE	• To test endurance, the test may be repeated 10 times.
RELIABILITY/SPECIFICITY/ SENSITIVITY	Unknown

SPECIAL TEST FOR FIRST RIB MOBILITY

Relevant Special Test

First rib mobility test

Definition

First rib mobility refers to joint impairment or dysfunction of the first rib. First rib impairments can be minor, such as a lack of mobility, or they can be more significant, such as a gross fracture of the rib itself. It is important that the examiner be aware that these impairments can result in upper quarter and cervical spine symptoms that can be local or radicular in nature.

Suspected Injury

First rib hypermobility
First rib hypomobility
First rib fracture
First rib dysfunction

Epidemiology and Demographics

First rib motion or mobility impairments may be more common, but their actual prevalence is not known. Exact numbers for first rib fractures were not found in the literature, but clinically they are quite rare. Nevertheless, with both shoulder and cervical injuries (especially lower cervical injuries), mobility of the ribs should be tested, because rib dysfunction may go hand in hand with lower cervical or shoulder dysfunction.

Relevant History

The past history may be unremarkable, although a history of a motor vehicle accident or trauma to the cervical spine, thorax, or shoulder may predispose a patient to altered mechanics in the region. The ROM of the cervical spine may be affected. In addition, altered respiratory patterns, along with an inability to expand the chest or engage the diaphragm, may force overwork of the accessory muscles of respiration, which also affect cervical spine and shoulder motion. These muscles attach to the first rib and may be a source of altered first rib mechanics.

Relevant Signs and Symptoms

- Upper thoracic and/or cervicothoracic pain
- Cervical tightness or pain (muscle spasm)
- Symptoms that can be exacerbated by breathing
- Symptoms that radiate into the upper extremity, including numbness, tingling, skin pallor, and changes in skin temperature
- Neurological or vascular symptoms in the upper quarter region (thoracic outlet syndrome/brachial plexus injury)

Mechanism of Injury

The condition may manifest as thoracic outlet syndrome, brachial plexus injury, or limited cervical or shoulder motion. Clinically, first rib dysfunction or first rib mobility limitations are more commonplace. Lindgren[71] postulated that the first rib is "susceptible to subluxation because it lacks a superior supporting ligament." Subluxation of the first rib may be due to the pull of the scalene muscles. If an accessory movement pattern is seen with respiration or if the scalene muscles are guarding injured cervical tissue, the mobility of the first rib may be affected. Fracture of the first rib may result from direct blows to the rib, but actual fractures are rare. This may be due partly to the smaller size of this rib compared with the other ribs and its protected position behind the clavicle. When they occur, fractures of the first rib can cause subsequent trauma to the arteries, veins, and nerves of the upper extremity. First rib dysfunction also may result from automobile accidents, which may cause either compressive or tensile forces on the first rib.

FIRST RIB MOBILITY TEST

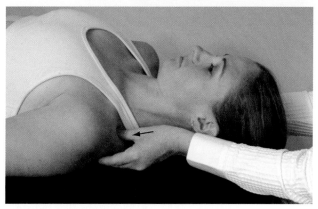

Figure 2–22
Testing the mobility of the first rib (anterior aspect).

PURPOSE	To assess the mobility and position of the first rib.
SUSPECTED INJURY	First rib dysfunction (hypomobility or hypermobility)
PATIENT POSITION	The patient is supine.
EXAMINER POSITION	The examiner is positioned at the head of the table.
TEST PROCEDURE	The examiner palpates the first rib bilaterally lateral to T1 and places the fingers along the path of the patient's ribs just posterior to the clavicles and anterior but very close to the trapezius muscle. One hand is placed on the first rib, and the other hand is used to support the patient's head. While palpating the ribs, the examiner observes the movement of both first ribs, noting any asymmetry as the patient takes a deep breath in and out. (Deep breathing involves the scalenes as accessory muscles of respiration. With deep breathing, the scalenes should pull the first rib in a cephalad direction.) Using the thumb, which may be reinforced by the other thumb, the examiner pushes the rib caudally, noting the amount of movement, the end feel, and whether pain results. The other first rib is tested in a similar fashion, and the two sides are compared. Normally, a firm tissue stretch is felt with no pain, except possibly where the examiner's thumbs are compressing soft tissue against the rib. Testing the pain-free side first, the examiner palpates the first rib and side-flexes the head to the opposite side until the rib is felt to move up. The range of neck side flexion is noted. The side flexion then is repeated on the painful side, and the results from the two sides are compared.
INDICATIONS OF A POSITIVE TEST	Asymmetry in motion between the two sides indicates a positive test result. Asymmetry may be caused by hypomobility of the first rib or tightness of the scalene muscles on the same side.
CLINICAL NOTES/CAUTIONS	• This test also may be performed with the patient prone. With the patient in the prone position, the examiner again palpates and pushes the first rib caudally. • Although the first rib normally is included in the assessment of the thoracic spine or shoulder, the examiner should always test for mobility of the first rib when examining the cervical spine, especially if side flexion is limited and pain or tenderness is present in the area of the first rib, T1, or scalenes.
RELIABILITY/SPECIFICITY/ SENSITIVITY	Unknown

JOINT PLAY MOVEMENTS

ANTERIOR-POSTERIOR GLIDE[13]

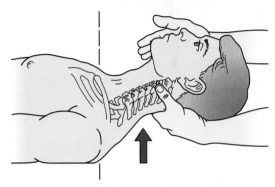

Figure 2–23
Anterior glide of the cervical spine.

PATIENT POSITION	The patient is supine.
EXAMINER POSITION	The examiner is seated or standing at the patient's head.
TEST PROCEDURE	The examiner holds the patient's head with one hand around the occiput and the other hand around the chin, making sure the patient is not choked. The examiner draws the head forward (upward) in the same plane as the shoulders for anterior glide and backward (downward) for posterior glide.
INDICATIONS OF A POSITIVE TEST	As the joint play movements are performed, the examiner should note any decreased ROM, pain, or difference in end feel. Variations or reproduction of symptoms is considered a positive test result.
CLINICAL NOTE/CAUTION	• Care should be taken to draw the head straight forward and straight backward. A common mistake is to flex and extend the head rather than to impart a direct anterior and posterior force.

SIDE GLIDE[72]

DVD

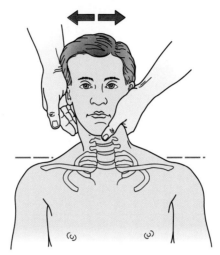

Figure 2–24
Side glide of the cervical spine (glide to the right is shown).

PATIENT POSITION	The patient is supine.
EXAMINER POSITION	The examiner is seated or standing at the patient's head.
TEST PROCEDURE	The examiner cups and supports the patient's head with both hands and then moves the head from side to side (laterally), keeping the head parallel to the shoulders.
INDICATIONS OF A POSITIVE TEST	As the movements are performed, the examiner should note any decreased ROM, pain, or difference in end feel. Variations or reproduction of symptoms is considered a positive test result.
CLINICAL NOTE/CAUTION	• While doing these movements, the examiner must prevent flexion, extension, and side bending of the head.

TRACTION GLIDE[73]

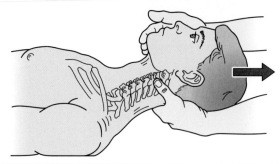

Figure 2–25
Traction glide of the cervical spine.

PATIENT POSITION	The patient is supine.
EXAMINER POSITION	The examiner is seated or standing at the patient's head.
TEST PROCEDURE	The examiner places one hand around the patient's chin and the other hand on the occiput. Traction then is applied in a straight longitudinal direction, with most of the pull occurring through the occiput.
INDICATIONS OF A POSITIVE TEST	As the movement is performed, the examiner should note any decreased ROM, pain, or difference in end feel. Variations or reproduction of symptoms is considered a positive test result.
CLINICAL NOTE/CAUTION	• While doing these movements, the examiner must keep the head in a neutral alignment.

POSTERIOR-ANTERIOR CENTRAL VERTEBRAL PRESSURE (PACVP)[74]

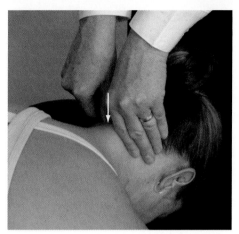

Figure 2–26
Posterior-anterior central vertebral pressure on the tip of a spinous process.

PATIENT POSITION	The patient is prone.
EXAMINER POSITION	The examiner stands at the patient's head.
TEST PROCEDURE	The examiner places the tips of both thumbs on the spinous process of the test segment (e.g., C4). Starting at the C2 spinous process and working downward to the T2 spinous process, pressure is applied through the thumbs, with the examiner pushing carefully from the shoulders. The targeted vertebra is pushed forward. The examiner must take care to apply pressure slowly, with carefully controlled movements, to "feel" the movement, which actually is minimal. This "springing test" may be repeated several times to determine the quality of the movement and the end feel.
INDICATIONS OF A POSITIVE TEST	End range can be determined by feeling the adjacent spinous process (above or below). When the adjacent spinous process begins to move, the end range of the vertebral motion for the targeted spinal segment has been reached. As the joint play movements are performed, the examiner should note any decreased ROM, pain, or difference in end feel. Variations or reproduction of symptoms is considered a positive test result.
CLINICAL NOTE	• This technique is specific to each vertebra and is applied to each vertebra in turn. • The movement of the affected vertebrae can be compared with that of the unaffected vertebrae.

POSTERIOR-ANTERIOR UNILATERAL VERTEBRAL PRESSURE (PAUVP)[74]

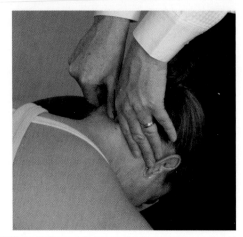

Figure 2–27
Posterior-anterior unilateral vertebral pressure on the posterior aspect of a transverse process.

PATIENT POSITION	The patient is prone.
EXAMINER POSITION	The examiner is standing at the patient's head.
TEST PROCEDURE	The examiner places the tips of both thumbs on the lamina or transverse process of the targeted spinal segment. This is about 2 to 3 cm (1 to 1.5 inches) lateral to the spinous process of each cervical vertebra. The examiner slowly and gently pushes through the soft tissue until the harder end feel of the bone or joint is felt. Starting at C1 and working downward to T2, the examiner applies pressure through the thumbs, pushing carefully from the shoulders, and the vertebra is pushed forward. The examiner must take care to apply pressure slowly, with carefully controlled movements, to "feel" the movement, which actually is minimal. This "springing test" may be repeated several times to determine the quality of the movement and the end feel.
INDICATIONS OF A POSITIVE TEST	The posterior-anterior unilateral pressure causes a minimal rotation of the vertebral body. If the spinous process were palpated during this technique, the spinous process would be felt to move to the side to which the pressure is applied. Similarly, end range can be determined by feeling the adjacent spinous process (above or below). When the adjacent spinous process begins to rotate, the end range of the vertebra to which the pressure is being applied has been reached. The two sides should be compared. As the joint play movements are performed, the examiner should note any decreased ROM, pain, or difference in end feel. Variations or reproduction of symptoms is considered a positive test result.
CLINICAL NOTE/CAUTION	• Testing of C1 often is difficult because it is tucked beneath the occiput. Unilateral pressure on C1 requires the examiner to direct the pressure in a more cephalad (45°) direction. • The movement of the affected vertebrae can be compared with that of the unaffected vertebrae.

TRANSVERSE VERTEBRAL PRESSURE (TVP)[74]

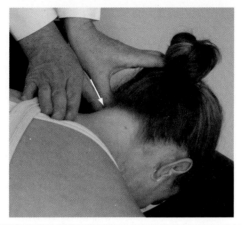

Figure 2–28
Transverse vertebral pressure on the side of a spinous process.

PATIENT POSITION   The patient is prone.

EXAMINER POSITION   The examiner stands at the patient's head.

TEST PROCEDURE   The examiner places the thumbs along the side of the spinous process of the cervical spine. Starting at C2 and working downward to T2, the examiner applies a transverse, springing pressure to the side of the spinous process, feeling for the quality of movement. Care must be taken to apply pressure slowly, with carefully controlled movements, to "feel" the movement, which actually is minimal. This "springing test" may be repeated several times to determine the quality of the movement and the end feel.

INDICATIONS OF A POSITIVE TEST   The transverse pressure causes rotation of the vertebral body, and end range can be determined by feeling for rotation of the adjacent spinous process. As the joint play movements are performed, the examiner should note any decreased ROM, pain, or difference in end feel. Variations or reproduction of symptoms is considered a positive test result.

CLINICAL NOTE/CAUTION   • This technique also can be performed with the patient in the side-lying position; however, care must be taken to maintain neutral alignment of the cervical spine. This can be accomplished through the use of pillows or a folded towel.
• The movement of the affected vertebrae can be compared with that of the unaffected vertebrae.

References

1. Youdas JW, Garrett TR, Suman VJ et al: Normal range of motion of the cervical spine: an initial goniometric study, *Phys Ther* 72:770-780, 1992.

2. Dvorak J, Antinnes JA, Panjabi M et al: Age and gender related normal motion of the cervical spine, *Spine* 17:S393-S398, 1992.

3. Neumann DA: *Kinesiology of the musculoskeletal system: foundations for physical rehabilitation,* St Louis, 2002, Mosby.

4. Dutton M: *Orthopedic examination, evaluation and intervention,* New York, 2004, McGraw Hill.

5. Petty NJ, Moore AP: *Neuromusculoskeletal examination and assessment: a handbook for therapists,* London, 1998, Churchill Livingstone.

6. Reese NB: *Muscle and sensory testing,* Philadelphia, 1999, Saunders.

7. Janda V: Muscles and cervicogenic pain syndrome. In Grant R (ed): *Physical therapy of the cervical and thoracic spine,* New York, 1988, Churchill Livingstone.

8. Kapandji IA: *The physiology of joints,* vol 3, *The trunk and the vertebral column,* New York, 1974, Churchill Livingstone.

9. Ishii T, Mukai Y, Hosono N et al: Kinematics of the cervical spine in lateral bending in vivo three-dimensional analysis, *Spine* 31:155-160, 2006.

10. Hall T, Robinson K: The flexion-rotation test and active cervical mobility: a comparative measurement study in cervicogenic headache, *Man Ther* 9:147-202, 2004.

11. Magarey ME: Examination of the cervical and thoracic spine. In Grant R (ed): *Physical therapy of the cervical and thoracic spine,* New York, 1988, Churchill Livingstone.

12. Elvey RL: The investigation of arm pain. In Boyling JD, Palastanga N (eds): *Grieve's modern manual therapy: the vertebral column,* ed 2, Edinburgh, 1994, Churchill Livingstone.

13. Magarey ME: Examination of the cervical spine. In Grieve GP (ed): *Modern manual therapy of the vertebral column,* Edinburgh, 1986, Churchill Livingstone.

14. Cyriax J: *Textbook of orthopaedic medicine,* vol 1, *Diagnosis of soft tissue lesions,* London, 1982, Baillière Tindall.

15. Wainner RS, Fritz JM, Boninger M et al: Reliability and diagnostic accuracy of the clinical examination and patient self-report measures for cervical radiculopathy, *Spine* 28:52-62, 2003.

16. Viikari-Juntura E, Porras M, Laasonen EM: Validity of clinical tests in the diagnosis of root compression in cervical disc disease, *Spine* 14:253-257, 1989.

17. Sandmark H, Nisell R: Validity of five common manual neck pain provoking tests, *Scand J Rehab Med* 27:131-136, 1995.

18. Heide BVD, Zusman AM: Pain and muscular responses to a neural tissue provocation test in the upper limb, *Man Ther* 6:154-162, 2001.

19. Coppieters M, Stappaerts K, Janssens K, Jull G: Reliability of detecting "onset of pain" and "submaximal pain" during neural provocation testing of the upper quadrant, *Physiother Res Int* 7:146-156, 2002.

20. Kleinrensink GJ, Stoeckart R, Mulder PG et al: Upper limb tension tests as tools in the diagnosis of nerve and plexus lesions: anatomical and biomechanical aspects, *Clin Biomech* 15:9-14, 2000.

21. Spurling RG, Scoville WB: Lateral rupture of the cervical intervertebral disc, *Surg Gynecol Obstet* 78:350-358, 1944.

22. Bradley JP, Tibone JE, Watkins RG: History, physical examination, and diagnostic tests for neck and upper extremity problems. In Watkins RG (ed): *The spine in sports,* St Louis, 1996, Mosby.

23. Mendel T, Wink CS, Zimny ML: Neural elements in human cervical intervertebral discs, *Spine* 17:132-135, 1992.

24. Wells P: Cervical dysfunction and shoulder problems, *Physiotherapy* 68:66-73, 1982.

25. Foreman SM, Croft AC: *Whiplash injuries: the cervical acceleration/deceleration syndrome,* Baltimore, 1988, Williams & Wilkins.

26. Butler DS: *Mobilisation of the nervous system,* Melbourne, 1991, Churchill Livingstone.

27. Slater H, Butler DS, Shacklock MO: The dynamic central nervous system: examination and assessment using tension tests. In Boyling JD, Palastanga N (eds): *Grieve's modern manual therapy: the vertebral column,* ed 2, Edinburgh, 1994, Churchill Livingstone.

28. Davidson RI, Dunn EJ, Metzmaker JN: The shoulder abduction test in the diagnosis of radicular pain in cervical extradural compressive monoradiculopathies, *Spine* 6:441-446, 1981.

29. Evans RC: *Illustrated essentials in orthopedic physical assessment,* St Louis, 1994, Mosby.

30. Farmer JC, Wisneski RJ: Cervical spine nerve root compression: an analysis of neuroforaminal pressure with varying head and arm positions, *Spine* 19:1850-1855, 1994.

31. Childs JD, Flynn TW, Fritz JM et al: Screening for vertebrobasilar insufficiency in patients with neck pain: manual therapy decision making in the presence of uncertainty, *J Orthop Sports Phys Ther* 35:300-306, 2005.

32. Kuether TA, Nesbit GM, Clark WM, Barnwell SL: Rotational vertebral artery occlusion: a mechanism of vertebrobasilar insufficiency, *Neurosurgery* 41:427-432, 1997.

33. Mitchell JA: Changes in vertebral artery blood flow following normal rotation of the cervical spine, *J Manip Physiol Ther* 26:347-351, 2003.

34. Davis JM, Zimmerman RA: Injury of the carotid and vertebral arteries, *Neuroradiology* 25:55-69, 1983.

35. Husni EA, Storer J: The syndrome of mechanical occlusion of the vertebral artery: further observations, *Angiology* 18:106-116, 1967.

36. Savitz SI, Caplan LR: Vertebrobasilar disease, *N Engl J Med* 352:2618-2626, 2005.

37. Licht PB, Christensen HW, Hoilund Carlsen PF: Is there a role for premanipulative testing before cervical manipulation? *J Manip Physiol Ther* 23:175-179, 2000.

38. Licht PB, Christensen HW, Hoilund-Carlsen PF: Carotid artery blood flow during premanipulative testing, *J Manip Physiol Ther* 25:568-572, 2002.

39. Yi-Kai L, Yun-Kun Z, Cai-Mo L, Shi-Zhen Z: Changes and implications of blood flow velocity of the vertebral artery during rotation and extension of the head, *J Manip Physiol Ther* 22:91-95, 1999.

40. Terrett A: *Current concepts in vertebrobasilar complications following spinal manipulation,* West Des Moines, Iowa, 2001, NCMIC Group.
41. Grant R: Vertebral artery testing: the Australian Physiotherapy Association protocol after 6 years, *Man Ther* 1:149-153, 1996.
42. Kunnasmaa KT, Thiel HW: Vertebral artery syndrome: a review of the literature, *J Orthop Med* 16:17-20, 1994.
43. Bolton PS, Stick PE, Lord RS: Failure of clinical tests to predict cerebral ischemia before neck manipulation, *J Manip Physiol Ther* 12:304-307, 1989.
44. Magarey ME, Rebbeck T, Coughlan B et al: Premanipulative testing of the cervical spine: review, revision and new clinical guidelines, *Man Ther* 9:95-108, 2004.
45. Rivett DA, Sharples KJ, Milburn PD: Effects of premanipulative test on vertebral artery and internal carotid artery blood flow: a pilot study, *J Manip Physiol Ther* 22:368-375, 1999.
46. Thiel H, Rix G: Is it time to stop functional premanipulation testing of the cervical spine? *Man Ther* 10:154-158, 2005.
47. Taylor AJ, Kerry R: Neck pain and headache as a result of internal carotid artery dissection: implications for manual therapists, *Man Ther* 10:73-77, 2005.
48. Arnold C, Bourassa R, Langer T, Stoneham G: Doppler studies evaluating the effect of a physical therapy screening protocol on vertebral artery blood flow, *Man Ther* 9:13-21, 2004.
49. Fast A, Zinicola DF, Marin EL: Vertebral artery damage complicating cervical manipulation, *Spine* 12:840-842, 1987.
50. Golueke P, Sclafani S, Phillips T et al: Vertebral artery injury: diagnosis and management, *J Trauma* 27:856-865, 1987.
51. Australian Physiotherapy Association: Protocol for premanipulative testing of the cervical spine, *Aust J Physiother* 34:97-100, 1988.
52. Wadsworth CT: Manual examination and treatment of the spine and extremities, Baltimore, 1988, Williams & Wilkins.
53. Maitland GD: Vertebral manipulation, London, 1973, Butterworths.
54. Ombregt L, Bisschop P, ter Veer HJ, Van de Velde T: A system of orthopedic medicine, London, 1995, Saunders.
55. Anderson LD, D'Alonzo RT: Fractures of the odontoid process of the axis, *J Bone Joint Surg Am* 56:1663-1674, 1974.
56. Levine AM, Edwards CC: Traumatic lesions of the occipitoatlantoaxial complex, *Clin Orthop Relat Res* 239:53-68, 1989.
57. Moon MS, Moon JL, Sun DH, Moon YW: Treatment of dens fractures in adults: a report of thirty-two cases, *Bull Hosp Jt Dis* 63:108-112, 2006.
58. Craig E: Rheumatoid arthritis of the spine: cervical spine trauma—upper and lower cervical spine injury, Clinical Orthopaedics, New York, 1999, Lippincott Williams & Wilkins.
59. Dvorak J, Schneider E, Saldinger P, Rahn B: Biomechanics of the craniocervical region: the alar and transverse ligaments, J Orthop Res 6:452-461, 1988.
60. Lincoln J: Case report: clinical instability of the upper cervical spine, *Man Ther* 5:41-46, 2000.
61. Uitvlugt G, Indenbaum S: Clinical assessment of atlantoaxial instability using the Sharp-Purser test, *Arthr Rheum* 31(7):918-922, 1988.
62. Aspinall W: Clinical testing for the craniovertebral hypermobility syndrome, *J Orthop Sports Phys Ther* 12:47-54, 1990.
63. Meadows JJ, Magee DJ: An overview of dizziness and vertigo for the orthopedic manual therapist. In Boyling JD, Palastanga N (eds): *Grieve's modern manual therapy: the vertebral column,* ed 2, Edinburgh, 1994, Churchill Livingstone.
64. Pettman E: Stress tests of the craniovertebral joints. In Boyling JD, Palastanga N (eds): *Grieve's modern manual therapy: the vertebral column,* ed 2, Edinburgh, 1994, Churchill Livingstone.
65. Meadows JT: *Orthopedic differential diagnosis in physical therapy: a case study approach,* New York, 1999, McGraw Hill.
66. Olson KA, Paris SV, Spohr C, Gorniak G: Radiographic assessment and reliability study of the craniovertebral side bending test, *J Man Manip Ther* 6:87-96, 1998.
67. Fejer R, Kyvik KO, Hartvigsen J: The prevalence of neck pain in the world population: a systematic critical review of the literature, *Eur Spine J* 15:834-848, 2006.
68. Falla DL, Jull GA, Hodges PW: Patients with neck pain demonstrate reduced electromyographic activity of the deep cervical flexor muscles during performance of the craniocervical flexion tests, *Spine* 29:2108-2114, 2004.
69. Jull GA: Physiotherapy management of neck pain of mechanical origin. In Giles LG, Singer KP (eds): *Clinical anatomy and management of cervical spine pain,* London, 1998, Butterworth-Heinemann.
70. Jull G, Barrett C, Magee R, Ho P: Further clinical clarification of the muscle dysfunction in cervical headache, *Cephalalgia* 19:179-185, 1999.
71. Lindgren KA: Conservative treatment of thoracic outlet syndrome: a 2-year follow-up, *Arch Phys Med Rehabil* 78:373-378, 1997.
72. Mennell JM: *Joint pain,* Boston, 1964, Little, Brown.
73. Schneider R, Gosch H, Norrell H et al: Vascular insufficiency and differential distortion of brain and cord caused by cervicomedullary football injuries, *J Neurosurg* 33:363-375, 1970.
74. Maitland GD: *Vertebral mobilization,* London, 1986, Butterworths.

CHAPTER 3

TEMPOROMANDIBULAR JOINT

Selected Movements
Active Movements
Functional Opening (Knuckle) Test
Resisted Isometric Movements

Précis of the Temporomandibular Joint Assessment*

History
Observation
Examination
Active movements
Neck flexion
Neck extension
Neck side flexion (left and right)
Neck rotation (left and right)
Extend neck by opening mouth
Assess functional opening (knuckle test)
Assess freeway space
Open mouth
Closed mouth (occlusion)
Measure protrusion of mandible
Measure retrusion of mandible
Measure lateral deviation of mandible (left and right)
Measure mandibular length

Swallowing and tongue position
Cranial nerve testing (if necessary)
Passive movements (as in active movements, if necessary)
Resisted isometric movements
Open mouth
Closed mouth (occlusion)
Lateral deviation of jaw
Special tests
Reflexes and cutaneous distribution
Joint play movements
Palpation
Diagnostic imaging

*The entire assessment usually is done with the patient sitting. After any examination, the patient should be warned that symptoms may be exacerbated as a result of the assessment.

SELECTED MOVEMENTS

ACTIVE MOVEMENTS[1]

DVD

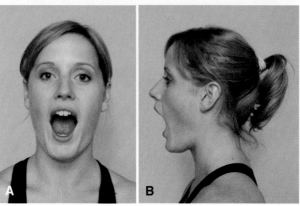

Figure 3–1
Active opening of the mouth. **A,** Anteroposterior view. **B,** Side view.

PURPOSE These movements assess the mobility and motion of the temporomandibular joint (TMJ).

SUSPECTED INJURY Temporomandibular joint dysfunction

PATIENT POSITION The patient is sitting.

EXAMINER POSITION The examiner stands or sits in front of the patient so as to observe mouth motion and range.

Mouth Opening and Closing

TEST PROCEDURE The patient is asked to open the mouth as far as possible. The first phase of opening is rotation while maintaining the tongue against the roof (hard palate) of the mouth. The second phase is translation and rotation as the condyles move along the slope of the eminence; this phase begins when the tongue loses contact with the roof of the mouth.

INDICATIONS OF A POSITIVE TEST Normally, the mandible should open and close in a straight line, provided the bilateral action of the muscles is equal and the inert tissues have normal pliability. If deviation to the left (a C-type curve) or to the right (a reverse C-type curve) occurs on opening, hypomobility is evident toward the side of the deviation; this is caused either by a displaced disc without reduction or by unilateral muscle or collagen hypomobility. If the deviation is an S-type or reverse S-type curve, the problem probably is muscular imbalance or medial displacement as the condyle "walks around" the disc on the affected side. The chin deviates toward the affected side, usually because of spasm of the pterygoid or masseter muscles or an obstruction in the joint. Early deviation on opening usually is caused by muscle spasm, whereas late deviation on opening usually is the result of capsulitis or a tight capsule. Pain or tenderness, especially on closing, indicates posterior capsulitis.

The mouth should be able to open approximately 35 to 55 mm. Generally, females have slightly more range of motion than males. Males have an average opening of 40 to 45 mm, while females have an average opening of 45 to 55 mm. If the patient has pain on opening, the examiner should also measure the amount of opening to the point of pain and compare this distance with the functional opening. If the space is less than 35 to 55 mm, the temporomandibular joints are said to be hypomobile.

ACTIVE MOVEMENTS[1]—*cont'd*

CLINICAL NOTES	• To observe any asymmetries, the examiner must make sure the patient opens and closes the mouth slowly. • Most clicking sensations occur during the second phase. Clicking is often an indication of the disc displacing as the condyle rolls and glides within the fossa. • The functional or full active opening is determined by having the patient try to place two or three flexed proximal interphalangeal joints within the mouth opening (see Functional Opening [Knuckle] Test later in the chapter). • Normally, only about 25 to 35 mm of opening is needed for everyday activity. • Kropmans et al.[2] have pointed out that for treatment purposes, at least 6 mm of change is required for a detectable difference when more than one measurement is taken or to determine the effect of treatment.

Protrusion of the Mandible

TEST PROCEDURE	The patient is asked to protrude (jut out) the lower jaw past the upper teeth.
INDICATIONS OF A POSITIVE TEST	The patient should be able to protrude without difficulty. Normal movement is greater than 7 mm, measured from the resting position to the protruded position.
CLINICAL NOTE	• Normal values vary, depending on the degree of overbite (greater movement) or underbite (less movement).

Retrusion of the Mandible

TEST PROCEDURE	The patient is asked to retrude (pull in or back) the lower jaw as far as possible
INDICATIONS OF A POSITIVE TEST	Normal movement is 3 to 4 mm.
CLINICAL NOTE	• In full retention or centric relation, the temporomandibular joint is in a close packed position. Pain with retrusion may be an indication of retrodiscal fat pad irritation.

Lateral Deviation or Excursion of the Mandible

TEST PROCEDURE	For lateral deviation, the teeth are slightly disoccluded and the patient moves the mandible laterally, first to one side and then to the other.
INDICATIONS OF A POSITIVE TEST	With the joints in the resting position, two points are picked on the upper and lower teeth that are at the same level. When the mandible is laterally deviated, the two points, which have moved apart, are measured, giving the amount of lateral deviation. Normal lateral deviation is 10 to 15 mm each way.
CLINICAL NOTES/CAUTIONS	• During lateral deviation, the opposite condyle moves forward, down, and toward the motion side. The condyle on the motion side (i.e., left condyle on left lateral deviation) remains relatively stationary (rotating/spinning in place) and becomes more prominent. • Any lateral deviation from the normal opening position or abnormal protrusion to one side indicates that the lateral pterygoid, masseter, or temporalis muscle; the disc; or the lateral ligament on the opposite side is affected.
RELIABILITY/SPECIFICITY/SENSITIVITY	Unknown

FUNCTIONAL OPENING (KNUCKLE) TEST[3-5]

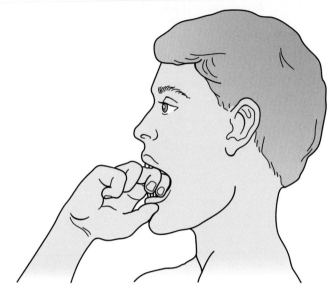

Figure 3–2
Functional opening (knuckle) test.

PURPOSE	To assess whether the patient's mouth can be opened a functional distance.
PATIENT POSITION	The patient is sitting.
EXAMINER POSITION	The examiner is positioned immediately in front of the patient so as to observe the patient's jaw motion and range of opening.
TEST PROCEDURE	The functional or full active opening is determined by having the patient try to place two or three flexed proximal interphalangeal joints (knuckles) within the mouth opening.
INDICATIONS OF A POSITIVE TEST	The opening should be approximately 35 to 55 mm. If the patient has pain on opening, the examiner should also measure the amount of opening to the point of pain and compare this distance with the functional opening. If the space is less than 35 to 55 mm, the temporomandibular joint range of motion should be considered restricted.
CLINICAL NOTES	• Normally, only about 25 to 35 mm of opening is needed for everyday activity. • Kropmans et al.[2] have pointed out that for treatment purposes, at least 6 mm of change is required for a detectable difference when more than one measurement is taken or to determine the effect of treatment
RELIABILITY/SPECIFICITY/ SENSITIVITY	Unknown

RESISTED ISOMETRIC MOVEMENTS

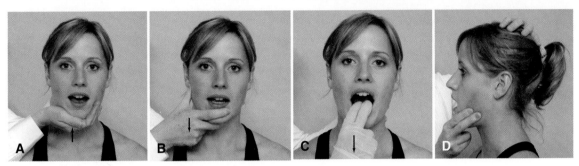

Figure 3–3

Resisted isometric movements for the muscles controlling the temporomandibular joint. **A,** Opening of the mouth (depression). **B,** Closing of the mouth (elevation or occlusion). **C,** Closing of the mouth (alternative method). **D,** Lateral deviation of the jaw.

PURPOSE	To assess the strength and endurance of the muscles controlling the temporomandibular joint.
PATIENT POSITION	The patient is sitting. The jaw should be in the resting position (tongue on the roof of the mouth). During the testing, the examiner asks the patient to hold this position and says, "Do not let me move you." The examiner then applies a firm pressure so the patient resists the pressure, which is in the opposite direction to the desired movement. No movement should occur.
EXAMINER POSITION	The examiner is positioned directly in front of the patient.
TEST PROCEDURE	**Opening of the mouth (depression).** Upward resistance is applied at the chin while the other hand rests behind the head or neck (or over the forehead) to stabilize the head.
	Closing of the mouth (elevation or occlusion). The examiner places one hand over the back of the head or neck to stabilize the head. The other hand is placed under the chin, with the patient's mouth slightly open. A downward force is placed upon the chin as the patient resists this motion. The examiner may alternatively place a gloved hand over the teeth and provide the downward force to the teeth.
	Lateral deviation of the jaw. The examiner places one hand over the side of the head above the temporomandibular joint to stabilize the head. The other hand is placed along the jaw of the patient's slightly open. mouth, and the patient pushes out against it. Each side is tested individually.
INDICATIONS OF A POSITIVE TEST	Weakness of the muscles is indicated by failure of the patient to hold the test position. Pain is not a positive test result, although it may indicate muscle tenderness. The clinician must be careful not to misinterpret the symptoms; contraction of the muscle also can compress the temporomandibular joint, causing pain and tenderness.
CLINICAL NOTE/CAUTION	• Resisted isometric movements of the temporomandibular joint are relatively difficult to test.
RELIABILITY/SPECIFICITY/ SENSITIVITY	Unknown

References

1. Boreadis AG, Gershon-Cohen J: Luschka joints of the cervical spine, *Radiology* 66:181-187, 1956.
2. Kropmans T, Dijkstra P, Stegenga B et al: Smallest detectable difference of maximal mouth opening in patients with painful restricted temporomandibular joint function, *Eur J Oral Sci* 108:9-13, 2000.
3. Friedman M, Weisberg J: Screening procedures for temporomandibular joint dysfunction, *Am Fam Physician* 25:157-160, 1982.
4. Dimitroulis G, Dolwick MF, Gremillion HA: Temporomandibular disorders: clinical evaluation, *Aust Dent J* 40:301-305, 1995.
5. House JW, Brackmann DE: Facial nerve grading system, *Otolaryngol Head Neck Surg* 93:146-147, 1985.

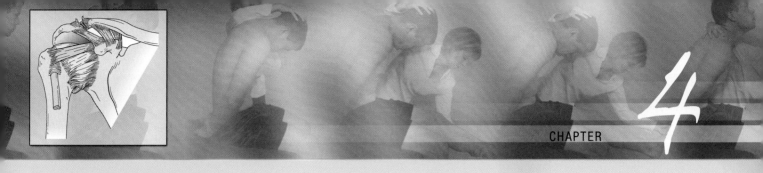

SHOULDER

Précis of the Shoulder Assessment*

History (sitting)
Observation (sitting or standing)
Examination
  Active movements (sitting or standing)
    Elevation through forward flexion of the arm
    Elevation through scaption of the arm
    Elevation through abduction of the arm
    Medial rotation of the arm
    Lateral rotation of the arm
    Extension of the arm
    Adduction of the arm
    Horizontal adduction and abduction of the arm
    Circumduction of the arm
    Scapular retraction/protraction
    Apley's scratch test, neck reach, back reach
  Passive movements (sitting)
    Elevation through abduction of the arm
    Elevation through forward flexion of the arm
    Elevation through abduction at the glenohumeral
      joint only
    Lateral rotation of the arm
    Medial rotation of the arm
    Extension of the arm
    Adduction of the arm
    Horizontal adduction and abduction of the arm
    Posterior capsular tightness
  Special tests (sitting or standing)
    Instability tests
      Load and shift test (anterior and posterior)
      Rockwood test
      Sulcus sign
      Feagin test
      Posterior apprehension or stress test
    Impingement tests
      Neer impingement test
      Hawkins-Kennedy impingement test
      Posterior internal impingement test
    Labral tears
      Clunk test (Bankart)
      Anterior slide test (Bankart)
      Active compression test of O'Brien (SLAP)
      Biceps tension test (SLAP)
      Labral crank test
      SLAP prehension test
    Scapular stability
      Lateral scapular slide test
      Scapular load test
      Scapular retraction test
      Wall (floor) push up
    Other shoulder joint tests
      Acromioclavicular crossover, cross-body, or
        horizontal adduction test
    Muscle/tendon pathological conditions
      Speed's test (biceps)
      Yergason's test (biceps)
      Empty can test (supraspinatus)
      Abdominal compression (Napoleon) test
      Bear hug test
      Lift-off sign (subscapularis)
      Medial rotation spring-back or lag test
        (subscapularis)

    Lateral rotation spring-back or lag test
      (infraspinatus/teres minor)
    Serratus anterior weakness
    Latissimus dorsi weakness
    Thoracic outlet test
    Roos test
  Reflexes and cutaneous distribution (sitting)
    Reflexes
    Sensory scan
    Peripheral nerves
      Axillary nerve
      Suprascapular nerve
      Musculocutaneous nerve
      Long thoracic nerve
      Spinal accessory nerve
  Palpation (sitting)
  Resisted isometric movements (supine lying)
    Forward flexion of the shoulder
    Extension of the shoulder
    Abduction of the shoulder
    Adduction of the shoulder
    Medial rotation of the shoulder
    Lateral rotation of the shoulder
    Flexion of the elbow
    Extension of the elbow
  Special tests (supine lying)
    Instability tests
      Crank apprehension/relocation test (anterior)
      Fulcrum test
      Norwood test (posterior)
      Push-pull test (posterior)
    Labral tears
      Biceps load test
      Clunk test
    Muscle/tendon pathological conditions
      Trapezius weakness—three positions (prone lying)
      Rhomboid weakness (prone lying)
      Pectoralis minor tightness (supine lying)
      Pectoralis major tightness (supine lying)
    Neurological tests
      Upper limb tension tests
  Joint play movements (supine lying)
    Backward glide of the humerus
    Forward glide of the humerus
    Lateral distraction of the humerus
    Long arm traction
    Backward glide of the humerus in abduction
    Anteroposterior and cephalocaudal movements of
      the clavicle at the acromioclavicular joint
    Anteroposterior and cephalocaudal movements of
      the clavicle at the sternoclavicular joint
    General movement of the scapula to determine
      mobility
  Diagnostic imaging

---

*This assessment is shown in an order that limits the amount of
movement the patient must do but ensures that all necessary
structures are tested. After any examination, the patient should
be warned that symptoms may be exacerbated as a result of the
assessment.

SELECTED MOVEMENTS

ACTIVE MOVEMENTS[1-21]

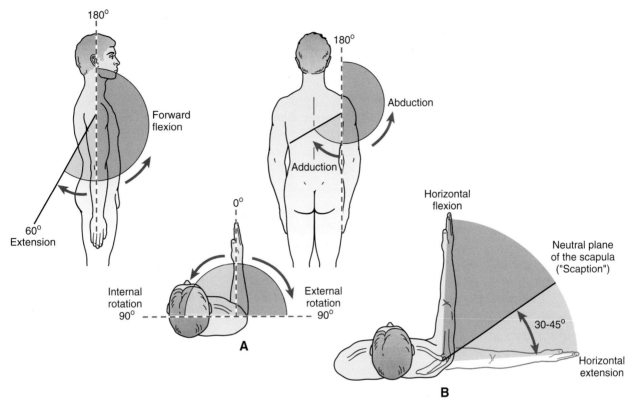

Figure 4-1

Movement in the shoulder complex. **A,** Range of motion (ROM) of the shoulder. **B,** Axes of arm elevation. (Modified from Perry J: Anatomy and biomechanics of the shoulder in throwing, swimming, gymnastics, and tennis, *Clin Sports Med* 2:255, 1983.)

GENERAL INFORMATION	The first movements to be assessed in any examination are the active movements. These movements usually are done in such a way that the painful movements are performed last so that pain does not carry over to the next movement. It also is essential to be able to differentiate between scapular movement and glenohumeral movement during active movements. Scapular movement often compensates for restricted glenohumeral movement, leading to weak and often lengthened scapular control muscles.
PATIENT POSITION	The patient may be tested in the standing or sitting position.
EXAMINER POSITION	The examiner is positioned directly in front or in back of the patient so as to instruct the patient, observe motion, and apply overpressure as needed. The movements must be observed from the front and from the back.

Elevation Through Forward Flexion

TEST PROCEDURE	The patient is instructed to raise his or her arm into forward flexion as far as possible with the arm/elbow straight (*A*).
INDICATIONS OF A POSITIVE TEST	Active elevation through forward flexion normally is 160° to 180°. Inability to attain this range of motion (ROM) and/or pain during the performance of this test is considered a positive test result.
CLINICAL NOTE	• At the extreme of the ROM, the arm is in the same position as for active elevation through abduction.

Continued

ACTIVE MOVEMENTS[1-21]—*cont'd*

Elevation Through Scaption

TEST PROCEDURE   The patient is instructed to raise the arm in the scapular plane as far as possible with the arm/elbow straight (*B*).

INDICATIONS OF A POSITIVE TEST   Active elevation (170° to 180°) through the plane of the scapula (30° to 45° of forward flexion, or *scaption*) is the most natural and functional motion of elevation. The exact angle is determined by the contour of the chest wall on which the scapula rests. Failure to attain this position and/or pain during testing indicates a positive test result. Also, the total elevation in scaption is about 170°, with scapular rotation being about 65° and humeral abduction about 105°.

CLINICAL NOTES
- Elevation in this position is sometimes called *neutral elevation.*
- Patients with weakness spontaneously choose this plane when elevating the arm.
- During elevation through scaption, scapulohumeral rhythm is similar to that of abduction, although there is greater individual variability.
- Often, movement into elevation is less painful in this position than elevation through abduction, when the glenohumeral joint is actually in extension, or elevation in forward flexion.
- Movement in the plane of the scapula puts less stress on the capsule and surrounding musculature and is the position in which most of the functions of daily activity are commonly performed.

Elevation Through Abduction

TEST PROCEDURE   The patient is instructed to raise the arm into abduction as far as possible with the arm/elbow straight (*A*).

INDICATIONS OF A POSITIVE TEST   Active abduction normally is 160° to 180°. Inability to attain this ROM and/or pain during the performance of this test is considered a positive test result. Altered mechanics during motion also may be an indication of a pathological condition.

When examining the movement of elevation through abduction, the examiner must take time to observe the scapulohumeral rhythm of the shoulder complex both anteriorly and posteriorly. During 180° of abduction, there is roughly a 2:1 ratio of movement of the humerus to the scapula, with 120° of movement occurring at the glenohumeral joint and 60° at the scapulothoracic joint. However, the examiner must keep in mind that a great deal of variability exists among individuals and may depend on the speed of movement; also, authors do not completely agree on the exact amounts of each movement.[18-20]

In the unstable shoulder, the scapulohumeral rhythm commonly is altered because of incorrect dynamic functioning of the scapular or humeral stabilizers or both. This may be related to incorrect arthrokinematics at the glenohumeral joint. Kibler[21] pointed out that watching the movement of the scapula in both the ascending and descending phases of abduction is especially important. Commonly, weakness of the scapular control muscles is more evident during descent as many of the muscles are required to work eccentrically. An instability jog, hitch, or jump may occur when the patient loses control of the scapula.

CLINICAL NOTES   This movement occurring simultaneously at the four joints involves three phases. There is variability regarding the amount of motion and the timing of motion that occurs at each phase of movement. Other authors will give values for the amount of each movement that differ from those noted here.
- In the first phase of 30° of elevation through abduction, the scapula is said to be "setting." This means that the scapula moves minimally during this stage—rotating slightly in, rotating slightly out, or not moving at all. Therefore, there is no 2:1 ratio

ACTIVE MOVEMENTS[1-21]—*cont'd*

of movement during this phase. The angle between the scapular spine and the clavicle also may increase up to 5° at the sternoclavicular and acromioclavicular joints when elevating the arm; however, this depends on whether the scapula moves during this phase.

- During the next 60° of upper extremity elevation (second phase), the scapula rotates about 20°, and the humerus elevates 40° with minimal protraction or elevation of the scapula. Therefore, there is a 2:1 ratio of scapulohumeral movement. During phase 2, the clavicle elevates because of the scapular rotation, but the clavicle still does not rotate or does so minimally.

- During the final 90° of motion (third phase), the 2:1 ratio of scapulohumeral movement continues and the angle between the scapular spine and the clavicle increases an additional 10°. Therefore, the scapula continues to rotate and now begins to elevate. The amount of protraction continues to be minimal when the abduction movement is performed. During this stage, the clavicle rotates posteriorly 30° to 50° on a long axis and elevates up to a further 15°. Also during this final stage, the humerus laterally rotates 90° so that the greater tuberosity of the humerus avoids the acromion process.

- During the second and third phases, rotation of the scapula (total, 60°) is possible because of the 20° of motion at the acromioclavicular joint and 40° at the sternoclavicular joint.

Medial Rotation

TEST PROCEDURE   The patient is instructed to reach the hand up behind the back as far as possible.

INDICATIONS OF A POSITIVE TEST   Active medial rotation normally is 60° to 100°. This usually is assessed by measuring the height of the "hitchhiking" thumb (thumb in extension) reaching up the patient's back. Common reference points include the greater trochanter, buttock, waist, and spinous processes, with T5 to T10 representing the normal degree of medial rotation. Failure to attain this position and/or pain during testing indicates a positive test result.

CLINICAL NOTES
- When the test is done in this fashion, the examiner must be aware that the range measured is not actually that of the glenohumeral joint alone. In fact, much of the range is gained by winging the scapula, or protraction of the scapula so when the patient does the movement, the examiner should watch for movement in the scapula. As soon as the scapula begins to move, it is usually the end of glenohumeral rotation.
- With tight medial glenohumeral motion, greater winging and protraction of the scapula occur.
- If the patient can abduct to 90°, it is often easier to measure medial rotation from this positon.
- Measurement may also be taken by measuring the height of the patient's radial styloid process as it reaches up the back. This eliminates variability in thumb position.

Lateral Rotation

TEST PROCEDURE   The patient is instructed to keep the elbow at the side and to rotate the hand outward as far as possible (*A*). Alternately, the patient's lateral rotation ROM can be tested at 90° of shoulder abduction if the patient's shoulder can achieve this position.

INDICATIONS OF A POSITIVE TEST   Active lateral rotation normally is 80° to 90° but may be greater in some athletes, such as gymnasts and baseball pitchers. If glenohumeral lateral rotation is limited, the patient compensates by retracting the scapula. Failure to attain this position and/or pain during testing indicates a positive test result.

Continued

ACTIVE MOVEMENTS[1-21]—*cont'd*

CLINICAL NOTES/CAUTIONS
- Care must be taken when applying overpressure with this movement, because it could lead to anterior subluxation/dislocation of the glenohumeral joint, especially in individuals with recurrent dislocation problems.
- It is important to compare medial and lateral rotation, especially in active people who use their dominant arm at extremes of motion and under high load situations. The examiner should note any glenohumeral internal (medial) rotation deficit (GIRD), which is the difference in medial rotation between the patient's two shoulders. Normally, the difference should be within 20°. This may also be compared with the glenohumeral external (lateral) rotation gain (GERG). If the GIRD/GERG ratio is greater than 1, the patient will often develop shoulder problems.

Extension

TEST PROCEDURE
The patient is asked to reach the hand backward as far as possible while keeping the arm/elbow straight.

INDICATIONS OF A POSITIVE TEST
Active extension normally is 50° to 60°. The examiner must make sure the movement is in the shoulder and not in the spine, because some patients may flex the spine or bend forward, giving the appearance of increased shoulder extension. Similarly, retraction of the scapula increases the appearance of glenohumeral extension. Failure to attain this position and/or pain during testing indicates a positive test result.

CLINICAL NOTE
- Weakness of full extension commonly implies weakness of the posterior deltoid in one arm. It is sometimes called the *swallow tail sign,* because the two arms do not extend the same amount, indicating an injury to the muscle itself or to the axillary nerve.

Adduction

TEST PROCEDURE
The patient is instructed to adduct the hand across the body.

INDICATIONS OF A POSITIVE TEST
Adduction normally is 50° to 75° when the arm is brought in front of the body.

Horizontal Adduction/Cross Flexion

TEST PROCEDURE
The patient is instructed to abduct the arm to shoulder level (90°) and then is asked to bring the hand/arm across the body (*B*).

INDICATIONS OF A POSITIVE TEST
Horizontal adduction, or cross flexion, normally is 130°. Failure to attain this position and/or pain during testing indicates a positive test result, most commonly a pathological condition of or localized pain in the acromioclavicular joint or sternoclavicular joint.

CLINICAL NOTE/CAUTION
- To assess glenohumeral horizontal adduction instead of total shoulder horizontal adduction, the patient's scapula can be stabilized into scapular retraction and the patient's shoulder horizontally adducted. Alternatively, the clinician can assess when the scapula begins to move during the horizontal adduction motion. Movement of the scapula in either case indicates the end of glenohumeral motion and the beginning of scapulothoracic motion.

Horizontal Abduction

TEST PROCEDURE
The patient is instructed to abduct the shoulders to shoulder level (90°); from this position, the patient is instructed to move both arms backward, comparing the amount of movement.

ACTIVE MOVEMENTS[1-21]—cont'd

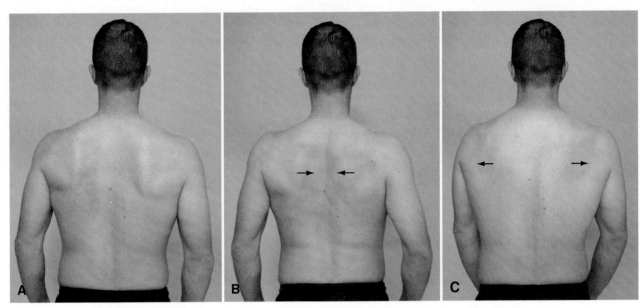

Figure 4–2
A, Resting position. **B,** Scapular retraction. **C,** Scapular protraction.

INDICATIONS OF A POSITIVE TEST   Horizontal abduction, or cross extension, is approximately 45°. Failure to attain this position and/or pain during testing indicates a positive test result.

CLINICAL NOTE   • During horizontal adduction and abduction, the examiner should note the difference in the relative amount of scapular movement between the normal side and the affected side. If movement is limited in the glenohumeral joint, greater scapular movement occurs.

Circumduction

TEST PROCEDURE   The patient is instructed to move the arm in a circle in the vertical plane.

INDICATIONS OF A POSITIVE TEST   Circumduction normally is approximately 200°. Failure to attain this position and/or pain during testing indicates a positive test result.

CLINICAL NOTE   • Circumduction requires multiple planes of motion and is a good indicator of functional mobility.

Scapular Retraction and Protraction

TEST PROCEDURE   **Scapular retraction.** The examiner asks the patient to squeeze the shoulder blades (scapulae) together.
Scapular protraction. The examiner instructs the patient to try to bring the shoulders together anteriorly so the scapulae move away from each other.

INDICATIONS OF A POSITIVE TEST   **Scapular retraction.** Normally, the medial borders of the scapulae remain parallel to the spine but move toward the spine with the soft tissue bunching up between them. Ideally, the patient is able to do this movement without excessive contraction of the upper trapezius muscles.
Scapular protraction. Normally, the scapulae move away from the midline; the inferior angle of the scapula commonly moves laterally more than the superior angle,

Continued

ACTIVE MOVEMENTS[1-21] —*cont'd*

resulting in some lateral rotation of the inferior angle. Commonly the two scapulae are tested simultaneously so that the examiner can visualize the difference between the two shoulders. A difference between the two sides indicates a positive test result.

CLINICAL NOTES
- If the serratus anterior muscle is weak or paralyzed, the scapula "wings" away from the thorax on its medial border. The serratus anterior also assists upward rotation of the scapula during abduction. Therefore, injury to the muscle (serratus anterior) or its nerve (long thoracic nerve) may limit abduction.
- Similarly, weakness of the trapezius muscle, especially the lower part, can alter scapular mechanics, resulting in anterior secondary impingement.
- The protraction/retraction cycle may cause a clicking or snapping near the inferior angle or supramedial corner, a condition sometimes called a "snapping scapula," which is caused by the scapula rubbing over the underlying ribs.

APLEY'S SCRATCH TEST[22]   DVD

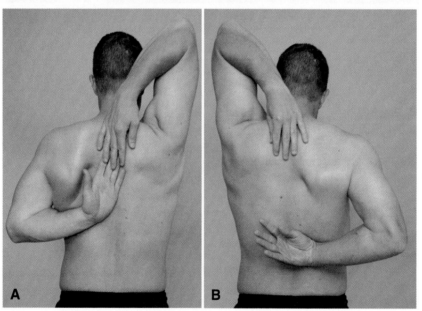

Figure 4–3
Apley's scratch test. **A,** The right arm is in lateral rotation, flexion, and abduction; the left arm is in medial rotation, extension, and adduction. **B,** The left arm is in lateral rotation, flexion, and abduction; the right arm is in medial rotation, extension, and adduction. Note the difference in medial rotation in the right arm compared with the left arm in *A*.

PURPOSE   Apley's scratch test combines medial rotation with adduction and lateral rotation with abduction. It is used to show combined movement patterns that may be limited, resulting in functional movement loss.

PATIENT POSITION   The patient may be sitting or standing.

APLEY'S SCRATCH TEST[22]—*cont'd*

EXAMINER POSITION   The examiner is positioned so as to observe the scapular motion and the amount of motion in the shoulder. The examiner often must move to different vantage points during the test to gain a full picture of shoulder motion and compensations.

TEST PROCEDURE   The patient is asked to reach upward and over the head to scratch the middle of the back with one hand. With the other hand, the patient is asked to reach backward behind the low back to scratch the back.

INDICATIONS OF A POSITIVE TEST   This test has no exact normal measurement. Instead, motion is compared with the opposite arm. A difference in ROM between the two sides and/or the production of symptoms indicates a positive test result.

CLINICAL NOTES
- Often the dominant shoulder shows greater restriction than the nondominant shoulder, even in the absence of a pathological condition. An exception would be individuals who continually use their arms at the extremes of motion (e.g., baseball pitchers). Because of the extra ROM developed over time doing the activity, the dominant arm may show greater ROM. However, the examiner must always be aware that shoulder movements include movements of the scapula and clavicle, as well as the glenohumeral joint. Many glenohumeral joint problems actually are scapular muscle control problems, which may secondarily lead to glenohumeral joint problems, especially in people under 40 years of age.
- The scapular reach test (neck and back) is a similar test in which the patient does medial rotation and adduction (back reach) of both arms at the same time, then lateral rotation and adduction (neck reach) of both arms at the same time. By having the patient do the combined movements, the examiner gets some idea of the individual's functional capacity and can easily see differences between the two sides. (See Figure 5-29 in Magee DJ: *Orthopedic Physical Assessment,* ed. 5.)

PASSIVE MOVEMENTS[22-26]   DVD

PATIENT POSITION   The patient is supine.

EXAMINER POSITION   The examiner stands adjacent to the patient's shoulder on the side being tested.

TEST PROCEDURE   Starting with the unaffected side, the examiner grasps the patient's forearm with one hand and places the other hand on the patient's shoulder to monitor shoulder compensation (i.e., movement at the glenohumeral joint, scapulothoracic joint, and acromioclavicular joint) while watching the sternoclavicular joint. While palpating the shoulder, the examiner passively lifts the patient's arm sequentially into flexion, then abduction, then scaption or brings it backward to assess shoulder extension.

The examiner then can assess passive medial and lateral rotation by bringing the patient's elbow to the side and medially or laterally rotating the arm. Rotation also can be assessed at varying degrees of shoulder abduction (most commonly, 90°).

Finally, the shoulder can be brought to 90° of shoulder abduction, provided the patient can achieve 90°. From this starting point, the shoulder can be brought across the body to assess shoulder horizontal adduction or extended backward to assess shoulder horizontal abduction.

INDICATIONS OF A POSITIVE TEST   The examiner assesses for scapular compensations that occur during passive motion, end feels at the end of shoulder motion, and the ROM available with each motion. Reproduction of symptoms is also noted. A positive test result is indicated by differences in motion compared with the contralateral side, significant differences from established norms, or symptom reproduction.

CLINICAL NOTES
- Passive movements may reveal the presence of a capsular pattern. The end feel of capsular tightness is different from the tissue stretch end feel or muscle tightness. Capsular tightness has a more hard and elastic feel to it, and it usually occurs earlier in the ROM.
- If unsure of the end feel, the examiner can have the patient contract the muscles acting in the opposite direction 10% to 20% of the maximum voluntary contraction (MVC) and then relax. The examiner then attempts to move the limb farther into range. If the range increases, the problem was muscular, not capsular.

POSTERIOR CAPSULAR TIGHTNESS TEST

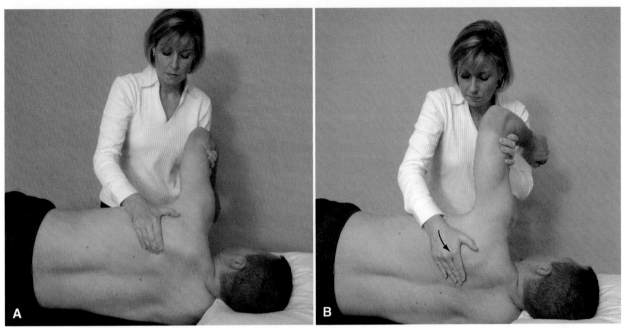

Figure 4–4

Testing for posterior capsular tightness. **A,** Starting position for the posterior shoulder flexibility measurement; the patient is positioned correctly on his side. **B,** Maximum passive ROM of the posterior shoulder tissues. Note the scapular stabilization with the torso perpendicular to the examining table. As soon as the scapula begins to move, the examiner stops.

PURPOSE	To assess for posterior capsular tightness in the shoulder.
SUSPECTED INJURY	Posterior capsular tightness
PATIENT POSITION	The patient should be suitably undressed (no shirt for men, only bra for women) to visualize the motion and position of the scapula. The patient is positioned in a supine/ side-lying position with body weight placed upon the scapula in order to stabilize the scapula upon the table.
EXAMINER POSITION	The examiner stands at the patient's side and holds the patient's arm above the epicondyles of the elbow.
TEST PROCEDURE	Starting with the unaffected side, the examiner uses one hand to abduct the patient's arm to 90° while maintaining the shoulder in neutral rotation. With the other hand, the examiner pushes the humeral head down to further stabilize the scapula and then, while holding the humeral head down, medially rotates the shoulder, noting the available ROM. The two sides are compared.
INDICATIONS OF A POSITIVE TEST	The available medial rotation is compared between the unaffected and affected shoulders. A tight posterior capsule limits the amount of medial rotation.
CLINICAL NOTE	• Capsular tightness should correlate well with decreased medial rotation, provided the scapula is not allowed to move in compensation.

RESISTED ISOMETRIC MOVEMENTS

DVD

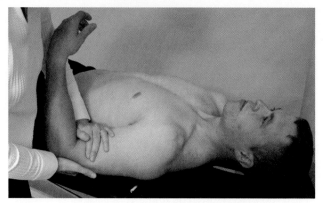

Figure 4–5

Positioning of the patient for resisted isometric movements.

PURPOSE	To assess the strength of the shoulder musculature.
PATIENT POSITION	The patient may be sitting or supine. The examiner positions the patient's arm at the side with the elbow flexed to 90°.
EXAMINER POSITION	If the patient is sitting, the examiner is positioned directly in front of the person. If the patient is supine, the examiner is positioned directly adjacent to the patient's shoulder.
TEST PROCEDURE	The muscles of the shoulder are tested isometrically, with the examiner positioning the patient and saying, "Don't let me move you." Pressure and force should be increased slowly and gradually. From this position, the examiner tests shoulder flexion, extension, abduction, adduction, medial rotation, and lateral rotation, as well as elbow flexion (biceps) and extension (triceps).

Flexion. The examiner places the palm of one hand on the anterior distal humerus to provide resistance near the elbow and uses the other hand to support the patient's hand at the wrist.

Extension. The examiner places the palm of one hand on the posterior distal humerus to provide resistance near the elbow and uses the other hand to support the patient's hand at the wrist.

Abduction. The examiner places the palm of one hand on the lateral distal humerus to provide resistance near the elbow and uses the other hand to support the patient's hand at the wrist.

Adduction. The examiner places the palm of one hand on the medial distal humerus to provide resistance near the elbow and uses the other hand to support the patient's hand at the wrist.

Medial rotation. The examiner places the palm of one hand on the distal forearm at the palmar aspect of the wrist to provide resistance, and the other hand just above the elbow.

Lateral rotation. The examiner places the palm of one hand on the distal forearm at the posterior aspect of the wrist to provide resistance and the other hand just above the elbow.

Elbow flexion. The examiner places the palm of one hand near the anterior wrist to provide resistance and uses the other hand to support the elbow.

Elbow extension. The examiner places the palm of one hand near the posterior wrist to provide resistance and uses the other hand to support the elbow.

RESISTED ISOMETRIC MOVEMENTS—*cont'd*

INDICATIONS OF A POSITIVE TEST   A positive test result is indicated by weakness and/or symptom reproduction noted when the affected side is compared with the contralateral (normal) side. During testing, the examiner will find differences in the relative strengths of the various muscle groups around the shoulder if pathology is present and affecting the muscles.

CLINICAL NOTES
- The disadvantage of testing shoulder isometrics with the patient in the supine position is that the examiner cannot observe the stabilization of the scapula during the testing. Normally, the scapula should not move during isometric testing. Scapular protraction, winging, or tilting during isometric testing indicates weakness of the scapular control muscles.
- Although all the muscles around the shoulder can be tested with the patient in the supine lying position, some recommend testing the muscles in more than one position (e.g., different amounts of abduction or forward flexion) to determine the mechanical effect of the contraction in different situations.
- If the patient history includes a complaint of pain in one or more positions, these positions also should be tested. If the initial position causes pain, other positions (e.g., position of injury, position of mechanical advantage) may be tried to further differentiate the specific contractile tissue that has been injured.
- The relative percentages for isometric testing will be altered if tests are performed at faster speeds and in different planes.
- If the patient history includes a complaint that concentric, eccentric, or econcentric (biceps and triceps) movements are painful or cause symptoms, these movements should be tested with loading or no loading as required.
- When testing isometric elbow flexion, the examiner should watch for the possibility of a third-degree strain (rupture) of the long head of the biceps tendon ("Popeye muscle").

SPECIAL TESTS FOR ANTERIOR GLENOHUMERAL INSTABILITY[27-37]

General Information

Two types of anterior instability may be found in the shoulder. Type I, which is more closely related to muscle weakness and labral tears, can be found in any part of the ROM (translational instability). Type II, which is related to end-range instability and trauma will typically present with apprehension when tested at end ROM. Type II instability is often associated with tearing of the labrum and/or capsule.

Relevant Special Tests

Load and shift test—anterior
Crank apprehension test (relocation test)
Rockwood test (modification of the crank test)
Fulcrum test (modification of the crank test)

Definition

Anterior glenohumeral instability is characterized by laxity in the anterior aspect of the shoulder joint, which makes it difficult for the humeral head to maintain its articulation and normal arthrokinematics within the glenoid.

Suspected Injury

- Unidirectional anterior instability.
- If the instability is the result of anterior dislocation or subluxation, injuries that may be present include a Hill-Sachs lesion, fracture of the anterior glenoid rim, or a Bankart lesion.
- Incorrect forward head posture, with rounded shoulders and protracted scapulae.
- Any of the peripheral nerves arising from the brachial plexus could be compromised. Damage can range from minor numbness or tingling to complete palsy of the nerve. The axillary nerve is especially susceptible.
- Anterior laxity often is accompanied by damage to the labrum, glenoid, anterior capsule, and/or brachial plexus.
- Vascular damage can occur with a shoulder dislocation. The brachial artery may be injured as it runs through the anterior shoulder complex.

Epidemiology and Demographics

Athletes who play overhead sports (e.g., tennis, volleyball, baseball) and patients with a history of dislocations or subluxations are more likely to have anterior shoulder instability. Several factors make the younger athlete more susceptible to anterior shoulder instability, such as poor technique and inadequate strength. Some researchers speculate that, in addition, adolescents' immature collagen makeup makes them more susceptible to anterior shoulder instability and laxity.[37]

A wide array of incidences has been proposed in studies on anterior shoulder instability. Most patients initially dislocate the shoulder in their 20s or 30s, and 85% to 95% of dislocations in the shoulder are anterior. One fourth of all patients with dislocations have a family history of the same problem. The patient's age at the time of dislocation has a significant impact on the recurrence rate. Reported recurrence rates in patients younger than age 20 vary from 70% to 100%.[37]

Relevant History

The patient may or may not have a history of a pathological condition of or an injury to the involved shoulder. Athletes may have a history of repetitive overhead activities.

Relevant Signs and Symptoms

Translational Instability

- The patient may complain of generalized or anterior shoulder pain that can radiate down into the deltoid region of the shoulder, especially when the arm is above shoulder height.
- The patient may also complain of weakness in the shoulder that may be accompanied by clicking or grinding with shoulder motion.
- The patient often has a subjective feeling of instability, dislocation, or apprehension.
- The patient may complain that the shoulder does not "feel right," especially when it is loaded above shoulder height.
- The results of unloaded active and passive movement and/or resisted isometric testing in neutral may be normal.
- Sensory loss, numbness or tingling, weakness, or complete palsy within a peripheral nerve distribution may be present in some cases.
- Coldness or weakness may be present if the vascular structures are compromised through the brachial region.

End-Range Instability

- Severe pain and restricted ROM are noted with dislocation.
- Severe muscle spasm may be present.
- The arm is held in 20° of abduction.
- Loss of shoulder roundness is seen.
- The humeral head may be palpated in the axilla.
- Once the dislocation has been reduced or if it has previously subluxed, apprehension predominates over pain.
- In individuals under age 35, anterior shoulder instability is commonly associated with scapular instability and a tight posterior capsule, both of which must be addressed for successful treatment.

Mechanism of Injury

Unidirectional anterior instability usually is the result of repetitive overhead use, such as from throwing, swimming, or playing tennis (type I), or of trauma (type II). For type II injuries, the most common position of injury is with the arm abducted to 90° and laterally rotated to end range.

Trauma that involves forced lateral rotation/abduction with a posterior force at the glenohumeral joint results in shoulder anterior dislocation or subluxation. Other mechanisms of injury include traction on the arm in an anterior direction and a fall onto an outstretched hand (FOOSH) with the arm abducted and laterally rotated.

Reliability/Specificity/Sensitivity/Comparison[27-30,32,33,36]

	Validity	Interrater Reliability	Intrarater Reliability	Specificity	Sensitivity	Positive Likelihood	Negative Likelihood Ratio
Anterior Crank Test	Unknown	Unknown	Unknown	56% to 100%	35% to 91%	1.05 (SLAP) 1.48 (Other)	0.91 (SLAP) 0.82 (Other)
Crank/Relocation Test	Unknown	0.31 (pain) 0.47 (apprehension) 0.44 (pain or apprehension)	Unknown	98.91	52.78	48.42	0.48
Fulcrum Test	Unknown	Unknown	Unknown	Unknown	Unknown	Unknown	Unknown
Load and Shift Test	Unknown	0.72 (anterior) 0.42 (posterior) 0.65 (inferior) 0.60 (sulcus)	Unknown	Unknown	Unknown	Unknown	Unknown
Rockwood Test	Unknown	Unknown	Unknown	Unknown	Unknown	Unknown	Unknown

LOAD AND SHIFT TEST—ANTERIOR[22,38-49]

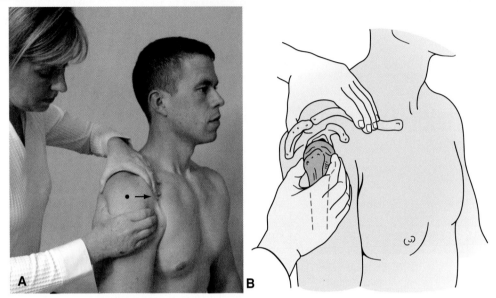

Figure 4–6

A, Load and shift test with the patient in the seated starting position. Note that the humerus first is loaded, or "centered," in the glenoid. The examiner then shifts the humerus anteriorly. **B,** The position of the examiner's hands in relation to the bones of the shoulder. Note that the examiner's left thumb holds the spine of the scapula for stability while the fingers stabilize the clavicle.

PURPOSE

The anterior load and shift test is designed to assess the anterior stability and mobility of the glenohumeral joint. Positive test results are related more to arthrokinematic instability (type I instability, related to muscle weakness) than to end-range (type II) instability. It is often combined with the posterior load and shift to compare the relative amount of movement in each direction.

RELEVANT HISTORY

The patient may have a history of subjective feelings of instability or two or more episodes of dislocation/subluxation. Each subsequent episode of dislocation/subluxation generally is easier to provoke than the previous episode. Persistent popping, clicking, or clunking may occur, with or without pain.

RELEVANT SIGNS AND SYMPTOMS

- Generalized shoulder pain may be present that can radiate down into the deltoid region of the shoulder on testing.
- The patient commonly complains of weakness in the shoulder and may complain of clicking or grinding with shoulder motion.
- Neural irritation may occur in conjunction with shoulder instability. Sensory loss, numbness or tingling, weakness, or complete palsy within a peripheral nerve distribution may be seen.

MECHANISM OF INJURY

Either trauma (e.g., injury to the labrum or capsule) or lack of muscular control can produce shoulder instability. Unidirectional instability of the shoulder typically occurs after shoulder dislocation or subluxation as a result of trauma (type II instability), or it may be the result of poor muscle function (type I instability). In most cases, laxity is felt in the anterior aspect of the joint. Multidirectional shoulder instability often is the result of a genetic predisposition to joint laxity combined with overuse of the shoulder, especially in the elevated position. Generally with multidirectional shoulder instability, laxity may be experienced in both shoulders and in other joints in the body.

LOAD AND SHIFT TEST—ANTERIOR[22,38-49]—cont'd

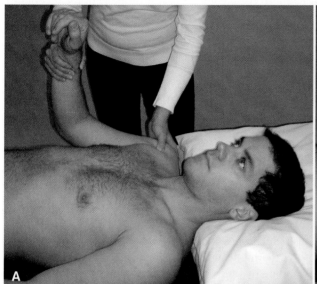

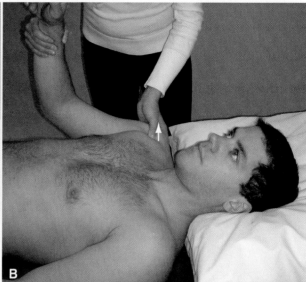

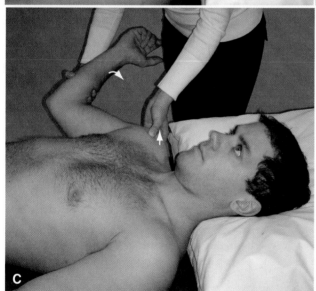

Figure 4–7

A, Initial position for load and shift test for anterior instability of the shoulder with the patient in the supine lying position. The examiner grasps the patient's upper arm with the fingers posterior. The examiner's arm positions the patient's arm and controls its rotation. The arm is placed in the plane of the scapula, abducted 45° to 60°, and maintained in 0° of rotation. The examiner's arm places an axial load on the patient's arm through the humerus. The examiner's fingers then shift the humeral head anteriorly and anteroinferiorly over the glenoid rim. **B,** The second position for the load and shift test for anterior stability is as described in *A* for the initial position, except that the arm is progressively laterally rotated in 10°- to 20°-increments while the anterior translation force is alternatively applied and released. **C,** The examiner compares the normal and abnormal shoulders for this difference in translation with the humeral rotation. The degree of rotation required to reduce the translation is an indicator of the functional laxity of the anterior inferior capsular ligaments.

PATIENT POSITION The patient may be tested in the seated or the supine lying position. If tested in sitting, the patient should be tested with no back support and with the hand of the test arm resting on the thigh.

EXAMINER POSITION The examiner stands or sits slightly behind the patient and stabilizes the shoulder with one hand over the clavicle and scapula. With the other hand, the examiner grasps the head of the humerus with the thumb over the posterior humeral head and the fingers over the anterior humeral head.

Continued

LOAD AND SHIFT TEST—ANTERIOR[22,38-49]—cont'd

TEST PROCEDURE

The humerus is gently pushed into the glenoid to seat it properly in the glenoid fossa so that the humeral head sits in neutral. This is the "load" portion of the test, and this seating of the humerus allows true translation to occur. If the load is not applied to put the head in neutral, the amount of movement found will not indicate the true amount of translation, and the end feel will be altered.

Next, the humeral head is pushed anteriorly to test for anterior instability or posteriorly to test for posterior instability, and the amount of translation is noted. This is the "shift" portion of the test. The affected side and the normal side should be compared for differences. Differences between the two sides and reproduction of symptoms often are considered more important than the amount of movement obtained.

INDICATIONS OF A POSITIVE TEST

Translation of 25% of the humeral head diameter or less anteriorly from the neutral position is considered normal. Hawkins and Mohtadi[39] proposed a three-grade system of anterior translation. Normally, the head translates 0 to 25% of the diameter of the humeral head. Up to 50% of humeral head translation, with the head riding up to the glenoid rim and spontaneous reduction, is considered a grade I anterior translation. In a grade II anterior translation, the humeral head has more than 50% translation, and the head feels as though it is riding over the glenoid rim, but it spontaneously reduces. Grade III is a dislocation with no spontaneous reduction.

The affected side and the normal side should be compared for the amount of translation and the ease with which it occurs. This comparison, along with reproduction of symptoms, often is considered more important than the amount of movement obtained. If the patient has multidirectional instability, both anterior and posterior translation may be excessive on the affected side compared with the normal side.

CLINICAL NOTES/CAUTIONS

• Normally, the head of the humerus should translate anteriorly 0% to 25% of the diameter of the humeral head. The head of the humerus should translate posteriorly equal if not more than the anterior translation (25% to 50% of the diameter of the humerus). (Authors vary with regard to the amount of movement possible.)

• The load and shift test is designed to test for clinical symptoms more than any particular pathological condition. Many types of pathological conditions can result in instability of the shoulder. The load and shift test can be used as an assessment tool for both multidirectional and unidirectional instability. Multidirectional instability usually is the result of a genetic predisposition to laxity in the joints. Unidirectional instability is the result of trauma or repetitive use. Shoulder dislocations/subluxations/labral tears (type II instability) and general joint laxity (type I instability) are examples of pathological conditions that can be detected with this test.

• It is important to note that a positive test result is not specific for any one pathological condition; rather, it helps to guide the clinician in the reasoning process. Instability may be a contributing factor in the development of the ultimate pathological condition. Other factors that may contribute to instability include muscle weakness of the rotator cuff and/or weakness of the scapular control muscles.

**RELIABILITY/SPECIFICITY/
SENSITIVITY[33]**

Reliability intrarater range: k = 0.34-0.79
Reliability interrater range: k = 0.09-0.31

CRANK APPREHENSION TEST (RELOCATION TEST)[27-30,36,41,50-61]

PURPOSE
- To determine whether the humerus will sublux or dislocate anteriorly out of the glenoid.
- To differentiate between dislocation/subluxation (apprehension) and impingement (pain).
- To differentiate between instability and impingement (relocation part of the test).

SUSPECTED INJURY
Anterior shoulder subluxations
Anterior instability
Spontaneously reduced dislocation

RELEVANT HISTORY
The patient may have a history of a FOOSH injury or of one or more dislocations or subluxations of the glenohumeral joint.

RELEVANT SIGNS AND SYMPTOMS
- If the shoulder has not been reduced, the patient will be in pain, will be supporting the arm, and will be hesitant to move it.
- If the shoulder has been reduced, the patient may have a generalized ache or pain that may radiate down into the deltoid region of the shoulder.
- Weakness in the shoulder may be noted, and the patient may complain of clicking or grinding with shoulder motion.
- Neural irritation is not uncommon in conjunction with shoulder instability. Sensory loss, numbness or tingling, weakness, or complete palsy within a peripheral nerve distribution (usually the axillary nerve) may be seen.
- If brachial vessels have been compromised, the patient may complain of weakness, coldness, or heaviness in the hand and arm.
- The patient often has a subjective feeling of instability, dislocation, or apprehension in the shoulder (especially with lateral rotation).

MECHANISM OF INJURY
The condition can arise from a FOOSH injury in which some lateral rotation levers the head of the humerus onto or over the rim of the glenoid cavity. The most common position of the FOOSH injury is with the arm abducted to 90° or more and laterally rotated to end range. Trauma that involves forced lateral rotation/abduction with posterior force at the glenohumeral joint results in shoulder anterior dislocation or subluxation. Another mechanism of injury is traction on the arm in the anterior direction.

PATIENT POSITION
The patient lies supine with the test arm close to the edge of the plinth.

EXAMINER POSITION
The examiner stands at the patient's side, facing the shoulder to be tested.

TEST PROCEDURE
Step 1—the crank test. The examiner places one hand beneath the elbow to support the upper extremity. The other hand grasps the wrist and is responsible for movement of the shoulder into lateral rotation. The examiner flexes the elbow to 90°, abducts the arm to 90°, and laterally rotates the shoulder slowly, watching for apprehension. The shoulder is laterally rotated as far as possible. The hand supporting the elbow then is moved to the anterior aspect of the humeral head. The examiner should maintain the amount of lateral rotation without releasing pressure.

Step 2—the relocation test. The examiner applies a posterior stress to the humeral head and assesses whether the patient loses the apprehension, the pain decreases, and further lateral rotation is possible before the apprehension returns. This relocation sometimes is referred to as the Fowler sign or Fowler test or the Jobe relocation test.[39,56] The hand pressure on the humeral head is removed, and symptoms are reassessed. For most patients, lateral rotation should be released before the posterior stress is released.

Continued

CRANK APPREHENSION/RELOCATION TEST[27-30,36,41,50-61]—*cont'd*

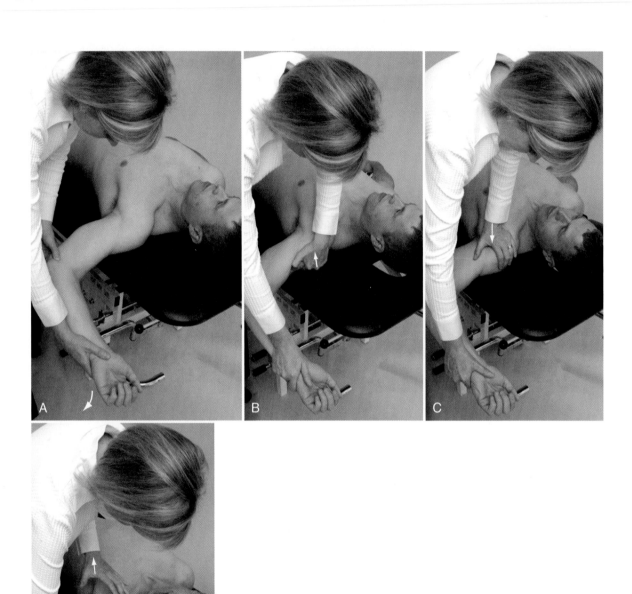

Figure 4–8

Crank apprehension/relocation test. **A,** Abduction and lateral rotation (crank test). **B,** Abduction and lateral rotation combined with anterior translation of the humerus, which may cause anterior subluxation or posterior joint pain. **C,** Abduction and lateral rotation combined with posterior translation of the humerus (relocation test). **D,** Surprise test.

CRANK APPREHENSION/RELOCATION TEST[27-30,36,41,50-61]—cont'd

INDICATIONS OF A POSITIVE TEST

Apprehension test. A positive test result is indicated if the patient becomes apprehensive as the arm is laterally rotated and begins to contract the muscles to stop the lateral rotation (apprehension predominates). The patient may say that the feeling resembles what it felt like when the shoulder was dislocated.

Relocation test. The patient's apprehension in the laterally rotated position disappears with the posterior translation. The examiner may find that lateral rotation will increase and apprehension will return as the lateral rotation increases. The test result is considered positive if pain decreases during the relocation maneuver, even if the patient felt no apprehension. If the arm is released ("surprise" test) in the new acquired range (step 3), pain and forward translation of the head are noted as positive test results.[40,56,57]

CLINICAL NOTES

- If pain rather than apprehension increases on lateral rotation, the problem is more likely to be impingement, and impingement tests should be performed.
- Hawkins and Bokor[58] state that the examiner should note the amount of lateral rotation present when the patient becomes apprehensive.
- With the relocation test, lateral rotation should be released before the posterior stress is released.
- If the patient's symptoms decrease or are eliminated during the relocation test, the diagnosis is glenohumeral instability, subluxation, dislocation, or impingement.
- If apprehension predominates during the crank test and disappears with the relocation test, the diagnosis is glenohumeral instability, subluxation, or dislocation.
- If pain predominates during the crank test and disappears with the relocation test, the diagnosis is pseudolaxity or anterior instability at either the glenohumeral joint or the scapulothoracic joint, with secondary impingement, or a posterior labral lesion.
- Kvitne and Jobe[59] advocate applying a mild, anteriorly directed force to the posterior humeral head when it is in the test position to see whether apprehension or pain increases. An increase in posterior pain may indicate a posterior internal impingement.
- Hamner et al[60] have suggested that if a posterior internal impingement is suspected, the relocation test should be done in 100° to 120° of abduction.
- In patients with a primary impingement, the relocation test does not alter the pain. A decrease in posterior pain when the relocation test is done posteriorly is a positive test result for posterior internal impingement.
- If the joint is normal, translation of the humeral head in the glenoid is less than with other tests, because the crank test takes the joint into the close packed position.
- If the arm is released (anterior release, or "surprise," test) in the newly acquired range of the relocation test, a positive test result is indicated by pain and forward translation of the head.
- The release maneuver (surprise test) should be done with care, because it often causes apprehension and distrust in the patient, and it could cause a dislocation.[40,56,57]
- The pain that results from the release maneuver (surprise test) may be caused by anterior shoulder instability, a labral lesion (Bankart or SLAP lesion), or bicipital peritenonitis or tendinosus.[40,56,57] Most often this pain is related to anterior instability, because it is temporarily produced by the anterior translation. The surprise test also has been reported to cause pain in older patients with a pathological condition of the rotator cuff and no instability.[61]

RELIABILITY/SPECIFICITY/ SENSITIVITY[27-30,32]

Specificity range: 56% to 100%
Sensitivity range: 35% to 91%

ROCKWOOD TEST (MODIFICATION OF THE CRANK TEST)[62]

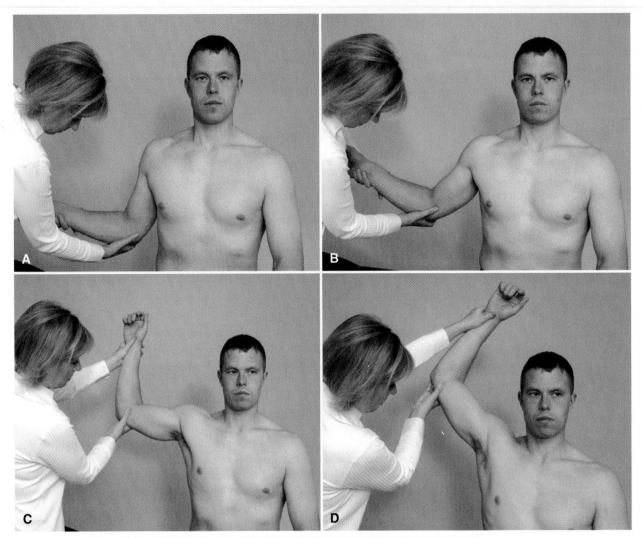

Figure 4–9
Rockwood test for anterior instability. **A,** Arm at the side. **B,** Arm at 45°. **C,** Arm at 90°. **D,** Arm at 120°.

PURPOSE	To assess for anterior instability of the glenohumeral joint.
PATIENT POSITION	The patient sits with no back support and with the hand of the test arm resting on the thigh.
EXAMINER POSITION	The examiner stands behind or to the side of the patient. The examiner should stand close enough to the involved shoulder to control the shoulder and allow for proper examiner body mechanics.
TEST PROCEDURE	The examiner places one hand beneath the elbow to provide support and stability and grasps the patient's wrist with the other hand. With the arm at the patient's side and the elbow flexed to 90°, the examiner laterally rotates the shoulder. The arm then is abducted to 45°, and passive lateral rotation is repeated. Lateral rotation is repeated at 90° (this part of the test is similar to the crank test) and 120° of abduction.

ROCKWOOD TEST (MODIFICATION OF THE CRANK TEST)[62]—*cont'd*

INDICATIONS OF A POSITIVE TEST   A positive test result is indicated if the patient shows marked apprehension with posterior pain when the arm is tested at 90°. At 45° and 120° of abduction, the patient will show some uneasiness and some pain; at 0°, apprehension is rarely seen.

CLINICAL NOTES/CAUTIONS

- It is imperative that this test be done slowly. If it is done too quickly, the humerus may dislocate, especially in patients who have had recurrent dislocations.
- The different positions of the arm are tested because different passive stabilizers of the shoulder come into play with changes in the angle of abduction.

RELIABILITY/SPECIFICITY/ SENSITIVITY   Unknown

FULCRUM TEST (MODIFICATION OF THE CRANK TEST)[50,54,56]

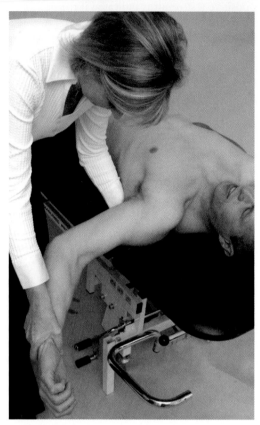

Figure 4–10
Fulcrum test, with the left fist pushing the head of the humerus anteriorly.

PURPOSE	To assess for anterior instability of the glenohumeral joint.
PATIENT POSITION	The patient lies supine.
EXAMINER POSITION	The examiner stands directly adjacent and slightly caudal to the shoulder region on the side closest to the test arm.
TEST PROCEDURE	The examiner places one hand under the posterior aspect of the glenohumeral joint to act as a fulcrum and grasps the patient's distal wrist with the other hand. The shoulder is abducted to 90°, and the elbow is flexed to 90°. The examiner then horizontally abducts and laterally rotates the arm gently over the fulcrum.
INDICATIONS OF A POSITIVE TEST	A positive test result for anterior stability is indicated by a look of apprehension on the patient's face or an increase in pain. Posterior pain may indicate a posterior internal impingement.
CLINICAL NOTE/CAUTION	• It is imperative that this test be done slowly. If it is done too quickly, the humerus may dislocate, especially in patients who have had recurrent dislocations.
RELIABILITY/SPECIFICITY/ SENSITIVITY	Unknown

SPECIAL TESTS FOR POSTERIOR GLENOHUMERAL INSTABILITY

Relevant Special Tests

Load and shift test—posterior
Norwood stress test
Posterior apprehension or stress test

Definition

Posterior glenohumeral instability is defined as laxity of the posterior aspect of the shoulder joint that makes it difficult for the humeral head to maintain its articulation and normal arthrokinematics within the glenoid.

Suspected Injury

The suspected injury is unidirectional instability; laxity in this direction often is accompanied by damage to the posterior rotator cuff muscles, posterior joint capsule, and possibly the posterior superior labrum.

Epidemiology and Demographics

Recurrent posterior instability of the glenohumeral joint is less common than anterior instability. The frequency of occurrence is less than 5% of shoulder dislocations in most series.[63] Other studies report that the rate of incidence is 2% to 12% of all cases of shoulder instability.[64]

Relevant History

The patient may or may not have a history of a pathological condition of or an injury to the involved shoulder. Posterior instability more often is related to trauma than to overuse.

Relevant Signs and Symptoms

- The patient may complain of generalized or posterior shoulder pain that may radiate down into the deltoid region of the shoulder.
- The patient may complain of weakness in the shoulder that may be accompanied by clicking or grinding with shoulder motion.
- Neural irritation is not common with posterior shoulder instability.
- The patient often has subjective feelings of instability, dislocation, or apprehension.
- The patient may complain that the shoulder "doesn't feel right," especially when it is loaded above shoulder height.
- The results of unloaded active and passive movement and resisted isometric testing may be normal.

Mechanism of Injury

The most common position of injury is with the arm flexed to 90° and slightly adducted. Blunt trauma to the shoulder in an anterior to posterior direction can cause posterior instability.

Clinical Note/Caution

- Posterior dislocations of the glenohumeral joint can be easily missed, even on x-ray films. Therefore, it is important to test all active and passive movements and compare the two sides before doing the instability test. Limited rotation may indicate that the dislocation has not been reduced.

LOAD AND SHIFT TEST—POSTERIOR[38-44,47-49,65]

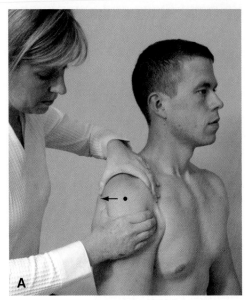
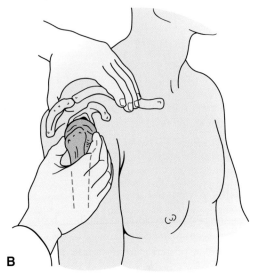

Figure 4–11

A, Load and shift test with the patient in the seated starting position. Note that the humerus first is loaded, or "centered," in the glenoid. The examiner then shifts the humerus posteriorly. **B,** The position of the examiner's hands in relation to the bones of the shoulder. Note that the examiner's left thumb holds the spine of the scapula for stability.

PURPOSE	To assess the posterior stability and mobility of the glenohumeral joint.
PATIENT POSITION	The patient sits with no back support and with the hand of the test arm resting on the thigh.
EXAMINER POSITION	The examiner stands or sits slightly behind the patient.
TEST PROCEDURE	The examiner stabilizes the shoulder with one hand over the clavicle and scapula. The other hand grasps the head of the humerus with the thumb over the posterior humeral head and the fingers over the anterior humeral head (right shoulder). The humerus then is gently pushed into the glenoid to seat it properly in the glenoid fossa so that the humeral head sits in neutral. This is the load portion of the test; seating the humerus centers it in the glenoid so that the amount of posterior motion from the neutral position can be determined. The examiner then pushes the humeral head posteriorly, noting the amount of translation. This is the shift portion of the test.
INDICATIONS OF A POSITIVE TEST	Differences between the two sides and reproduction of symptoms are considered more important than the amount of movement obtained. Posterior movement is often compared with anterior translation. Normally, posterior movement is equal to or greater than anterior movement.

LOAD AND SHIFT TEST—POSTERIOR[38-44,47-49,65]—cont'd

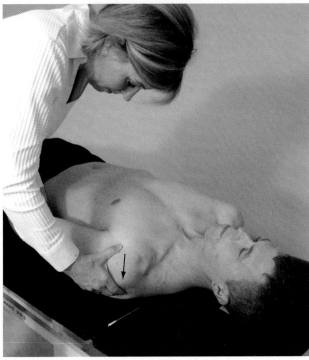

Figure 4–12

Load and shift test for posterior instability of the shoulder with the patient in the supine-lying position. The patient is supine on the examining table. The arm is brought into approximately 90° of forward elevation in the plane of the scapula. A posteriorly directed force is applied to the humerus with the arm in varying degrees of lateral rotation.

CLINICAL NOTES

- If the load is not applied to put the head in neutral position, the amount of movement found will not indicate the true amount of translation posteriorly, and the end feel will be altered.
- Normally, the head of the humerus should translate 25% to 50% of the diameter of the humeral head.
- Posterior translation of the humeral head is generally greater than anterior translation. (Authors vary on the amount of movement possible, but normally, posterior movement is never less than anterior movement.)
- The test also may be done with the patient in the supine-lying position. It is important to note that a positive test result is not specific for any one pathological condition; rather, it helps guide the clinician in the reasoning process.

RELIABILITY/SPECIFICITY/ SENSITIVITY[33]

Reliability range: k = 0.53-0.79

NORWOOD STRESS TEST[66,67]

DVD

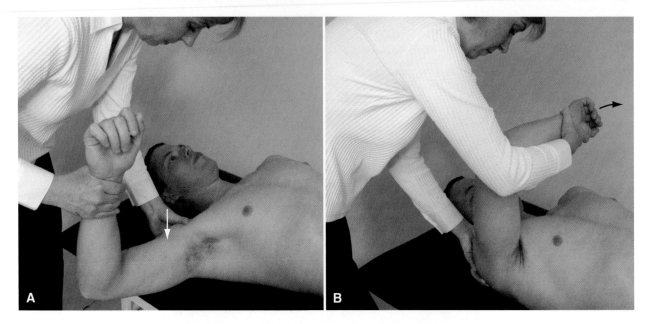

Figure 4–13
Norwood stress test for posterior shoulder instability. **A,** Arm abducted 90°. **B,** The arm is horizontally adducted to the forward flexed position.

PURPOSE	To assess the posterior stability and mobility of the glenohumeral joint.
PATIENT POSITION	The patient lies supine.
EXAMINER POSITION	The examiner stands directly adjacent and slightly cephalad to the shoulder region on the side closest to the test arm and should be facing the patient's feet.
TEST PROCEDURE	The examiner places the left hand as illustrated on the shoulder joint to support and stabilize the scapula. With the right hand, the examiner abducts the shoulder 60° to 100° and laterally rotates it 90°, with the elbow flexed to 90° so that the arm is horizontal. The examiner palpates the posterior humeral head with the fingers of the left hand and stabilizes the upper limb by holding the forearm and elbow at the elbow with the right hand. The examiner then brings the arm into 90° of forward flexion with the right hand.
	To perform the test, the examiner horizontally adducts the abducted arm across the patient's body with the right arm and at the same time pushes the humeral head posteriorly with the thumb of the left hand. As the humeral head is pushed posteriorly with the thumb, the examiner palpates the posterior humeral head with the fingers of the left hand to feel how far it slides posteriorly. The test first is performed on the unaffected shoulder and then the affected one, and the two sides are compared.
INDICATIONS OF A POSITIVE TEST	A positive test result is seen if the humeral head slips (subluxes) posteriorly over the rim of the glenoid. The patient confirms that the sensation felt is the same as that felt during activities. The arm is returned to the starting position, and the humeral head is felt to reduce. A clicking sound, caused by the passage of the humeral head over the glenoid rim, may accompany either subluxation or reduction.

NORWOOD STRESS TEST[66,67]—cont'd

CLINICAL NOTES/CAUTIONS	• Cofield and Irving[67] recommend medially rotating the forearm approximately 20° after the forward flexion and then pushing the elbow posteriorly to enhance the effect of the test.
	• Care must be taken with this test, because it does not cause apprehension in the patient, but it may cause subluxation or dislocation.
RELIABILITY/SPECIFICITY/ SENSITIVITY	Unknown

POSTERIOR APPREHENSION OR STRESS TEST[41,49,63,68,69]

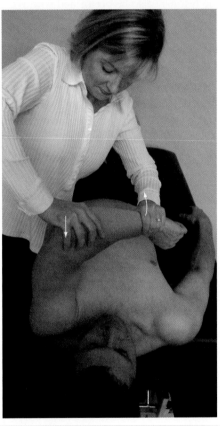

Figure 4–14
Posterior apprehension test with the patient supine.

PURPOSE	To assess the posterior stability and mobility of the glenohumeral joint.
PATIENT POSITION	The patient lies supine with the test arm close to the edge of the plinth.
EXAMINER POSITION	The examiner stands directly adjacent and slightly distal to the shoulder on the side closest to the test arm.

Continued

POSTERIOR APPREHENSION OR STRESS TEST[41,49,63,68,69]—*cont'd*

TEST PROCEDURE

The examiner grasps the patient's elbow with one hand and holds the distal wrist with the other. The patient's shoulder is forward-flexed in the plane of the scapula to 90°. A posterior force then is applied to the elbow. While applying the axial load to the elbow, the examiner horizontally adducts and medially rotates the arm. The examiner palpates the head of the humerus with one hand while the other hand pushes the head of the humerus posteriorly.

INDICATIONS OF A POSITIVE TEST

A positive test result is indicated by a look of apprehension or alarm on the patient's face and resistance to further motion or by reproduction of symptoms. In either case, if the humeral head moves posteriorly more the 50% of its diameter, posterior instability is evident. The movement may be accompanied by a clunk as the humeral head passes posteriorly over the glenoid rim.

CLINICAL NOTES/CAUTIONS

- The test may also be performed with the arm in 90° of abduction.
- The test also may be done with the patient in the sitting position, but the scapula must be stabilized.
- It is important to note that a positive test result is not specific for any one pathological condition; rather, it helps guide the clinician in the reasoning process. Instability may be a contributing factor in the development of the ultimate pathological condition.
- Pagnani and Warren[69] reported that a positive test result is more likely to be marked by pain than by apprehension. They reported that with atraumatic multidirectional (inferior) instability, the test result is negative.

RELIABILITY/SPECIFICITY/ SENSITIVITY

Unknown

SPECIAL TESTS FOR INFERIOR GLENOHUMERAL INSTABILITY

Relevant Special Tests

Sulcus sign
Feagin test

Definition

Inferior glenohumeral instability is defined as laxity of the inferior aspect of the shoulder joint that makes it difficult for the humeral head to maintain its articulation and normal arthrokinematics within the glenoid.

Suspected Injuries

Unidirectional instability
Multidirectional instability

Epidemiology and Demographics

Athletes who play overhead sports (e.g., tennis, volleyball, baseball) and patients with a history of dislocations or subluxations are more likely to have multidirectional instability of the shoulder. Several factors make the younger athlete more susceptible to multidirectional shoulder instability. Younger athletes have a tendency to have poor shoulder mechanics (incorrect techniques) and inadequate strength. In addition, some researchers speculate that adolescents' immature collagen makeup leaves them more susceptible to shoulder instability and laxity.[37,70-77]

Relevant History

The patient may or may not have a history of a pathological condition of or an injury to the affected shoulder. Many patients have joint hypermobility in other areas (e.g., elbow or knee hyperextension). The symptoms of instability are insidious and include progressive increases in popping, clicking, or clunking in the shoulder. The patient may complain of weakness and paresthesia in the shoulder and upper extremity, or the person may have a recent history of stroke (involuntary instability).

Relevant Signs and Symptoms

- The patient may have subjective feelings of instability, dislocation, or apprehension.
- The patient may complain that the shoulder "doesn't feel right," especially when it is loaded above shoulder height.
- Test results with unloaded active and passive movement and resisted isometric testing may be normal.

Mechanism of Injury

Shoulder instability may be the result of trauma, repetitive use, or a genetic joint laxity. Multidirectional instability may be the result of a genetic predisposition to joint laxity. Generally, genetic laxity occurs in both shoulders and in other joints. It is believed that if a patient demonstrates inferior instability, multidirectional instability also is present; therefore, a patient with inferior instability also will demonstrate anterior or posterior instability, or both.

SULCUS SIGN[50,69,78-82]

DVD

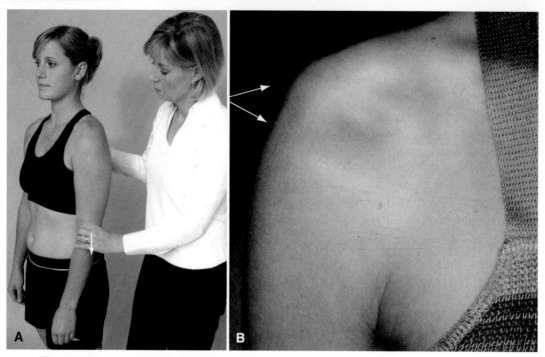

Figure 4–15
A, Test for inferior shoulder instability (sulcus test). **B,** Positive sulcus sign *(arrows)*.

PURPOSE	To assess inferior laxity within the glenohumeral joint.
PATIENT POSITION	The patient stands with the arm by the side and the shoulder muscles relaxed.
EXAMINER POSITION	The examiner stands beside the patient.
TEST PROCEDURE	The examiner stabilizes the scapula with one hand over the clavicle and scapula. With the other hand, the examiner grasps the patient's arm above the elbow and pulls the arm distally (applies traction), looking for a sulcus at the end of the acromion.
INDICATIONS OF A POSITIVE TEST	The presence of a sulcus under the acromion indicates inferior instability or glenohumeral laxity. The sulcus sign may be graded by measuring from the inferior margin of the acromion to the humeral heads (Table 4-1).

Table 4-1
Grading of the Sulcus Sign

Grading	Measurement
+1	<1 cm
+2	1-2 cm
+3	>2 cm

SULCUS SIGN[50,69,78-82]—cont'd

CLINICAL NOTE

- Some researchers have reported that the best position for testing for inferior instability is at 20° to 50° of abduction with neutral rotation.[48] Therefore, the examiner should consider testing more than one position. Depending on the history, the examiner should test the patient in the position in which the sensation of instability is reported

RELIABILITY/SPECIFICITY/ SENSITIVITY

Unknown

FEAGIN TEST[62]

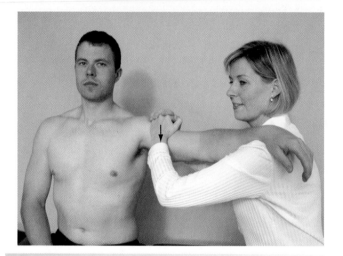

Figure 4–16
Feagin test.

PURPOSE	To assess inferior laxity within the shoulder glenohumeral joint.
PATIENT POSITION	The patient stands or sits.
EXAMINER POSITION	The examiner stands beside the test arm.
TEST PROCEDURE	The examiner abducts the patient's arm to 90° with the elbow extended and holds the arm so that it is fully supported, with the arm against the examiner's body. The examiner places the other hand just lateral to the acromion over the humeral head. Making sure that the shoulder musculature is relaxed, the examiner pushes the head of the humerus down and forward. Performing the test in this manner gives the examiner greater control of the arm.
INDICATIONS OF A POSITIVE TEST	A positive test result is indicated by a look of apprehension on the patient's face and the presence of anteroinferior instability. In addition, a sulcus may be seen above the coracoid process.
CLINICAL NOTES/CAUTIONS	• The Feagin test is a modification of the sulcus test with the arm abducted to 90° instead of being at the patient's side. Some authors consider the Feagin test the second part of the sulcus test.[80] • This test position also puts more stress on the inferior glenohumeral ligament. • Positive results on both the sulcus sign and the Feagin test point more decisively to multidirectional instability, rather than just laxity.
RELIABILITY/SPECIFICITY/ SENSITIVITY	Unknown

SPECIAL TESTS FOR IMPINGEMENT

Relevant Special Tests

Hawkins-Kennedy impingement test
Neer impingement test
Posterior internal impingement test

Definition

Shoulder impingement syndrome is a generalized term used to describe the compression of and resultant damage to soft tissue structures within the shoulder region, most commonly anteriorly and superiorly. Shoulder impingement is not in itself a pathological condition, but rather the action that may result in such a condition. Classically, the term *impingement* has been used to define the compression of tissue in the subacromial space or under the coracoacromial ligament; however, in reality the term can be used to define compression between or pinching of any structures in the shoulder.

Suspected Injuries

Rotator cuff tendinopathy
Subacromial bursitis
Bicipital tendinopathy

Epidemiology and Demographics[83]

Neer has described three stages of impingement (Table 4-2).

Relevant History

A patient with anterior impingement may or may not have a history of shoulder injury or pain; in most cases, impingement is the result of a gradual progressive process. Patients with a history of shoulder dislocation or subluxation also may have a posterior labral lesion as a result of the injury. A patient with posterior impingement may complain of pain posteriorly in the late cocking and early acceleration phase of throwing or similar overhead activities.

Relevant Signs and Symptoms

- Pain under the acromion and over the coracoacromial ligament
- Lateral deltoid/arm pain
- Point tenderness over greater tubercle of humerus
- Diffuse upper trapezius pain
- Diffuse thoracic/interscapular pain
- Anteromedial shoulder pain

Mechanism of Injury[84-88]

Anterior shoulder impingement. Regardless of its cause (e.g., pathological condition of the rotator cuff, bicipital paratenonitis/tendinosis, scapular or humeral instability, labral pathology), anterior shoulder impingement most commonly results when structures are compressed in the anterior aspect of the humerus between the head of the humerus and the coracoid process, under the acromion process and under the coracoacromial ligament. These injuries may be acute or degenerative. An acute injury produces a sudden onset of shoulder pain after a specific activity. The aggravating activity commonly is an overhead maneuver, such as throwing or painting. Trauma, such as a fall onto an outstretched hand (FOOSH injury), also can result in shoulder impingement. Because of the progressive nature of subacromial impingement, patients with degenerative-type impingement often complain of several bouts of shoulder pain over a number of years. Each subsequent episode generally is worse than the previous one. The patient often reports that the latest episode did not resolve and has increasing loss of ROM.

Posterior shoulder impingement. Posterior impingement occurs when the rotator cuff impinges against the

Table 4-2
Neer's Grades of Shoulder Impingement[83]

Grade	Pathology	Symptoms	Range of Motion and Strength
Grade I	Subacromial bursitis/ tendonitis	Local pain; mild swelling, ecchymosis, tenderness Mild tightness or spasm locally	Minimal loss of ROM and strength
Grade II	Partial rotator cuff tear	Symptoms similar to grade I but symptoms more pronounced	Moderate loss of ROM and strength
Grade III	Full-thickness rotator cuff tear	Significant swelling and ecchymosis	Severe loss of ROM and strength

posterosuperior edge of the glenoid when the arm is abducted, extended, and laterally rotated. The result is a "kissing" labral lesion posteriorly. The resulting impingement occurs between the rotator cuff and greater tuberosity on one side and the posterior glenoid and labrum on the other side. This type of impingement often accompanies anterior instability or pseudolaxity, and deltoid activity increases to compensate for weakened rotator cuff muscles.

Reliability/Specificity/Sensitivity/Comparison[89]

	Validity	Interrater Reliability	Intrarater Reliability	Specificity	Sensitivity
Hawkins-Kennedy Impingement Test	Unknown	Unknown	Unknown	25%	92%
Neer Impingement Test	Unknown	Unknown	Unknown	30.5%	88.7%
Posterior Internal Impingement Test	Unknown	Unknown	Unknown	Unknown	Unknown

HAWKINS-KENNEDY IMPINGEMENT TEST[87,89-99]

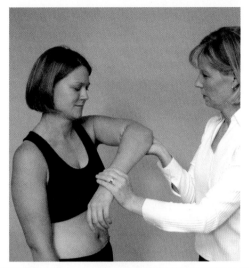

Figure 4–17
Hawkins-Kennedy impingement test demonstrates the impingement sign by forcibly medially rotating the proximal humerus when the arm is forward flexed to 90°.

PURPOSE	The Hawkins-Kennedy impingement test is designed to reduce the space between the inferior aspect of the acromial arch and the superior surface of the humeral head. The additional compressive forces subsequently put pressure on the supraspinatus tendon, the tendon of the long head of the biceps, the subacromial bursa, and/or the coracoacromial ligament.
PATIENT POSITION	The patient may be standing or sitting.
EXAMINER POSITION	The examiner stands adjacent and slightly to the front of the shoulder to be tested.
TEST PROCEDURE	The examiner puts one hand on the patient's elbow for support and stabilization and grasps the wrist with the other hand. The examiner flexes the elbow to 90°, forward-flexes the arm to 90°, and then forcibly medially rotates the shoulder. This movement pushes the supraspinatus tendon against the anterior surface of the coracoacromial ligament and coracoid process.
INDICATIONS OF A POSITIVE TEST	Pain is a positive test result for supraspinatus paratenonitis/tendinosis or secondary impingement often associated with scapular control problems.
CLINICAL NOTES/CAUTIONS	• The test also may be performed in different degrees of forward flexion (vertically "circling the shoulder") or horizontal adduction (horizontally circling the shoulder). • McFarland et al.[96] described the coracoid impingement sign, which is the same as the Hawkins-Kennedy test but involves horizontally adducting the arm across the body 10° to 20° before doing the medial rotation. This is more likely to approximate the lesser tuberosity of the humerus and the coracoid process. • The Yocum test is a modification of the Hawkins-Kennedy test in which the patient's hand is placed on the opposite shoulder and the examiner elevates the elbow.[97,98] • Park et al.[99] found that combining tests gave better results. They found that the Hawkins-Kennedy test, the painful arc sign, and a positive result on the infraspinatus test gave the best probability of detecting impingement, whereas the painful arc sign, drop arm test, and infraspinatus test were best for detecting full-thickness rotator cuff tears.
RELIABILITY/SPECIFICITY/ SENSITIVITY[89,93-95]	Specificity range: 25% to 66% Sensitivity range: 47% to 92%

NEER IMPINGEMENT TEST[89,90,95,99-102]

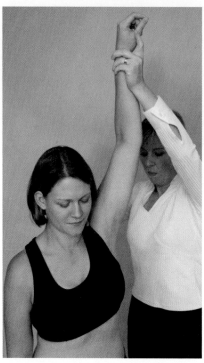

Figure 4–18
A positive result for the Neer impingement test is indicated by pain and its resulting facial expression when the arm is forcibly flexed forward by the examiner, jamming the greater tuberosity against the anteroinferior surface of the acromion.

PURPOSE	The Neer impingement test is designed to reduce the space between the inferior aspect of the acromial arch and the superior surface of the humeral head. The compressive forces subsequently put pressure on the supraspinatus tendon, the tendon of the long head of the biceps, the subacromial bursa, and/or the coracoacromial ligament.
PATIENT POSITION	The patient may be standing or sitting.
EXAMINER POSITION	The examiner stands lateral and slightly behind the shoulder to be tested.
TEST PROCEDURE	The examiner places one hand over the patient's clavicle and scapula to help stabilize the scapula and the other hand around the wrist or forearm. The examiner passively and forcibly elevates the arm fully in the scapular plane and then medially rotates the arm. This passive stress causes the greater tuberosity to jam against the anteroinferior border of the acromion.
INDICATIONS OF A POSITIVE TEST	A positive test result is indicated by an expression of pain on the patient's face.
CLINICAL NOTES/CAUTIONS	• A positive test result may indicate an overuse injury to the supraspinatus muscle and sometimes to the biceps tendon; these injuries often are associated with scapular control problems. • If the test result is positive when the test is done with the arm laterally rotated, the examiner should check the acromioclavicular joint (acromioclavicular differentiation test).
RELIABILITY/SPECIFICITY/ SENSITIVITY[89,95,99,102]	Specificity range: 30.5% to 68% Sensitivity range: 59% to 89%

POSTERIOR INTERNAL IMPINGEMENT TEST[55,103-106]

DVD

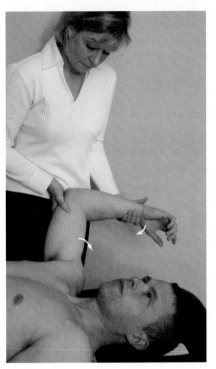

Figure 4–19
Posterior internal impingement test.

PURPOSE	To test for a lesion on the posterior of the shoulder labrum and rotator cuff.
SUSPECTED INJURY	• Posterior labral lesion • Posterior rotator cuff lesion
RELEVANT HISTORY	The patient often has a history of repetitive overuse through overhead activities (e.g., throwing or tennis). A patient with a history of shoulder dislocation or subluxation also may have a posterior labral lesion as a result of the injury.
RELEVANT SIGNS AND SYMPTOMS	The patient complains of pain posteriorly in the late cocking and early acceleration phase of throwing or similar overhead activities.
MECHANISM OF INJURY	Posterior impingement occurs when the rotator cuff impinges against the posterosuperior edge of the glenoid when the arm is abducted, extended, and laterally rotated. The result is a "kissing" labral lesion posteriorly. The resulting impingement is between the rotator cuff and greater tuberosity on one side and the posterior glenoid and labrum on the other side. The condition often accompanies anterior instability or pseudolaxity, and deltoid activity increases to compensate for weakened rotator cuff muscles.
PATIENT POSITION	The patient is in the supine-lying position.
EXAMINER POSITION	The examiner stands adjacent to the shoulder to be tested.

Continued

POSTERIOR INTERNAL IMPINGEMENT TEST[55,103-106]—*cont'd*

TEST PROCEDURE

The examiner places one hand under the patient's elbow for support and stability; the other hand grasps the patient's wrist and is responsible for shoulder rotation. The examiner passively abducts the shoulder to 90°, with 15° to 20° of forward flexion and maximum lateral rotation.

INDICATIONS OF A POSITIVE TEST

The test result is considered positive if it elicits localized pain in the posterior shoulder.

CLINICAL NOTE

- Posterior internal impingement is found primarily in athletes involved in overhead sports, although it may be found in others who hold the arm in the vulnerable position of full elevation and rotation.

RELIABILITY/SPECIFICITY/ SENSITIVITY

Unknown

SPECIAL TESTS FOR LABRAL TEARS OF THE GLENOHUMERAL JOINT

Relevant Special Tests

Active compression test of O'Brien
Anterior slide test
Biceps tension test
Clunk test
Biceps load test
Labral crank test
SLAP prehension test
Note: Parentis et al.[107] concluded that no one test can provide a definitive diagnosis of a labral lesion.

Definition

The labrum is a firm ring of cartilage that surrounds the shoulder joint. It serves two purposes: it increases the depth and size of the glenoid fossa, giving the joint greater stability and surface area, and it acts as a "chock block" to stop the humeral head from translating off the glenoid. The term *labral tear* is used to classify several types of labral injury, the most common of which are the Bankart lesion and the SLAP lesion (superior labrum anterior and posterior [to the biceps]).

Suspected Injuries

Labral tear
Labral lesion
Bankart lesion (in which the anteroinferior labrum is torn)
SLAP lesion (in which the anterior or posterior superior labrum may have been injured)

Epidemiology and Demographics

The most common cause of a labral tear is trauma from a dislocation. In addition, younger individuals are prone to labral injury with repetitive overhead motions, such as swimming, tennis, or throwing. Older people are more prone to degenerative lesions, which often are associated with poor vascular supply to the labral tissue.[54,74,108,109]

Relevant History

Injuries to the labrum are relatively common, especially in athletes involved in throwing and overhead sports; in these activities, the labrum plays a key role in glenohumeral stability. In the young, the tensile strength of the labrum is less than that of the capsule; consequently, the labrum is more prone to injury when anterior stress (e.g., anterior dislocation) is applied to the glenohumeral joint.

Relevant Signs and Symptoms

- Aching of the shoulder region
- A feeling of instability may be noted by the patient
- Clicking or popping with motion
- Catching in the shoulder with movement
- Weakness or pain (or both) with overhead motions
- Diffuse upper trapezius or thoracic pain (or both)
- Pain with activities that require biceps contraction
- Pain on palpation of the anterior joint line

Mechanism of Injury

Repetitive overhead activities, such as serving a tennis ball or throwing, can result in labral injury. Traumatic injuries also can damage the labrum, such as a FOOSH injury, catching a heavy object with forced biceps contraction, shoulder dislocation, and shoulder subluxation.

A Bankart lesion occurs most commonly with a traumatic anterior dislocation that leads to anterior instability. For example, if this type of injury occurs in the right shoulder, the labrum is detached anywhere from the 3 o'clock to the 7 o'clock position, resulting in both anterior and posterior structural injury. Not only is the labrum torn; the stability of the inferior glenohumeral ligament also is lost.

With a SLAP lesion, the labrum is detached from the glenoid (pulled or peeled, depending on the mechanism).

This detachment can occur anywhere from the 10 o'clock to the 2 o'clock position on the glenoid. This lesion often results from a FOOSH injury, occurs during deceleration when throwing, or arises when sudden traction is applied to the biceps. If the biceps tendon also detaches, the shoulder becomes unstable and the support of the superior glenohumeral ligament is lost.

Clinical Note/Caution

• Diagnosis of a SLAP lesion is based primarily on the history. The special tests are used to verify the suspected involvement of the labrum. The tests themselves should not be the sole source of diagnosis; they must correlate with the patient's subjective complaints.

RELIABILITY/SPECIFICITY/SENSITIVITY COMPARISON[27-29,110-112]

	Active Compression Test of O'Brien	Anterior Slide Test	Biceps Load Test	Biceps Tension Test	Clunk Test	Labral Crank Test	SLAP Prehension Test
Specificity	31% to 55%	84% to 91.5%	96.6%	Unknown	Unknown	56% to 100%	Unknown
Sensitivity	47% to 54%	8% to 78.4%	89.7%	Unknown	Unknown	46% to 91%	Unknown

ACTIVE COMPRESSION TEST OF O'BRIEN[29,30,32,53,102,103,110,111,113,114]

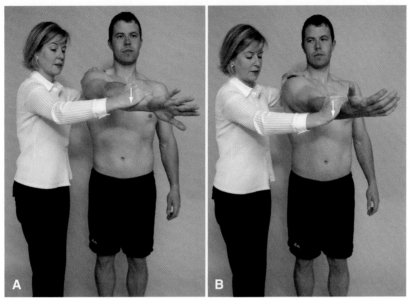

Figure 4–20

Active compression test of O'Brien. **A,** Position 1: The patient forward flexes the arm to 90° with the elbow extended and adducted 15° medial to the midline of the body and the thumb pointed down. The examiner applies a downward force to the arm, which the patient resists. **B,** Position 2: The test is performed with the arm in the same position, but the patient fully supinates the arm with the palm facing the ceiling. The maneuver is repeated. The test result is positive for a superior labral injury if pain is elicited in the first step (position 1) and reduced or eliminated in the second step (position 2).

PURPOSE	To assess the integrity of the superior aspect of the shoulder labrum.
PATIENT POSITION	The patient is standing with the arm forward flexed to 90° and the elbow fully extended.
EXAMINER POSITION	The examiner stands slightly behind and adjacent to the test shoulder.
TEST PROCEDURE	The examiner puts one hand on the patient's shoulder to stabilize the scapula and clavicle and the other hand on the forearm of the affected arm. The arm is horizontally adducted 10° to 15° (starting position) and medially rotated by the patient so that the thumb faces downward. The examiner applies a downward eccentric force to the arm. The arm is returned to the starting position, the palm is supinated, and the downward eccentric load is repeated.
INDICATIONS OF A POSITIVE TEST	If pain or painful clicking is produced inside the shoulder (not over the acromioclavicular joint) in the first part of the test (medial rotation) and eliminated or decreased in the second part (lateral rotation), the test result is considered positive for labral abnormalities.
CLINICAL NOTE/CAUTION	• This test also "locks and loads" the acromioclavicular joint in medial rotation; therefore, the examiner must take care to differentiate between labral and acromioclavicular pathological conditions.
RELIABILITY/SPECIFICITY/ SENSITIVITY[29,30,32,102,110,111]	Specificity range: 31% to 99% Sensitivity range: 54% to 00%

ANTERIOR SLIDE TEST[110,111,115,116]

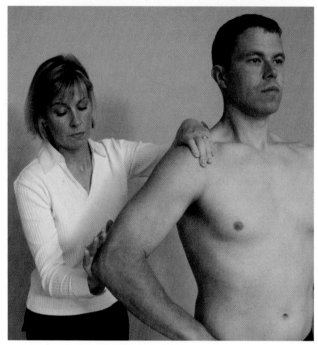

Figure 4–21
Anterior slide test. Note the position of the examiner's hands and the patient's arms.

PURPOSE	To assess the integrity of the anterior shoulder labrum.
PATIENT POSITION	The patient is sitting or standing with the hands on the waist, thumbs posterior.
EXAMINER POSITION	Standing behind the patient, the examiner stabilizes the scapula and clavicle with one hand and uses the fingers of the same hand to lightly palpate the anterior humeral head. The examiner places the other hand on the posterior aspect of the elbow.
TEST PROCEDURE	The examiner applies an anterosuperior force at the patient's elbow.
INDICATIONS OF A POSITIVE TEST	If the labrum is torn (SLAP lesion), the humeral head slides over the labrum with a pop or crack and the patient complains of anterosuperior pain. The pop or crack sometimes may be palpated if the examiner lightly places the fingers of the stabilizing hand over the anterior humeral head.
RELIABILITY/SPECIFICITY/ SENSITIVITY[110,111]	Specificity range: 85% to 91.5% Sensitivity range: 8% to 78%

BICEPS TENSION TEST

DVD

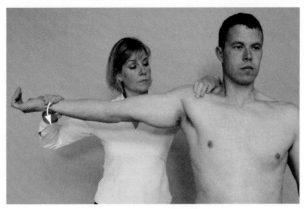

Figure 4–22
Biceps tension test. The patient's arm is abducted to 90° and laterally rotated. The examiner then applies an eccentric adduction force.

PURPOSE	To assess for a lesion of the superior labrum.
PATIENT POSITION	The patient, standing, abducts and laterally rotates the arm to 90° with the elbow extended and the forearm supinated.
EXAMINER POSITION	The examiner stands slightly behind and adjacent to the test shoulder.
TEST PROCEDURE	The examiner places one hand on the test shoulder to stabilize the scapula and clavicle and grasps the forearm with the other hand. The examiner then applies an eccentric adduction force to the straightened and supinated arm.
INDICATIONS OF A POSITIVE TEST	Reproduction of the patient's symptoms is a positive test result.
CLINICAL NOTES/CAUTIONS	• Speed's test should be done to rule out a biceps pathological condition. • Because SLAP lesions may involve the long head of the biceps tendon, any test stressing the long head of the biceps could stress the superior labrum. Several similar tests are designed to stress both structures, such as the biceps load test, biceps tension test, SLAP prehension test, and labral crank test.
RELIABILITY/SPECIFICITY/ SENSITIVITY	Unknown

CLUNK TEST[116,117]

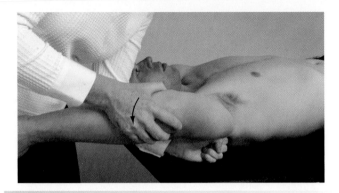

Figure 4–23
Clunk test.

PURPOSE	To assess the integrity of the anterior shoulder labrum.
PATIENT POSITION	The patient lies supine.
EXAMINER POSITION	The examiner stands adjacent and superior to the shoulder to be tested.
TEST PROCEDURE	The examiner places one hand under the posterior aspect of the shoulder so that it lies under the humeral head; the other hand holds the humerus above the elbow. The examiner fully abducts the arm over the patient's head. The examiner then pushes anteriorly with the hand under the humeral head (a fist may be used to apply more anterior pressure) while the other hand rotates the humerus into lateral rotation.
INDICATIONS OF A POSITIVE TEST	A clunk or grinding sound indicates both a positive test result and a labral tear. The test also may cause apprehension if anterior instability is present.
CLINICAL NOTES	• The examiner may position the arm in different amounts of abduction (vertically circling the shoulder) and perform the test in each position. This stresses different parts of the labrum. • Walsh[117] reported that if the examiner follows the abduction maneuvers with horizontal adduction that relocates the humerus, a clunk or click may be heard, indicating a labral tear.
RELIABILITY/SPECIFICITY/ SENSITIVITY	Unknown

BICEPS LOAD TEST[112,118]

DVD

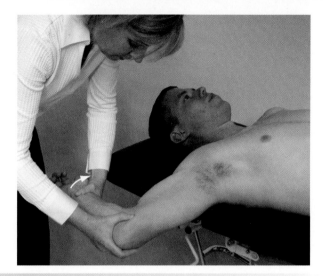

Figure 4–24
Biceps load test.

PURPOSE	To assess for a lesion of the superior labrum.
PATIENT POSITION	The patient lies supine with the shoulder abducted to 90° and laterally rotated, with the elbow flexed to 90° and the forearm supinated.
EXAMINER POSITION	The examiner stands slightly superiorly and adjacent to the test shoulder.
TEST PROCEDURE	The examiner holds the patient's elbow for support with one hand and grasps the wrist with the other hand. The examiner performs an apprehension test by taking the arm into full lateral rotation. If apprehension appears, the examiner stops lateral rotation and holds the position. The patient then is asked to flex the elbow against the examiner's resistance at the wrist.
INDICATIONS OF A POSITIVE TEST	If apprehension decreases or the patient feels more comfortable when the elbow is flexed, the test result is negative for a SLAP lesion. If the apprehension remains the same or the shoulder becomes more painful, the test result is considered positive.
SPECIFICITY/SENSITIVITY[112]	Specificity: 96.6% Sensitivity: 89.7%

LABRAL CRANK TEST[28]

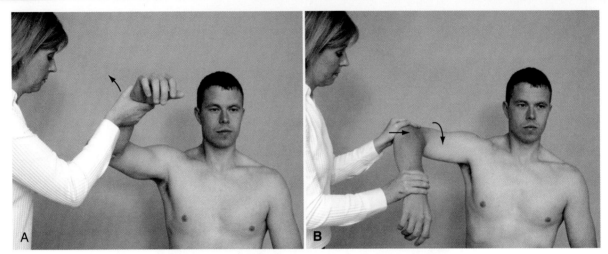

Figure 4–25
Labral crank test. **A,** Crank test, with the patient sitting, with lateral humeral rotation. **B,** Crank test, with the patient sitting, with medial humeral rotation.

PURPOSE	To assess for a lesion of the labrum of the shoulder.
PATIENT POSITION	The patient is in the supine-lying or sitting position.
EXAMINER POSITION	The examiner stands adjacent to the test shoulder.
TEST PROCEDURE	The examiner places one hand on the patient's elbow for support and stability and grasps the wrist with the other hand. The arm is elevated to 160° in the scapular plane. In this position, the examiner applies an axial load to the humerus with one hand while the other hand rotates the humerus medially and laterally.
INDICATIONS OF A POSITIVE TEST	A positive test result is indicated by pain on rotation, especially lateral rotation, with or without a click or reproduction of symptoms.
RELIABILITY/SPECIFICITY/ SENSITIVITY	Unknown

SLAP PREHENSION TEST[119]

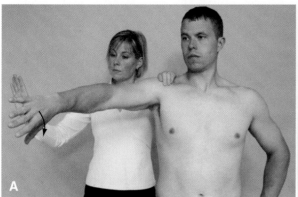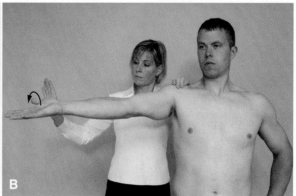

Figure 4–26

SLAP prehension test. **A,** Start position 1: The arm is abducted to 90° with the elbow extended and the forearm pronated. The patient then horizontally adducts the arm. **B,** Start position 2: This is the same as position 1, but forearm is supinated. The patient again horizontally adducts the arm. If position 1 is painful but position 2 is not, the test result is considered positive.

PURPOSE	To assess for a lesion of the superior labrum.
PATIENT POSITION	The patient is sitting or standing.
EXAMINER POSITION	The examiner stands behind and adjacent to the test shoulder.
TEST PROCEDURE	The examiner places one hand on the patient's shoulder to stabilize the scapula and clavicle and holds the wrist with the other hand. The examiner abducts the arm to 90° with the elbow extended and the forearm pronated (thumb down and shoulder medially rotated). The patient then is asked to adduct the arm horizontally. The movement is repeated with the forearm supinated (thumb up and shoulder laterally rotated).
INDICATIONS OF A POSITIVE TEST	If the patient feels pain in the bicipital groove with pronation but the pain lessens or is absent with supination, the test result is considered positive for a SLAP lesion.
RELIABILITY/SPECIFICITY/ SENSITIVITY	Unknown

SPECIAL TESTS FOR SCAPULAR STABILITY[15,120-123]

Relevant Special Tests

Lateral scapular slide test
Scapular load test
Scapular retraction test
Push up test

Definition

The muscles of the glenohumeral joint should work in a normal, coordinated fashion. For this to happen, the scapula must be stabilized by its muscles. A stable scapula provides a firm base for the glenohumeral muscles (primarily the rotator cuff) to function properly. The scapula not only must be stable in static positions, it also must move in correct patterns during dynamic motions. Scapular stability is the ability of the scapula to provide this solid base to enable arm motion. *Scapular dyskinesia* is the term used to describe the inability of the scapula to move and function normally during upper extremity motion.

Suspected Injuries

Dynamic winging (i.e., winging with movement) may be caused by a lesion of the long thoracic nerve, spinal accessory nerve, or suprascapular nerve; by muscle imbalance patterns; or by hypomobility either in the scapula or the glenohumeral joint.

Cervical radiculopathies, rhomboid weakness, multidirectional instability, and voluntary action also may result in abnormal scapular mechanics.

Scapular instability or dyskinesia may be the result of a pathological condition in other regions, such as rotator cuff tears, biceps tendinopathies, or rib dysfunction. The scapula may move abnormally to protect or compensate for such conditions.

Static winging (i.e., winging that occurs at rest) usually is caused by a structural deformity of the scapula, clavicle, spine, or ribs; by muscle weakness; or by hypomobility (collagen or muscular).

Epidemiology and Demographics

The epidemiology and demographics of scapular dyskinesia depend on the pathological condition causing the abnormal scapular mechanics. Nerve palsies (e.g., long thoracic nerve palsy, suprascapular nerve palsy, and spinal accessory nerve palsy) are not tied to a specific age or time frame; they more often are associated with activities or generalized laxity within the shoulder. Suprascapular nerve palsy is common in athletes involved in overhead sports and in patients with capsular laxity. The long thoracic nerve commonly is compressed by heavy backpacks or as a result of direct trauma; therefore, it is seen in students who carry backpacks, in military personnel, and in contact sports. Other causes, such as shoulder or cervical pathological conditions, vary in demographics based on the source of the patient's symptoms.

Relevant History

The patient may complain of tightness in the rhomboid region or a dull ache between the shoulder blades. The person also may notice clicking or catching beneath the shoulder blade with motion. The past history may include trauma or repetitive use. However, most patients do not seek medical attention for scapular dyskinesia. The poor scapular stability usually comes to light as a contributor to other symptoms or pathological conditions, such as anterior shoulder pain and anterior glenohumeral instability. Patients with a shoulder or cervical pathological condition often show scapular dyskinesia.

Relevant Signs and Symptoms

- Dull ache in the rhomboid region
- Catching, clicking, or popping beneath the scapula with upper extremity motion
- Scapular winging or tilting ("dumping")
- Cervical tightness or pain
- Shoulder pain
- Weakness in the shoulder
- Rib hypomobility

Mechanism of Injury

The spines of the scapulae, which begin medially at the level of the third thoracic vertebra (T3), should be at the same angle. The scapula itself should extend from the T2 or T3 spinous process to the T7 or T9 spinous process of the thoracic vertebrae.

Sobush et al.[122] developed the Lennie test, a method for measuring the scapular position. For this test, they measured from the spinous processes horizontally to three scapular positions: the medial aspect of the most superior point (superior angle), the root of the spine of the scapula, and the inferior angle. If the scapula sits lower than normal against the chest wall, its superior medial border may "washboard" over the ribs, causing a snapping or clunking sound (snapping scapula) during abduction and adduction. The inferior angles of the scapulae should be equidistant from the spine.

Kibler et al.[123] described four patterns of scapular dysfunction or dyskinesia.

- In *type I* dysfunction, the inferior medial border is prominent at rest, the inferior angle tilts dorsally with movement (scapular tilt), and the acromion tilts anteriorly over the top of the thorax. This type of dyskinesia may be seen at rest or during concentric or eccentric movements. Tilting of the inferior border away from the chest wall may indicate weak muscles (e.g., lower trapezius, latissimus dorsi, or serratus anterior) or a tight pectoralis minor or major that pulls or tilts the scapula forward from above (sometimes called *scapular dumping*).

- *Type II* dysfunction is the classic winging of the scapula; the whole medial border of the scapula is prominent and lifts away from the posterior chest wall both statically and dynamically. This pattern, too, may be seen at rest or during eccentric or concentric movements. It may indicate a SLAP lesion; weakness of the serratus anterior, rhomboids, or lower, middle, or upper trapezius; a long thoracic nerve problem; or tight humeral rotators.

- *Type III* dysfunction is marked by elevation of the superior border of the scapula at rest and during movement; a shoulder shrug initiates the movement, and winging is minimal. This deformity is seen with active movement and may result from overactivity of the levator scapula and upper trapezius, along with an imbalance in the upper and lower trapezius force couple. Type III dysfunction is associated with impingement and rotator cuff lesions.

- In *type IV* dysfunction, the two scapulae are symmetrical at rest and during motion; they rotate symmetrically upward, and the inferior angles rotate laterally away from the midline (rotary winging). This type of dysfunction is seen during movement and may indicate that the scapular control muscles are not stabilizing the scapula.

LATERAL SCAPULAR SLIDE TEST[6,124-127]

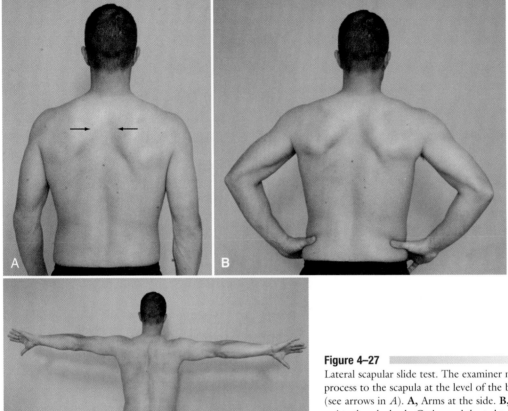

Figure 4–27

Lateral scapular slide test. The examiner measures from the spinous process to the scapula at the level of the base of the spine of the scapula (see arrows in *A*). **A,** Arms at the side. **B,** Arms abducted, hands on the waist, thumbs back. **C,** Arms abducted to 90°, arms medially rotated (thumbs down).

PURPOSE	To determine the static stability of the scapula with different glenohumeral positions.
PATIENT POSITION	The patient sits or stands with the arm resting at the side.
EXAMINER POSITION	The examiner stands behind the patient so as to observe the scapula.
TEST PROCEDURE	The examiner measures the distance from the base of the spine of the scapula to the spinous process of T2 or T3 (most common), from the inferior angle of the scapula to the spinous processes of T7 to T9, or from T2 to the superior angle of the scapula. The patient then is tested holding two or four other positions:

• 45° of abduction (hands on waist, thumbs posterior)
• 90° of abduction with medial rotation
• 120° of abduction
• 150° of abduction

INDICATIONS OF A POSITIVE TEST	Davies and Dickoff-Hoffman[6] and Kibler[127] stated that in each position, the distance measured should not vary more than 1 to 1.5 cm (0.5 to 0.75 inch) from the original measurement. However, increased distances may be noted above 90° as the scapula rotates during scapulohumeral rhythm. Minimal protraction of the scapula should occur during full elevation through abduction; therefore, it is important to look for asymmetry of position between the left and right sides when assessing scapular stability.

Continued

LATERAL SCAPULAR SLIDE TEST[6,124-127]—cont'd

CLINICAL NOTES
- The test also may be conducted with load variations placed on the arm or with eccentric movement (see scapular load tests).
- As a variation of the scapular load and lateral scapular slide tests, the examiner may use an eccentric force during the test. In the different positions, the examiner may test for scapular and humeral stability by performing an eccentric movement at the shoulder (i.e., by pushing the arm forward [eccentric hold test]). One arm is tested at a time, starting with the uninvolved side. The examiner should watch for winging of the scapula, which indicates scapular instability. As the arm is pushed forward eccentrically, the examiner should watch the relative movement at the scapulothoracic joint (protraction) and the glenohumeral joint (horizontal adduction). Normally, slightly more movement (relatively) occurs at the glenohumeral joint. If instability caused by muscle weakness is present at either joint, excessive movement is evident at that joint relative to the other joint.

RELIABILITY/SPECIFICITY/ SENSITIVITY[125,126]
Specificity range: 26.7% to 56%
Sensitivity range: 28% to 50%

SCAPULAR LOAD TEST[126]

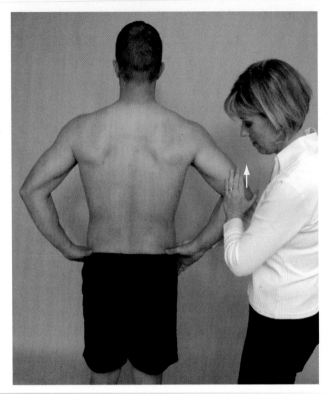

Figure 4–28
Scapular load test in 45° of abduction.

PURPOSE	To determine the stability of the scapula during glenohumeral movements when a load is placed on the arm.
PATIENT POSITION	The patient sits or stands with the arm in 45° of abduction (hands on waist, thumbs posterior).
EXAMINER POSITION	The examiner stands behind the patient so as to observe the motion of the scapula.
TEST PROCEDURE	The examiner applies a load to the arm (providing resistance) at 45° or greater abduction to see how the scapula stabilizes under dynamic load. This load may be applied to the arm anteriorly, posteriorly, inferiorly, or superiorly.
INDICATIONS OF A POSITIVE TEST	The scapula should not move more than 1.5 cm (0.75 inch). However, loading the scapula, either by the weight of the arm or by applying a load to the arm, indicates the stabilizing ability of the scapular control muscles and whether abnormal winging or abnormal movement patterns occur. Minimal protraction of the scapula should occur during full elevation through abduction; therefore, it is important to look for asymmetry of movement between left and right sides, as well as the amount of movement when assessing scapular stability.
CLINICAL NOTE/CAUTION	• For the muscles of the glenohumeral joint to work in a normal, coordinated fashion, the scapula must be stabilized by its muscles so that it can act as a firm base for the glenohumeral muscles. Therefore, when doing these tests, the examiner watches for the movement patterns of the scapula, as well as scapular dyskinesia. Loading the arm should amplify any scapular dysfunction seen.
RELIABILITY/SPECIFICITY/ SENSITIVITY	Unknown

SCAPULAR RETRACTION TEST[15,21,127-129]

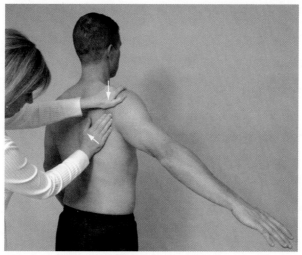

Figure 4–29
Scapular retraction test. The examiner uses the hands to stabilize the clavicle and scapula.

PURPOSE	To determine the static stability of the scapula during glenohumeral movements.
PATIENT POSITION	The patient is standing. The arm is straight for testing abduction.
EXAMINER POSITION	The examiner stands behind the patient.
TEST PROCEDURE	The examiner places the fingers of one hand over the clavicle with the heel of the hand over the spine of the scapula to stabilize the clavicle and scapula and to hold the scapula retracted. The examiner's other hand compresses the body and inferior angle of the scapula against the chest wall. The examiner then holds the scapula in the start position while the patient abducts the arm.
INDICATIONS OF A POSITIVE TEST	Holding the scapula in the start position provides a firm, stable base for the rotator cuff muscles to act, and often rotator cuff strength (if tested by a second examiner) improves and pain on movement will be less. The test result also may be positive in a patient who has had a positive result on the relocation test. If scapular retraction reduces the pain when the relocation test is performed, the weak scapular stabilizers must be addressed in the treatment.
CLINICAL NOTES	• The scapular retraction test also may be done with the patient supine. • In a patient who has scapular malposition, inferior medial border prominence, coracoid pain and malposition, or dyskinesis of scapular motion (a condition known as *SICK scapula*),[5] repositioning of the scapula improves forward flexion.
RELIABILITY/SPECIFICITY/ SENSITIVITY	Unknown

PUSH UP TEST[21,128,130]

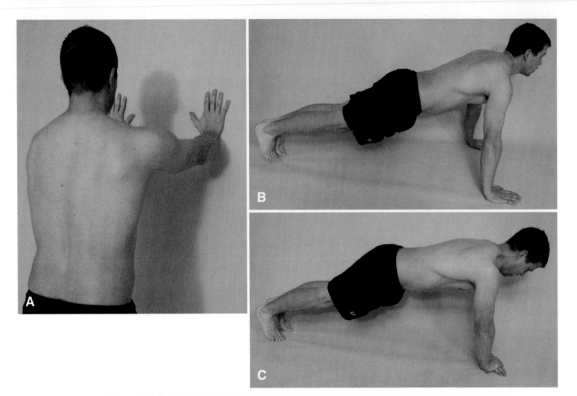

Figure 4–30

Push up test. **A,** Wall push up. **B,** Floor push up. **C,** Closed kinetic chain–upper extremity stability test showing patient touching the opposite hand.

PURPOSE	To test the stability of the scapula during dynamic closed chain glenohumeral movements.
PATIENT POSITION	The patient stands an arm's length from a wall with both palms flat on the wall.
EXAMINER POSITION	The examiner stands behind the patient to observe the scapula.
TEST PROCEDURE	The patient is asked to do a wall push up 15 to 20 times. If the patient is able to do this with no difficulty, progressions can include doing a push up from the end of a table (table push up) and then on the floor (floor push up).
INDICATIONS OF A POSITIVE TEST	Weakness of the scapular muscles or winging usually shows up with five to 10 push ups.
CLINICAL NOTE/CAUTION	• Goldbeck and Davies[130] have taken the push up test farther, describing a closed kinetic chain–upper extremity stability test. In this test, two markers (e.g., tape) are placed 91 cm (36 inches) apart. The patient assumes the push up position with one hand on each marker. When the examiner says "Go," the patient moves one hand to touch the other and returns it to the original position and then does the same with the other hand, repeating the motions for 15 seconds. The examiner counts the number of touches or crossovers made in the allotted time. The test is repeated three times, and the average is the test score. This test is designed primarily for young, active patients.
RELIABILITY/SPECIFICITY/ SENSITIVITY	Unknown

SPECIAL TEST OF THE ACROMIOCLAVICULAR AND STERNOCLAVICULAR JOINTS[131-133]

Relevant Special Test

Acromioclavicular crossover, cross-body, or horizontal adduction test

Definition

The acromioclavicular joint is the articulation between the acromion and the clavicle. *Acromioclavicular joint separation* is a disruption in the ligamentous integrity of the acromioclavicular joint. The ligaments that provide stability to the acromioclavicular joint are the superior and inferior acromioclavicular ligaments and the coracoclavicular (conoid and trapezoid) ligaments. Likewise, the sternoclavicular joint is stabilized by its ligaments—the anterior and posterior sternoclavicular ligaments, the costoclavicular ligaments, and the interclavicular ligament.

Epidemiology and Demographics

Acromioclavicular joint separation injuries occur more frequently in men than in women (approximately 5:1). They account for approximately 12% of shoulder girdle injuries seen in clinical practice, and the prevalence is estimated at 40% of all shoulder injuries in sports. The number actually may be higher, because patients with minor sprains are less likely to seek medical attention. The joint is most commonly injured in the first three decades of life, and these injuries frequently are seen in young adults involved in contact sports, such as football. They also are common in bicycle riding, soccer, rugby, hockey, gymnastics, martial arts, and skiing. Sternoclavicular dislocations are much more rare but have the potential to cause more problems, especially if they are displaced posteriorly because of the great vessels lying immediately behind them.

Relevant History

No prior history is associated with an acromioclavicular joint separation; it usually is the result of direct trauma. Acromioclavicular joints with dysfunction may have a past history of acromioclavicular joint separation or a fractured clavicle. Similarly, the sternoclavicular joint is most commonly injured by a direct blow.

Relevant Signs and Symptoms

- Localized pain over the joint
- Step-off deformity (with acromioclavicular joint separation)
- Aggravation of pain over the joint by forced horizontal adduction
- Edema (may or may not be present, depending on the acuteness of the injury)
- Local tenderness to palpation of the afftected joint
- "Piano key" sign (hypermobile clavicle) at the acromioclavicular joint

Mechanism of Injury

The injury typically occurs as a result of a fall involving a direct impact on the acromion or to the clavicle near the sternum. Falls onto an adducted shoulder also may produce acromioclavicular joint dysfunction. Spraining of the acromioclavicular and/or coracoclavicular ligaments may result from a fall onto an outstretched arm in which the force is transmitted through the humeral head to the acromion. The sternoclavicular joint is usually injured by a direct blow to the sternal end of the clavicle.

Reliability/Specificity/Sensitivity

Unknown

ACROMIOCLAVICULAR CROSSOVER, CROSS-BODY, OR HORIZONTAL ADDUCTION TEST[22,101,134-136]

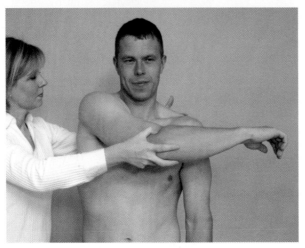

Figure 4–31

Acromioclavicular crossover, cross-body, or horizontal adduction test.

PURPOSE	To test for dysfunction by placing a shearing stress on the acromioclavicular joint or sternoclavicular joint.
PATIENT POSITION	The patient sits or stands with the arm at the side.
EXAMINER POSITION	The examiner stands directly adjacent to the test shoulder.
TEST PROCEDURE	The examiner places one hand on the contralateral shoulder for support and grasps the elbow of the involved arm with the other hand. The examiner passively forward flexes the arm to 90° and then horizontally adducts the arm as far as possible.
INDICATIONS OF A POSITIVE TEST	The test result is positive if the patient feels localized pain over the acromioclavicular joint or sternoclavicular joint.
CLINICAL NOTES/CAUTIONS	• The patient may also actively perform the test. • This technique also tests the sternoclavicular joint; the test result is positive for sternoclavicular dysfunction if localized pain is noted around the sternoclavicular joint.
RELIABILITY/SPECIFICITY/ SENSITIVITY	Unknown

SPECIAL TESTS FOR MUSCLE OR TENDON PATHOLOGY

Relevant Special Tests

Speed's test (biceps or straight arm test)

Yergason's test

Supraspinatus test ("empty can" or Jobe test)

Abdominal compression test (belly press or Napoleon test)

Bear hug test

Lift-off sign

Subscapularis spring-back, lag, or modified lift-off test

Lateral (external) rotation lag sign (ERLS) or drop test

Lateral (external) rotation test (infraspinatus spring-back test)

Testing for trapezius weakness

Testing for serratus anterior weakness

Testing for rhomboid weakness

Testing for latissimus dorsi weakness

Testing for pectoralis major and minor tightness or contracture

Definition

Injuries to muscle or tendon tissue are often viewed as two distinctly different types of injury. From a tissue standpoint, this is true. From a functional standpoint, however, differentiating between damage to the muscle or to the tendon often is difficult, because the two are part of the same functional unit. Both muscle and tendon are involved in producing motion through any joint.

Pathological conditions that involve the tendon often are referred to as *tendinopathies*. Acute injuries are classified as a *tendonitis*, and more chronic or degenerative injuries are classified as *tendinosis*. Injuries also can occur within the muscle, at the muscle-tendon interface, or at the myotendinous junction. The pathological classification commonly is based on the actual tissue that has been injured. Because most testing done in a clinical setting tests the entire muscle-tendon-bone functional unit, positive test results reflect damage to any one of these tissues.

Suspected Injuries

Muscle strains

Muscle tears

Tendinopathies (tendonitis, tendinosis)

Tendon rupture (third-degree strain)

Epidemiology and Demographics

The epidemiology and demographics for patients with muscle or tendon injuries vary greatly according to the location and the actual tissue damaged. In general, muscle strains occur in younger patients and in muscles with a higher prevalence of fast twitch muscle fibers. Pathological conditions of the tendons can occur in either younger or older patients.

Relevant History

The patient history varies. A patient with a muscle or tendon injury may have a history of previous shoulder pain that has progressed in both frequency and intensity. However, the patient also may report no previous history of shoulder pain.

Relevant Signs and Symptoms

Tendinitis/Tendinosis

- Point tenderness at the site of injury
- Pain that may radiate distally into the upper arm and forearm
- Pain that usually is exacerbated at the initial onset of activities
- Possible weakness or fatigue in the shoulder
- Nocturnal pain (common)

Tendon Ruptures

Tendon ruptures are rare but easy to assess. They are marked by loss of strength with overhead motions, poor strength and pain with use of the affected muscle, weakness on testing of the affected muscle, and possibly a bulge at the point of muscle retraction. In the shoulder, the biceps is most commonly ruptured at either the long head or the insertion. In older individuals, rotator cuff tears occur near the insertion. Often the patient reports feeling a "pop" in the arm with a lifting activity.

Muscle Strain/Tear (Third-Degree Strain)

With a muscle strain or tear, localized swelling and bruising at the site of injury initially may be seen. Over time, as the swelling spreads, the localized tenderness may become a more generalized or diffuse tenderness and achiness. Partial tears may still be strong with functional motions and on strength testing, but pain is elicited by contraction of the injured muscle. Full-thickness and complete tears, especially of the rotator cuff, present with weakness when the muscle is tested, but pain responses vary. Some full and complete tears elicit pain, whereas others are pain free.

General Signs and Symptoms

If the shoulder is irritable (i.e., inflamed), it may cause peripheral numbness or tingling as a result of impingement of nerves through the shoulder complex. Symptoms may have a peripheral nerve distribution and may correlate with shoulder irritability.

Mechanism of Injury

Acute injury. Any undue stress or strain on the tendon or muscle can cause muscle or tendon injury. Overhead throwing, a FOOSH injury, lifting of heavy objects, and sudden muscle contraction are common causes of injury to the muscles and tendons of the shoulder. Muscle and tendon injuries may be associated with other pathological conditions, such as fractures, dislocations, and subluxations.

Degenerative condition. Degenerative muscle and tendon pathological conditions often are associated with chronic and persistent subacromial impingement. Chronic and repetitive subacromial impingement can lead to a rotator cuff tear. As the shoulder joint degenerates, bone spurs may develop in the subacromial area, which may lead to increased impingement and further muscle and tendon injury. Other factors, such as forward shoulder posture, increased thoracic spine kyphosis, weakness in the rotator cuff, and a past history of shoulder problems all can contribute to a degenerative tear in the rotator cuff.

Activities that require repetitive overhead motions (e.g., painting ceilings, construction, and throwing overhead) can lead to repetitive trauma to the shoulder muscles and tendons. Repetitive overhead use or repetitive activities can cause the humeral head to translate anteriorly and superiorly, impinging the tendons and muscles. Common activities that cause this type of pathological condition include:

- Repetitive lifting overhead
- Repetitive carrying of objects, especially away from body
- Rowing
- Bench pressing
- Catching a heavy falling object
- Falling onto an outstretched hand (FOOSH injury)

RELIABILITY/SPECIFICITY/SENSITIVITY COMPARISON[89,99,137-142]

	Validity	Interrater Reliability	Intrarater Reliability	Specificity	Sensitivity
Speed's Test	56%	Unknown	Unknown	83.3%	38.3%
Yergason's Test	63%	Unknown	Unknown	79%	37%
Empty Can Test	Unknown	0.43	Unknown	Tendinitis: 6.9% Tear: 89.5%	Tendinitis: 25% Tear: 52.6%
Lift-Off Sign	Unknown	Unknown	Unknown	100%	17.6%
Subscapularis Lag Test	15/16 Patients	Unknown	Unknown	1	0.002%
Abdominal Compression Test	Unknown	Unknown	Unknown	97.9%	40% to 60%
Lateral Rotation Lag Test	15/16 Patients	Unknown	Unknown	1	0.002%
Drop Test	Unknown	Unknown	Unknown	97.2%	7.8%
Bear Hug Test	Unknown	Unknown	Unknown	Unknown	Unknown
Testing for Trapezius Weakness	Unknown	Unknown	Unknown	Unknown	Unknown
Testing for Serratus Anterior Weakness	Unknown	Unknown	Unknown	Unknown	Unknown
Testing for Rhomboid Weakness	Unknown	Unknown	Unknown	Unknown	Unknown
Testing for Latissimus Dorsi Weakness	Unknown	Unknown	Unknown	Unknown	Unknown
Testing for Pectoralis Major and Minor Tightness	Unknown	Unknown	Unknown	Unknown	Unknown

Note: Where a value of 1 is given, all patients tested were postive for the sign.

SPEED'S TEST (BICEPS OR STRAIGHT ARM TEST)[90,99,137,143,144]

DVD

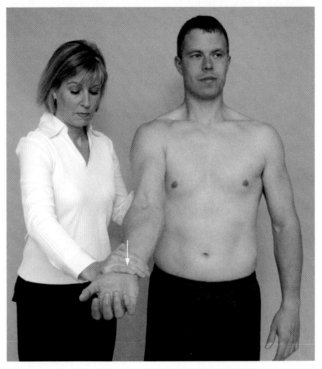

Figure 4–32
Speed's test (biceps or straight arm test).

PURPOSE	To test for a pathological condition of the biceps tendon and secondarily to test for labral SLAP lesions or strains of the distal biceps.
SUSPECTED INJURY	Long head of the biceps injury
PATIENT POSITION	The patient is sitting or standing.
EXAMINER POSITION	The examiner stands adjacent to the test arm.
TEST PROCEDURE	The examiner places one hand beneath the upper arm for support and stability; the other hand grasps the wrist and will deliver the resistance to the arm. The test may be done statically or dynamically (concentrically or eccentrically).

If the test is done statically, the examiner positions the patient in the forward flexed position at the angle at which the patient complained of symptoms. The patient is asked to hold the position isometrically while the examiner provides a downward isometric force at the wrist.

For dynamic testing, the examiner resists concentric shoulder forward flexion by the patient while the patient's forearm is first supinated and then pronated, and the elbow is completely extended. The test also may be performed by forward flexing the patient's arm to 90° or to the position of the complaint and then asking the patient to resist an eccentric movement into extension, first with the arm supinated and then with it pronated. The two sides are compared.

Continued

SPEED'S TEST (BICEPS OR STRAIGHT ARM TEST)[90,99,137,143,144]—*cont'd*

INDICATIONS OF A POSITIVE TEST	A positive test result is increased tenderness in the bicipital groove, especially with the arm supinated; this indicates bicipital paratenonitis or tendinosis.[144] If the injury is at the biceps insertion, the muscle is weak, and elbow flexion strength should be tested.
CLINICAL NOTES/CAUTIONS	• Speed's test has been reported to cause pain; therefore, the test result will be positive if the patient has a SLAP (type II) lesion.[90] • If profound weakness is found on resisted supination, a severe second- or third-degree (rupture) strain of the distal biceps should be suspected. • During dynamic movement, the humerus moves over the tendon; the tendon moves minimally.
RELIABILITY/SPECIFICITY/ SENSITIVITY[99,137]	Validity: 56% Specificity range: 55% to 87% Sensitivity range: 44% to 68%

YERGASON'S TEST[30,89,137,138,144-146]

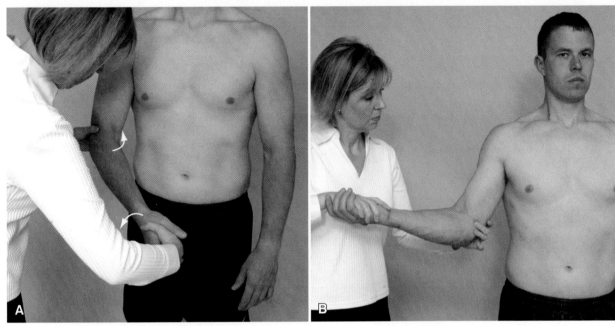

Figure 4–33
Yergason's test. **A,** Start position. **B,** End position.

PURPOSE	To check the ability of the transverse humeral ligament to hold the biceps tendon in the bicipital groove.
PATIENT POSITION	The patient is sitting or standing.
EXAMINER POSITION	The examiner stands adjacent to the test arm.
TEST PROCEDURE	The examiner places one hand beneath the upper arm for support and stability; the other hand grasps the wrist and will deliver the resistance to the arm. The examiner flexes the patient's elbow to 90° and stabilizes the patient's arm against the thorax with the forearm pronated. The examiner resists patient forearm supination while the patient also laterally rotates the arm against resistance. The two sides are compared.
INDICATIONS OF A POSITIVE TEST	If the examiner palpates the biceps tendon in the bicipital groove during the supination and lateral rotation movement, the tendon will be felt to "pop out" of the groove if the transverse humeral ligament is torn. Tenderness in the bicipital groove alone, without dislocation, may indicate bicipital paratenonitis/tendinosis.
RELIABILTY/SPECIFICITY/ SENSITIVITY[89,137,138]	Specificity range: 79% to 96% Sensitivity range: 9% to 43%

SUPRASPINATUS TEST ("EMPTY CAN" OR JOBE TEST)[99,137,139,147,148]

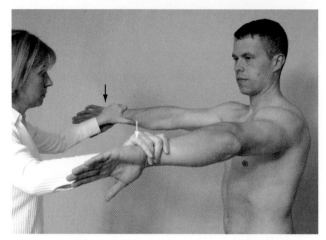

Figure 4–34
Supraspinatus ("empty can") test.

PURPOSE	To assess for tears of the supraspinatus tendon or muscle or for neuropathy of the suprascapular nerve.
PATIENT POSITION	The patient is standing or sitting.
EXAMINER POSITION	The examiner stands in front of the patient.
TEST PROCEDURE	Each of the examiner's hands grasps one of the patient's wrists. The patient's arms are abducted to 90° (actively by the patient or passively by the examiner) with neutral (no) rotation, and the examiner provides resistance to elevation. The patient's shoulders then are medially rotated and angled forward 30° (as if emptying a can) so that the patient's thumbs point toward the floor in the plane of the scapula; the examiner provides resistance to this scapular plane movement. The two sides are compared.
INDICATIONS OF A POSITIVE TEST	A positive test result is indicated by weakness or pain (or both) when resistance is delivered to the arm.
CLINICAL NOTE	• Some researchers contend that testing the arm with the thumb up ("full can") is best for maximum contraction of the supraspinatus.[148]
RELIABILITY/SPECIFICITY/ SENSITIVITY[99,139]	Reliability: k = 0.43 Specificity range: 62% to 89.5% Sensitivity range: 25% to 88%

ABDOMINAL COMPRESSION TEST (BELLY PRESS OR NAPOLEON TEST)[140,149-152]   DVD

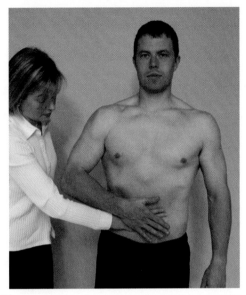

Figure 4–35
Abdominal compression test.

PURPOSE	To test for weakness of the subscapularis muscle, especially if the patient cannot medially rotate the shoulder enough to take the hand behind the back.
PATIENT POSITION	The patient is standing.
EXAMINER POSITION	The examiner stands to the side of and facing the patient.
TEST PROCEDURE	The examiner places a hand on the patient's abdomen so as to feel how much pressure the patient is applying to the abdomen. The patient places the hand of the test shoulder on the examiner's hand and pushes the hand as hard as possible into the stomach, causing medial shoulder rotation and pressure on the examiner's hand. The two sides are compared.
INDICATIONS OF A POSITIVE TEST	If the patient is unable to maintain the pressure on the examiner's hand while moving the elbow forward or extends the shoulder or flexes the wrist, the test result is positive for a tear of the subscapularis muscle. Burkhart et al.[152] outlined two possible positive results for this test: (1) If the patient flexes the wrist to about 80° and extends the shoulder by using the posterior deltoid, this indicates a nonfunctional subscapularis; (2) if the patient flexes the wrist 30° to 60° (which these researchers called an *intermediate Napoleon sign*), it indicates partial function of the subscapularis.
CLINICAL NOTE/CAUTION	• The examiner should pay close attention to the wrist, elbow, and shoulder positions, because the patient will attempt to compensate by changing the positions of these three joints to maintain the pressure on the examiner's hand.
RELIABILITY/SPECIFICITY/ SENSITIVITY[140]	Specificity: 97.9% Sensitivity: 40% to 60%

BEAR HUG TEST[140,152]

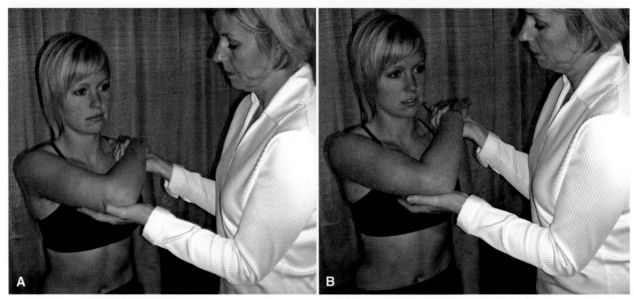

Figure 4–36
Bear hug test. **A,** Start position. **B,** Lifting hand off shoulder.

PURPOSE	To test for weakness of the subscapularis muscle.
PATIENT POSITION	The patient sits or stands with the test shoulder forward flexed and the elbow bent so that the patient's hand sits on top of the opposite shoulder and the fingers are extended.
EXAMINER POSITION	The examiner stands, facing the patient.
TEST PROCEDURE	The patient is instructed to resist the examiner's motion. The examiner lifts the patient's hand straight up off the shoulder. The two sides are compared.
INDICATIONS OF A POSITIVE TEST	If the examiner is able to lift the hand off the shoulder, the test result is considered positive for a tear of the upper subscapularis tendon.
RELIABILITY/SPECIFICITY/ SENSITIVITY[140]	Sensitivity: 60% Specificity: 91.7%

LIFT-OFF SIGN[140,141,146,148-150,153]   DVD

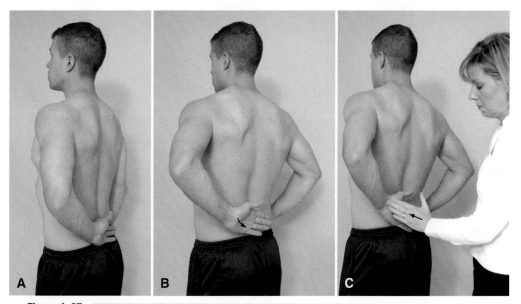

Figure 4–37

Lift-off sign. **A,** Start position. **B,** Lift-off position. **C,** The examiner provides resistance to lift off. The examiner tests the strength of the subscapularis and watches the positioning of the scapula.

PURPOSE	To test for weakness of the subscapularis muscle in patients who can get the arm behind the back.
PATIENT POSITION	The patient stands and places the dorsum of the hand on the opposite back pocket or against the midlumbar spine.
EXAMINER POSITION	The examiner stands directly behind the patient.
TEST PROCEDURE	The patient is asked to lift the hand away from the back. The two sides are compared.
INDICATIONS OF A POSITIVE TEST	Inability to lift the hand away from the back indicates weakness of the subscapularis muscle. Abnormal motion in the scapula during the test may indicate scapular instability, preventing proper subscapularis function. If the patient is able to take the hand away from the back, the examiner can apply a load to the palm, pushing the hand toward the back, to test the strength of the subscapularis and to test how the scapula acts under dynamic loading. With a torn subscapularis tendon, passive (and active) lateral rotation may increase. The technique also may be used to test the rhomboids; medial winging of the scapula during the test may indicate that the rhomboids are affected.
CLINICAL NOTES/CAUTIONS	• Stefko et al.[146] reported that maximum isolation of the subscapularis was achieved by placing the hand against the posteroinferior border of the scapula (maximum medial rotation test) and then attempting to lift the hand from the back. • In the other positions for lift off where the hand is not placed on the scapula, the teres major, latissimus dorsi, posterior deltoid, or rhomboids may compensate for a weak subscapularis.
RELIABILITY/SPECIFICITY/ SENSITIVITY[141]	Specificity: 100% Sensitivity: 17.6%

SUBSCAPULARIS SPRING-BACK, LAG, OR MODIFIED LIFT-OFF TEST[142,149,153,154]

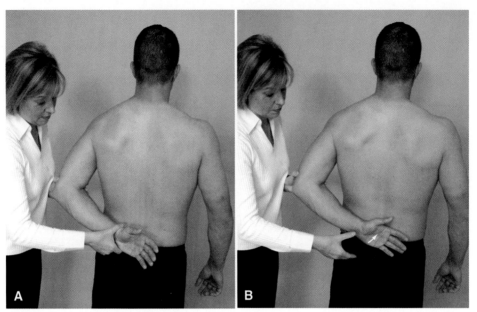

Figure 4–38

Subscapularis spring-back (lag) test. **A,** Start position. **B,** The patient is unable to hold the start position, and the hand springs back toward the lower back.

PURPOSE	To test for weakness of the subscapularis muscle; weakness of the rotator cuff and rhomboid muscles also may be assessed with this test.
PATIENT POSITION	The patient stands and places the dorsum of the hand on the back pocket or against the midlumbar spine.
EXAMINER POSITION	The examiner stands adjacent and slightly behind the test arm.
TEST PROCEDURE	The examiner places one hand (left hand as illustrated) on the patient's elbow for support and stability, and the other hand (right hand as illustrated) holds the wrist. The patient's arm is passively medially rotated as far as possible away from the back, and the patient is asked to hold the position. The two sides are compared.
INDICATIONS OF A POSITIVE TEST	A positive test result is indicated if the hand moves toward the back, because the subscapularis cannot hold the position as a result of weakness or pain. A small lag between maximum passive medial rotation and active medial rotation implies a partial tear (1° or 2°) of the subscapularis.
CLINICAL NOTES/CAUTIONS	• This modified test is reported to be more accurate for diagnosing rotator cuff tears. • The technique also may be used to test the rhomboids; medial border winging of the scapula during the test may indicate that the rhomboids are affected. • The amount of medial rotation achieved during this test is greater than for the lift-off test.
RELIABILITY/SPECIFICITY/ SENSITIVITY[142]	*Validity:* A lag of 10° to 15° was observed in all patients with infrascapularis, suprascapularis, and subscapularis weakness. *Specificity:* The internal rotation lag sign is as specific as the lift-off test ($p = 1$); the external rotation lag sign is as specific as the drop test, and both are more specific than the Jobe test ($p = 0.002$). *Sensitivity:* The internal rotation lag sign is more sensitive than the lift-off test ($p = 0.0002$); the external rotation lag sign is more sensitive than the drop test ($p = 0.0001$) and less sensitive than the Jobe test ($p = 0.05$)

LATERAL (EXTERNAL) ROTATION LAG SIGN (ERLS) OR DROP TEST[96,142,155]

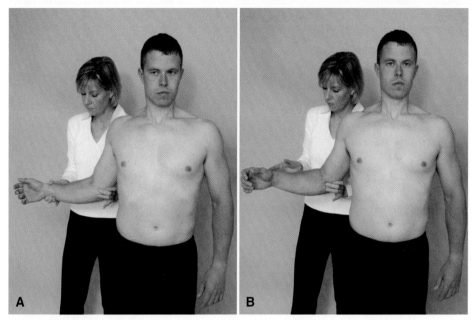

Figure 4–39
External rotation lag sign (drop test). **A,** Start position. **B,** Position with a positive test result.

PURPOSE	To test for injury of the infraspinatus, supraspinatus, and/or subscapularis muscles.
PATIENT POSITION	The patient is standing.
EXAMINER POSITION	The examiner stands directly behind the test shoulder.
TEST PROCEDURE	The examiner places one hand on the patient's elbow for support and stabilization. The other hand holds the patient's wrist. The patient's arm is abducted to 20° with the elbow flexed to 90°. The examiner maximally laterally rotates the patient's arm, and the patient is asked to hold the position. The two sides are compared.
INDICATIONS OF A POSITIVE TEST	If the arm falls, or "drops," into medial rotation, the test result is considered positive for tears of the rotator cuff, especially of the infraspinatus and supraspinatus and perhaps subscapularis muscles.
CLINICAL NOTE	• If the patient is able to hold the position, the strength of the infraspinatus can be graded as 3 or greater, depending on the resistance to the examiner's medially rotated force.
RELIABILITY/SPECIFICITY/ SENSITIVITY[142]	See subscapularis lag test.

LATERAL (EXTERNAL) ROTATION LAG TEST (INFRASPINATUS SPRING-BACK TEST)[80,96,141,142,153-156]

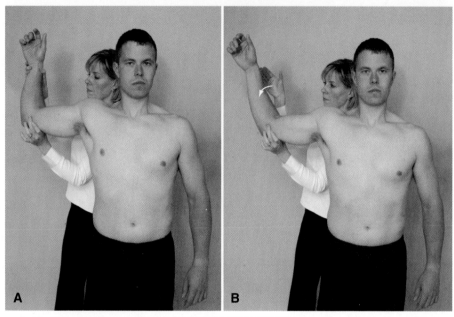

Figure 4–40

Lateral rotation lag test for the teres minor and infraspinatus. **A,** The arm is abducted 90°. **B,** Note how the hand springs forward when released by the examiner.

PURPOSE	To test for tears of or injury to the infraspinatus, teres minor, and/or supraspinatus muscle.
PATIENT POSITION	The patient is seated or standing with the arm by the side and the elbow flexed to 90°.
EXAMINER POSITION	The examiner stands directly behind the test shoulder.
TEST PROCEDURE	The examiner places one hand on the patient's flexed elbow (at 90°) for support and stabilization. The other hand holds the patient's wrist. The examiner passively abducts the arm to 90° in the scapular plane, laterally rotates the shoulder to end range (some authors say 45°),[155] and asks the patient to hold this position. The two sides are compared.
INDICATIONS OF A POSITIVE TEST	The test result is positive if the patient is unable to hold the position and the hand springs forward anteriorly toward the midline; this indicates that the infraspinatus and teres minor cannot hold the position because of weakness or pain. Also, passive medial rotation is increased on the affected side.
RELIABILITY/SPECIFICITY/ SENSITIVITY	Unknown

TESTING FOR TRAPEZIUS WEAKNESS[157-159]

DVD

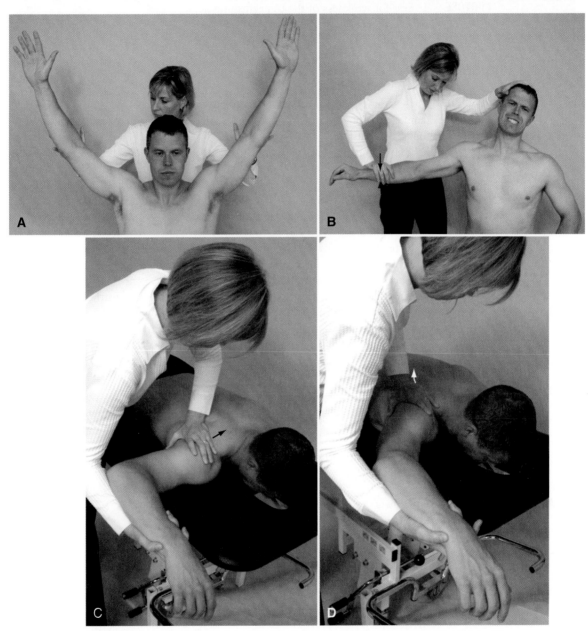

Figure 4–41
Test for trapezius weakness. **A,** All portions of the triceps. **B,** Upper trapezius **C,** Middle trapezius. **D,** Lower trapezius..

TESTING FOR TRAPEZIUS WEAKNESS[157-159]—*cont'd*

PURPOSE	To test for weakness of the trapezius muscle.
PATIENT POSITION	The patient sits and places the hands together over the head.
EXAMINER POSITION	The examiner stands directly adjacent and slightly behind the test shoulder.
TEST PROCEDURE	The examiner places one hand on the posterior aspect of the humeral head; the other hand grasps the forearm. From this starting position, the examiner pushes the elbow forward against resistance. Normally, the three parts of the trapezius contract to stabilize the scapula so that it does not move or wing.
	The upper trapezius can be tested separately by elevating the shoulder with the arm slightly abducted or by elevating the shoulder against resisted shoulder abduction and ipsilateral head side flexion simultaneously. If the shoulder is elevated with the arm by the side, the levator scapulae and rhomboids are more likely to be tested.
	The middle trapezius can be tested with the patient in a prone position with the arm abducted to 90° and laterally rotated. The examiner retracts the shoulder and then gives resistance over the scapula near the posterior glenoid. The examiner resists retraction of the shoulder by giving resistance over the scapula near the glenohumeral joint.
	For testing of the lower trapezius, the patient is placed in the prone lying position with the arm abducted to 120° and the shoulder laterally rotated. The examiner retracts the shoulder and then gives resistance to patient retraction over the scapula near the posterior glenoid.
	The two sides are compared
INDICATIONS OF A POSITIVE TEST	Retraction of the scapula when force is applied to the arm is a normal response. A positive test result is seen if the scapula protracts or wings/tilts when force is applied to the arm.
CLINICAL NOTE	• Greater than normal elevation of the scapula may indicate a tight trapezius or cervical torticollis.
RELIABILITY/SPECIFICITY/ SENSITIVITY	Unknown

TESTING FOR SERRATUS ANTERIOR WEAKNESS[120,157]

DVD

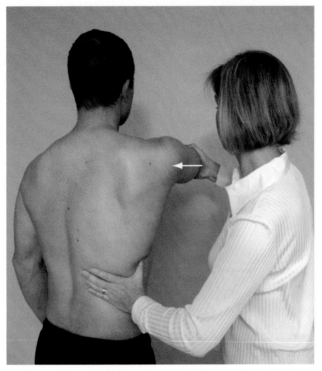

Figure 4–42
Test for serratus anterior weakness. Punch out test: The examiner applies a backward force.

PURPOSE	To test for weakness of the serratus anterior muscle.
PATIENT POSITION	The patient is standing.
EXAMINER POSITION	The examiner stands adjacent to and slightly behind the test shoulder.
TEST PROCEDURE	The patient forward flexes the arm to 90° and makes a fist. The examiner places one hand on the patient's upper arm or against the fist and the other hand on the posterolateral aspect of the lower thoracic region for stability. The examiner applies a backward force to the arm or fist. The two sides are compared.
INDICATIONS OF A POSITIVE TEST	The test result is positive for a weak or paralyzed serratus anterior muscle if the medial border of the scapula wings (classic winging).
CLINICAL NOTES	• With a weak serratus anterior muscle, the patient also will have difficulty abducting or forward flexing the arm above 90°; however, it still may be possible with lower trapezius compensation. • A similar positive test result may be obtained by having the patient do a wall, table, or floor push up.
RELIABILITY/SPECIFICITY/ SENSITIVITY	Unknown

TESTING FOR RHOMBOID WEAKNESS[80,157]

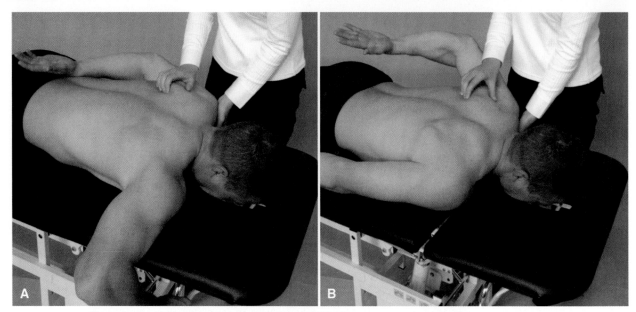

Figure 4–43

Test for rhomboid weakness. A, Start position. B, Test position.

PURPOSE	To test for weakness of the rhomboid muscles.
PATIENT POSITION	The patient is in a prone lying or sitting position with the test arm behind the body so that the hand is on the opposite side (opposite back pocket).
EXAMINER POSITION	The examiner stands directly adjacent to the test shoulder.
TEST PROCEDURE	The examiner places the fingers along and under the medial border of the scapula. The patient is asked to push the shoulder forward slightly against resistance to relax the trapezius and to allow the fingers to slip under or adjacent to the scapula. The patient then is asked to raise the forearm and hand away from the body. The two sides are compared.
INDICATIONS OF A POSITIVE TEST	If the rhomboids are normal, the fingers are pushed away from under the scapula or the examiner will feel the rhomboids contract. A positive test result is indicated if either of these responses do not occur.
RELIABILITY/SPECIFICITY/ SENSITIVITY	Unknown

TESTING FOR LATISSIMUS DORSI WEAKNESS[160]

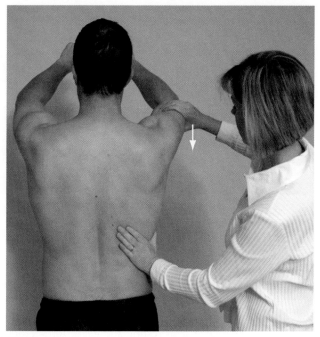

Figure 4–44
Test for latissimus dorsi weakness.

PURPOSE	To test for weakness of the latissimus dorsi muscle.
PATIENT POSITION	The patient stands with the arms elevated in the plane of the scapula to 160°.
EXAMINER POSITION	The examiner stands adjacent to and slightly behind the test arm.
TEST PROCEDURE	The examiner places one hand on the inferior aspect of the latissimus dorsi muscle and grasps the elbow with the other hand. While providing resistance, the examiner instructs the patient to medially rotate and extend the arm downward as if climbing a ladder.
INDICATIONS OF A POSITIVE TEST	A positive test result is indicated if weakness is noted when resistance is applied. The two sides are compared.
CLINICAL NOTE	• Scapular winging may occur as compensation for weakness of the latissimus dorsi muscle.
RELIABILITY/SPECIFICITY/ SENSITIVITY	Unknown

TESTING FOR PECTORALIS MAJOR AND MINOR TIGHTESS OR CONTRACTURE

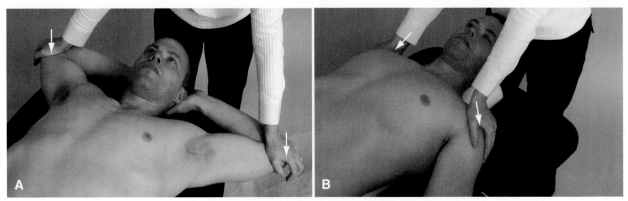

Figure 4–45
Test for tightness of the pectoralis major **(A)** and pectoralis minor **(B)**. The examiner is testing end feel.
Note the position of the examiner's hand on the humerus *(A)* and coracoid process *(B)*.

PURPOSE	To test for tightness of the pectoralis major or pectoralis minor muscles or both.
PATIENT POSITION	The patient lies supine and clasps the hands together behind the head (for pectoralis major) or with the arms resting abducted (for pectoralis minor).
EXAMINER POSITION	The examiner stands at the head of the table, facing the patient.
TEST PROCEDURE	**Pectoralis Major.** The examiner places a hand on each of the patient's elbows. The patient's bent arms are lowered until the elbows touch the examining table. The examiner then pushes posteriorly on the head of the humerus or the elbows.
	Pectoralis Minor. The examiner places a hand on the anterior aspect of each shoulder over the coracoid processes and then pushes the coracoid process toward the examining table (posteriorly). Normally, the posterior movement causes the patient no discomfort, and the scapula lies flat against the table.
	The two sides are compared.
INDICATIONS OF A POSITIVE TEST	A positive test result is indicated if the elbows do not reach the table (tight pectoralis major) or the scapulae do not lie flat (pectoralis minor). A positive test result also is indicated if tightness (muscle tissue stretch) is noted over the pectoralis major or minor muscle during the posterior movement.
RELIABILITY/SPECIFICITY/SENSITIVITY	Unknown

SPECIAL TEST FOR THORACIC OUTLET SYNDROME

Relevant Special Test

Roos test

Definition

The term *thoracic outlet syndrome* (TOS) encompasses numerous scenarios of compression (neurological and vascular) in the thoracic outlet region of the shoulder girdle. The syndrome can be divided into two subclassifications: TOS caused by neurological factors and TOS caused by vascular problems. Neurological and vascular conditions also may be observed together.

Suspected Injuries

- Arterial thoracic outlet syndrome
- Venous thoracic outlet syndrome
- Neurogenic thoracic outlet syndrome

Epidemiology and Demographics[161-168]

It is believed that in 98% of TOS cases, the resultant symptoms are neurogenic. Nonspecific neurogenic TOS is fairly common, although its prevalence is difficult to estimate because diagnosis is difficult. The condition often can be missed or overdiagnosed; it commonly is a diagnosis of exclusion, meaning that all other causes have been eliminated. Young and middle-aged adults are most susceptible to nonspecific neurogenic TOS.

With neurogenic TOS, symptom onset is most common in teenagers and young adults. Women are at least three times more likely than men to develop the disorder. Vascular TOS is rare and occurs more often in younger, very active individuals. Arterial TOS occurs equally among males and females. Venous TOS occurs most frequently in young men.

Relevant History

Although the exact mechanism behind thoracic outlet syndrome is unknown, several factors may contribute to the pathological condition, including whiplash, a direct or an indirect blow to the shoulder, repetitive strain through prolonged upper limb activity, accessory breathing, and/or poor posture.

Relevant Signs and Symptoms

Arterial Thoracic Outlet Syndrome

- Coldness in the arm
- Heaviness in the arm
- Diminshed or no pulses in the arm
- Pallor in the arm
- Loss of strength or fatigue with overuse of the arm
- True arm claudication during activity (particularly overhead activity)
- Weakened grip
- Reduced finger function (difficulty gripping and carrying bags)

Venous Thoracic Outlet Syndrome

- Swelling in the arm
- Edema in the arm
- Cyanosis in the arm
- Arm discomfort with activity

Neurogenic Thoracic Outlet Syndrome

- Clumsiness with fine hand activities
- Weakness on gripping
- Anterior or posterior shoulder pain that extends to the medial arm, forearm, and hand
- Pain in the clavicular region that extends to the occipital region and mastoid (headaches can be quite severe)
- Anterior chest pain

Mechanism of Injury

The most common cause of TOS is repetitive strain through prolonged or vigorous upper limb activity, often combined with abnormal posture. Activities or work that requires repetitive use of the hand and wrist can be a cause. Positions and postures that put increased strain on the vascular structures of the thoracic outlet include:

- Prolonged writing or use of a keyboard or telephone
- Poor posture (i.e., droopy shoulders or forward head posture)
- Prolonged overhead or reaching activities (e.g., styling hair, painting, playing musical instruments such as the violin or flute, swimming, playing tennis, and pitching)
- Excessive carrying of heavy objects, such as suitcases and shopping bags
- Wearing a heavy coat or backpack that depresses the shoulder

ROOS TEST[169-172]

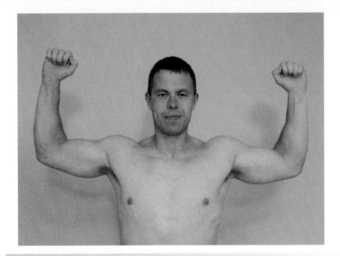

Figure 4–46
Roos test.

PURPOSE	To test for compromise of neurovascular structures through the brachium. This test also may be called the *positive abduction and external rotation (AER) position test*, the *"hands up" test*, or the *elevated arm stress test (EAST)*.
PATIENT POSITION	The patient is standing.
EXAMINER POSITION	The examiner may stand or sit near the patient so as to inquire about the person's symptoms. This is an observational test, and no handling of the limbs is required.
TEST PROCEDURE	The patient abducts the arms to 90°, laterally rotates the shoulder, and flexes the elbows to 90° so that the elbow is slightly behind the frontal plane. The patient opens and closes the hands slowly for 3 minutes.
INDICATIONS OF A POSITIVE TEST	Minor fatigue and distress are considered negative test results. A positive test result for TOS is indicated if the patient is unable to keep the arms in the starting position for 3 minutes or if the person has ischemic pain, arm heaviness, or profound weakness of the arm or numbness and tingling of the hand during the 3 minutes.
CLINICAL NOTES/CAUTIONS	• Thoracic outlet syndromes may combine neurological and vascular signs, or the signs and symptoms of neurological deficit, restriction of arterial flow, or restriction of venous flow may be seen individually. For this reason, a diagnosis of TOS usually is one of exclusion, meaning all other causes have been eliminated. • Neurogenic signs are rare in TOS, and poor correlation is seen between the vascular signs of the condition and neurological involvement.
RELIABILITY/SPECIFICITY/ SENSITIVITY	Unknown

JOINT PLAY MOVEMENTS

ANTERIOR-POSTERIOR GLIDE OF THE HUMERUS[173]

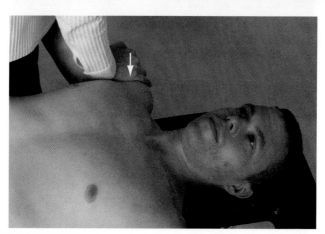

Figure 4–47
Backward glide of the humerus.

PATIENT POSITION	The patient is supine.
EXAMINER POSITION	The examiner stands adjacent to the patient's shoulder.
TEST PROCEDURE	The examiner holds the patient's upper limb, placing the palm of one hand over the anterior humeral head. The other hand grasps the humerus above and near the elbow. The examiner's arm holds the patient's hand against the examiner's thorax. The examiner then applies a posterior-directed force (similar to a posterior shift), keeping the patient's arm parallel to the body so that no rotation or torsion occurs at the glenohumeral joint. The two sides are compared.
INDICATIONS OF A POSITIVE TEST	The examiner compares the amount of available movement and the end feel on the affected side with the movement on the unaffected side and notes whether the movements affect the patient's symptoms. As the movements are performed, the examiner should note any decreased ROM, pain, or difference in end feel.
CLINICAL NOTE	• When the posterior force is applied to the humeral head, it is important that the examiner also lower the rest of the patient's arm so that the upper arm is kept parallel to the floor. If a posterior force is applied at the humeral head without the associated lowering of the arm, rotation torsion occurs at the glenohumeral joint instead of posterior translation.

POSTERIOR-ANTERIOR GLIDE OF THE HUMERUS[173]

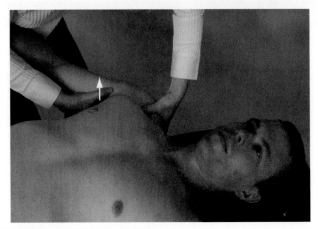

Figure 4–48
Forward glide of the humerus.

PATIENT POSITION	The patient is supine.
EXAMINER POSITION	The examiner stands adjacent to the patient's shoulder.
TEST PROCEDURE	The examiner grasps the patient's upper limb, placing one hand under the posterior humeral head and using the elbow of the same hand to support the patient's arm and hand. The other hand is placed around the upper shoulder to stabilize the scapula and clavicle. The examiner applies an anterior force (anterior shift), keeping the patient's arm parallel to the body so that no rotation or torsion occurs at the glenohumeral joint. The two sides are compared.
INDICATIONS OF A POSITIVE TEST	The examiner compares the amount of available movement and the end feel on the affected side with the movement on the unaffected side and notes whether the movements affect the patient's symptoms. As the joint play movements are performed, the examiner should note any decreased ROM, pain, or difference in end feel.
CLINICAL NOTE	• When the anterior force is applied to the humeral head, it is important that the examiner also raise the rest of the patient's arm so that the upper arm is kept parallel to the floor. If an anterior force is applied at the humeral head without the associated raising of the arm, rotation or torsion occurs at the glenohumeral joint instead of anterior translation.

LATERAL DISTRACTION OF THE HUMERUS[173]

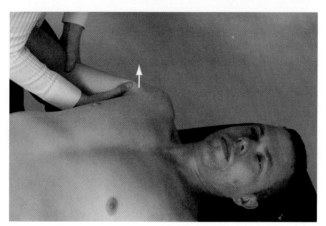

Figure 4–49
Lateral distraction of the humerus.

PATIENT POSITION	The patient is supine.
EXAMINER POSITION	The examiner stands adjacent to the patient's shoulder.
TEST PROCEDURE	The examiner places one hand in the patient's axilla and grasps the medial proximal humerus. The other hand grasps and supports the patient's elbow, forearm, and hand. The examiner applies a lateral distraction force to the glenohumeral joint, keeping the patient's arm parallel to the body so that no rotation or torsion occurs at the glenohumeral joint. The two sides are compared.
INDICATIONS OF A POSITIVE TEST	The examiner compares the amount of available distraction and the end feel on the affected side with the movement on the unaffected side and notes whether the movements affect the patient's symptoms. As the joint play movements are performed, the examiner should note any decreased ROM, pain, or difference in end feel.
CLINICAL NOTES/CAUTIONS	• Care must be taken to apply the lateral distraction force with the flat of the hand. Examiners sometimes have a tendency to turn the hand when applying force, such that the distraction is applied through the side of the index finger. This is uncomfortable for the patient. • It also is important that the proximal hand be placed as close to the glenohumeral joint as possible.

CAUDAL GLIDE (LONG ARM TRACTION) OF THE HUMERUS[173]

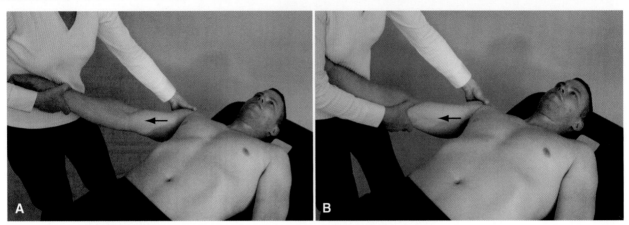

Figure 4–50
A, Long arm traction applied below the elbow. **B,** Long arm traction applied above the elbow.

PATIENT POSITION	The patient is supine.
EXAMINER POSITION	The examiner stands adjacent to the patient's shoulder.
TEST PROCEDURE	The examiner grasps just above the patient's wrist with one hand. With the other hand, the examiner palpates the upper part of the head of the humerus, below the distal spine of the scapula posteriorly, and below the distal clavicle anteriorly. The examiner then applies a traction force to the shoulder while palpating to see whether the head of the humerus drops down (moves distally) in the glenoid cavity as it should. This traction force is accomplished through a slight weight shift of the examiner away from the shoulder. The two sides are compared.
INDICATIONS OF A POSITIVE TEST	The examiner compares the amount of available movement and the end feel on the affected side with the movement on the unaffected side and notes whether the movements affect the patient's symptoms. As the joint play movements are performed, the examiner should note any decreased ROM, pain, or difference in end feel.
CLINICAL NOTE	• If the patient complains of pain in the elbow, the test may be done with the distal hand grasping above the elbow instead of at the wrist.

ANTERIOR-POSTERIOR GLIDE OF THE HUMERUS IN ABDUCTION[173]

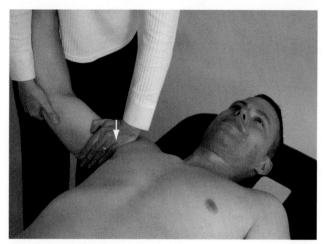

Figure 4–51
Backward glide of the humerus in abduction.

PATIENT POSITION	The patient is supine.
EXAMINER POSITION	The examiner stands adjacent to the patient's shoulder.
TEST PROCEDURE	With the patient's arm abducted to 90°, the examiner places one hand over the anterior humerus while grasping and stabilizing the patient's elbow with the other hand. The elbow also is held tightly against the examiner's body to stabilize the patient's hand against the thorax. The examiner applies a backward force (similar to a posterior shift), keeping the patient's arm parallel to the body so that no rotation or torsion occurs at the glenohumeral joint. The two sides are compared.
INDICATIONS OF A POSITIVE TEST	The examiner compares the amount of available movement and the end feel on the affected side with the movement on the unaffected side and notes whether the movements affect the patient's symptoms. As the joint play movements are performed, the examiner should note any decreased ROM, pain, or difference in end feel.
CLINICAL NOTE	• As in the anterior to posterior glide test in neutral position, the examiner must keep the upper arm parallel to the floor when applying the posterior force so the elbow is lowered as the humeral head is depressed.

ACROMIOCLAVICULAR AND STERNOCLAVICULAR JOINT MOBILITY

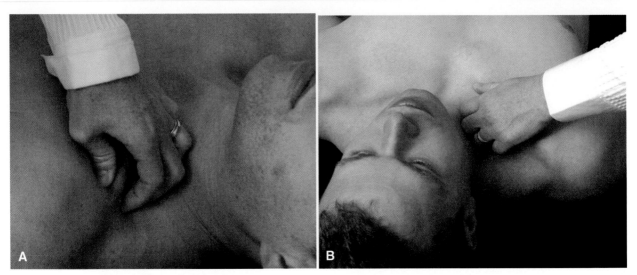

Figure 4–52
A, Joint play of the acromioclavicular joint. **B,** Joint play of the sternoclavicular joint.

PATIENT POSITION	The patient is supine.
EXAMINER POSITION	The examiner stands adjacent to the patient's shoulder.
TEST PROCEDURE	The examiner gently grasps the clavicle as close as possible to the joint to be tested (acromioclavicular or sternoclavicular joint). The examiner then moves the clavicle in and out or up and down while palpating the joint with the other hand. The two sides are compared.
INDICATIONS OF A POSITIVE TEST	The examiner compares the amount of available movement and the end feel on the affected side with the movement on the unaffected side and notes whether the movements affect the patient's symptoms. As the joint play movements are performed, the examiner should note any decreased ROM, pain, or difference in end feel.
CLINICAL NOTES/CAUTIONS	• Because the bone lies just under the skin, these techniques are uncomfortable for the patient where the examiner grasps the clavicle. The examiner should warn the patient before attempting this technique. • Care should be taken not to squeeze the clavicle, because this, too, may cause pain.

SCAPULOTHORACIC JOINT MOBILITY

DVD

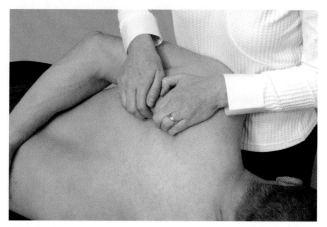

Figure 4–53
General movement of the scapula to determine its mobility.

PATIENT POSITION	The patient is assessed in the side-lying position, which fixates the thorax by placing the contralateral shoulder on the table. The upper (test) arm should be relaxed and resting behind the low back (the hand is by the opposite back pocket). The patient leans the upper shoulder into the examiner.
EXAMINER POSITION	The examiner stands in front of the patient's shoulder.
TEST PROCEDURE	The examiner uses his or her body to push the patient's uppermost shoulder backward to retract the shoulder. The examiner then grasps the medial border of the scapula with both hands; the lower hand is placed along the medial border, and the upper hand holds the upper (cranial) dorsal surface. The examiner moves the scapula medially, laterally, caudally, cranially, and away from the thorax. The two sides are compared.
INDICATIONS OF A POSITIVE TEST	The examiner compares the amount of available movement and the end feel on the affected side with the movement on the unaffected side and notes whether the movements affect the patient's symptoms. As the joint play movements are performed, the examiner should note any decreased ROM, pain, or difference in end feel.
CLINICAL NOTES/CAUTIONS	• In some patients, the scapulae are easy to assess because they wing readily; other patients require positioning and muscle relaxation to enable the examiner to grasp the scapula. • The examiner may also palpate various structures around the shoulder.

References

1. Payne LZ, Deng X-H, Craig EV et al: The combined dynamic and static contributions to subacromial impingement: a biomechanical analysis, *Am J Sports Med* 25:801-808, 1997.

2. Watson CJ, Schenkman M: Physical therapy management of isolated serratus anterior muscle paralysis, *Phys Ther* 75:194-202, 1995.

3. Kessel L, Watson M: The painful arc syndrome, *J Bone Joint Surg Br* 59:166-172, 1977.

4. Inman VT, Saunders M, Abbott LC: Observations on the function of the shoulder joint, *J Bone Joint Surg Br* 26:1-30, 1944.

5. Sugamoto K, Harada T, Machida A et al: Scapulohumeral rhythm: relationship between motion velocity and rhythm, *Clin Orthop Relat Res* 401:119-124, 2002.

6. Davies GJ, Dickoff-Hoffman S: Neuromuscular testing and rehabilitation of the shoulder complex, *J Orthop Sports Phys Ther* 18:449-458, 1993.

7. Lucas DB: Biomechanics of the shoulder joint, *Arch Surg* 107:425-432, 1973.

8. Freedman L, Munro RR: Abduction of the arm in the scapular plane: scapular and glenohumeral movements, *J Bone Joint Surg Am* 48:1503-1510, 1966.

9. Foo CL, Swann M: Isolated paralysis of the serratus anterior: a report of 20 cases, *J Bone Joint Surg Br* 65:552-556, 1983.

10. van Eisenhart-Rothe R, Matsen FA, Eckstein F et al: Pathomechanics in atraumatic shoulder instability, *Clin Orthop Relat Res* 433:82-89, 2005.

11. Perry J: Biomechanics of the shoulder. In Rowe CR (ed): *The shoulder,* Edinburgh, 1988, Churchill Livingstone.

12. Kapandji IA: *The physiology of joints,* vol 1, *Upper limb,* New York, 1970, Churchill Livingstone.

13. Matsen FA, Lippitt SB, Sidles JA et al: *Practical evaluation and management of the shoulder,* Philadelphia, 1994, Saunders.

14. Burkhart SS, Morgan CD, Kibler WB: The disabled throwing shoulder: spectrum of pathology. I. Pathoanatomy and biomechanics, *Arthroscopy* 19:404-420, 2003.

15. Burkhart SS, Morgan CD, Kibler WB: The disabled throwing shoulder: spectrum of pathology. III. The SICK scapula, scapular dyskinesia, the kinetic chain, and rehabilitation, *Arthroscopy* 19:641-661, 2003.

16. Nishijima N, Yamamuro T, Fujio K et al: The swallowtail sign: a test for deltoid function, *J Bone Joint Surg Br* 77:152-153, 1994.

17. Manske RC, Reiman MP, Stovak ML: Nonoperative and operative management of snapping scapula, *Am J Sports Med* 32:1554-1565, 2004.

18. Reid DC: The shoulder girdle: its function as a unit in abduction, *Physiotherapy* 55:57-59, 1969.

19. Saha SK: Mechanism of shoulder movements and a plea for the recognition of "zero position" of glenohumeral joint, *Clin Orthop* 173:3-10, 1983.

20. Boody SG, Freedman L, Waterland JC: Shoulder movements during abduction in the scapular plane, *Arch Phys Med Rehabil* 51:595-604, 1970.

21. Kibler WB: Evaluation and diagnosis of scapulothoracic problems in the athlete, *Sports Med Arthro Rev* 8:192-202, 2000.

22. Rudert M, Wulker M: Clinical evaluation. In Wulker N, Mansat M, Fu F (eds): *Shoulder surgery: an illustrated textbook,* London, 2001, Martin Dunitz.

23. Petersen CM, Hayes KW: Construct validity of Cyriax's selective tension examination: association of end feels with pain in the knee and shoulder, *J Orthop Sports Phys Ther* 30:512-521, 2000.

24. Tyler TF, Roy T, Nicholas SJ et al: Reliability and validity of a new method of measuring posterior shoulder tightness, *J Orthop Sports Phys Ther* 29:262-274, 1999.

25. Tyler TF, Nicholas SJ, Roy T et al: Quantification of posterior capsule tightness and motion loss in patients with shoulder impingement, *Am J Sports Med* 28:668-673, 2000.

26. Pagnani MJ, Galinat BJ, Warren RF: Glenohumeral instability. In De Lee JC, Drez D (eds): *Orthopedic sports medicine: principles and practice,* Philadelphia, 1994, Saunders.

27. Mimori K, Muneta T, Nakagawa T et al: A new pain provocation test for superior labral tears of the shoulder, *Am J Sports Med* 27:137-142, 1999.

28. Liu SH, Henry MH, Nuccion SL: A prospective evaluation of a new physical examination in predicting glenoid labral tears, *Am J Sports Med* 24:721-725, 1996.

29. Stetson WB, Templin K: The crank test, the O'Brien test, and routine magnetic resonance imaging scans in the diagnosis of labral tears, *Am J Sports Med* 30:806-809, 2002.

30. Guanche CA, Jones DC: Clinical testing for tears of the glenoid labrum, *Arthroscopy* 19:517-523, 2003.

31. Su KA, Johnson MP, Gracely EJ et al: Scapular rotation in swimmers with and without impingement syndrome: practice effects, *Med Sci Sports Exerc* 31:1117-1123, 2004.

32. Myers TH, Zemanovic JR, Andrews JR: The resisted supination external rotation test: a new test for the diagnosis of superior labral anterior posterior lesions, *Am J Sports Med* 33:1315-1320, 2005.

33. Tzannes A, Paxinos A, Callanan M et al: An assessment of the interexaminer reliability of tests for shoulder instability, *J Shoulder Elbow Surg* 13:18-23, 2004.

34. Jorgensen U, Bak K: Shoulder instability: assessment of anterior-posterior translation with a knee laxity tester, *Acta Orthop Scand* 66:398-400, 1995.

35. Pizzari T, Kolt GS, Remedios I: Measurement of anterior-to-posterior translation on the glenohumeral joint using the KT-1000, *J Orthop Sports Phys Ther* 29:602-608, 1999.

36. Lo IK, Nonweiler B, Woolfrey M et al: An evaluation of the apprehension, relocation, and surprise tests for anterior shoulder instability, *Am J Sports Med* 32:301-307, 2004.

37. Rowe CR: Prognosis in dislocations of the shoulder, *J Bone Joint Surg Am* 38:957-977, 1956.

38. Boublik M, Silliman JF: History and physical examination. In Hawkins RJ, Misamore GW (eds): *Shoulder injuries in the athlete,* New York, 1996, Churchill Livingstone.

39. Hawkins RJ, Mohtadi NG: Clinical evaluation of shoulder instability, *Clin J Sports Med* 1:59-64, 1991.
40. Silliman JF, Hawkins RJ: Classification and physical diagnosis of instability of the shoulder, *Clin Orthop* 291: 7-19, 1993.
41. Harryman DT, Sidles JA, Harris SL et al: Laxity of the normal glenohumeral joint: a quantitative in vivo assessment, *J Shoulder Elbow Surg* 1:66-76, 1992.
42. Borsa PA, Sauers EL, Herling DE: Patterns of glenohumeral joint laxity and stiffness in healthy men and women, *Med Sci Sports Exerc* 32:1685-1690, 2000.
43. Sauers EL, Borsa PA, Herling DE et al: Instrumented measurement of glenohumeral joint laxity and its relationship to passive range of motion and generalized joint laxity, *Am J Sports Med* 29:143-150, 2001.
44. Sauers EL, Borsa PA, Herling DE et al: Instrumental measurement of glenohumeral joint laxity: Reliability and normative data, *Knee Surg Sports Traumatol Arthros* 9:34-41, 2001.
45. Ellenbecker TS, Maltalino AJ, Elam E et al: Quantification of anterior translation of the humeral head in the throwing shoulder: manual assessment vs. stress radiography, *Am J Sports Med* 28:161-167, 2000.
46. Lintner SA, Levy A, Kenter K et al: Glenohumeral translation in the asymptomatic athlete's shoulder and its relationship to other clinically measurable anthropometric variables, *Am J Sports Med* 24:716-720, 1996.
47. Altchek DA, Warren RF, Skyhar MJ et al: T-plasty: a technique for treating multidirectional instability in the athlete, *J Bone Joint Surg Am* 73:105-112, 1991.
48. Matthews LS, Pavlovich LJ: Anterior and anteroinferior instability: diagnosis and management. In Iannotti JP, Williams CR (eds): *Disorders of the shoulder,* Philadelphia, 1999, Lippincott Williams & Wilkins.
49. Ramsey ML, Klimkiewicz JJ: Posterior instability: diagnosis and management. In Iannotti JP, Williams CR (eds): *Disorders of the shoulder,* Philadelphia, 1999, Lippincott Williams & Wilkins.
50. Matsen FA, Thomas SC, Rockwood CA: Glenohumeral instability. In Rockwood CA, Matsen FA (eds): *The shoulder,* Philadelphia, 1990, Saunders.
51. Jobe FW, Kvitne RS: Shoulder pain in the overhand or throwing athlete: the relationship of anterior instability and rotator cuff impingement, *Orthop Rev* 18:963-975, 1989.
52. Speer KP, Hannafin JA, Alteck DW et al: An evaluation of the shoulder relocation test, *Am J Sports Med* 22: 177-183, 1994.
53. Burkhart SS, Morgan CD, Kibler WB: The disabled throwing shoulder: spectrum of pathology. II. Evaluation and treatment of SLAP lesions in throwers, *Arthroscopy* 19:531-539, 2003.
54. Jobe CM: Superior glenoid impingement, *Orthop Clin North Am* 28:137-143, 1997.
55. Davidson PA, Elattrache NS, Jobe CM et al: Rotator cuff and posterior-superior glenoid labrum injury associated with increased glenohumeral motion: a new site of impingement, *J Shoulder Elbow Surg* 4:384-390, 1995.
56. Luime JJ, Verhagen AP, Miedema HS et al: Does this patient have instability of the shoulder or a labrum lesion? *JAMA* 292:1989-1999, 2004.
57. Gross ML, Distefano MC: Anterior release test: a new test for occult shoulder instability, *Clin Orthop Relat Res* 339:105-108, 1997.
58. Hawkins RJ, Bokor DJ: Clinical evaluation of shoulder problems. In Rockwood CA, Matsen FA (eds): *The shoulder,* Philadelphia, 1990, Saunders.
59. Kvitne RS, Jobe FW: The diagnosis and treatment of anterior instability in the throwing athlete, *Clin Orthop* 291:107-123, 1993.
60. Hamner DL, Pink MM, Jobe FW: A modification of the relocation test: arthroscopic findings associated with a positive test, *J Shoulder Elbow Surg* 9:263-267, 2000.
61. Kelley MJ: Evaluation of the shoulder. In Kelley MJ, Clark WA (eds): *Orthopedic therapy of the shoulder,* Philadelphia, 1995, JB Lippincott.
62. Rockwood CA: Subluxations and dislocations about the shoulder. In Rockwood CA Green, DP (eds): *Fractures in adults,* Philadelphia, 1984, JB Lippincott.
63. Pollock RG, Bigliani LU: Recurrent posterior shoulder instability: diagnosis and treatment, *Clin Orthop Relat Res* 291:85-96, 1993.
64. Wolf EM, Eakin CL: Arthroscopic capsular placation for posterior shoulder instability, *Arthroscopy* 14:153-163, 1998.
65. Sobush DC, Simoneau GG, Dietz KE et al: The Lennie test for measuring scapular position in healthy young adult females: a reliability and validity study, *J Orthop Sports Phys Ther* 23:39-50, 1996.
66. Norwood LA, Terry GC: Shoulder posterior subluxation, *Am J Sports Med* 12:25-30, 1984.
67. Cofield RH, Irving JF: Evaluation and classification of shoulder instability, *Clin Orthop* 223:32-43, 1987.
68. Davies GJ, Gould JA, Larson RL: Functional examination of the shoulder girdle, *Phys Sportsmed* 9:82-104, 1981.
69. Pagnani MJ, Warren RF: Multidirectional instability in the athlete. In Pettrone FA (ed): *Athletic injuries of the shoulder,* New York, 1995, McGraw Hill.
70. Burkhead WZ, Rockwood CA: Treatment of instability of the shoulder with an exercise program, *J Bone Joint Surg Am* 74:890-896, 1992.
71. Cordasco FA: Understanding multidirectional instability of the shoulder, *J Athl Train* 35:278-285, 2000.
72. Gross TP: Anterior glenohumeral instability, *Orthopaedics* 11:87-94, 1988.
73. Hawkins RJ, Bell RH, Hawkins RH, Koppert GJ: Anterior dislocation of the shoulder in the older patient, *Clin Orthop* 206:192-195, 1986.
74. Hayes K, Callanan M, Walton J et al: Shoulder instability: management and rehabilitation, *J Orthop Sports Phys Ther* 32:497-509, 2002.
75. Hovelius L, Eriksson K, Fredin H et al: Recurrences after initial dislocation of the shoulder, *J Bone Joint Surg Am* 65:343-349, 1983.
76. Lippitt S, Matsen F: Mechanisms of glenohumeral joint stability, *Clin Orthop* 291:20-28, 1993.
77. Walton J, Paxinos A, Tzannes A et al: The unstable shoulder in the adolescent athlete, *Am J Sports Med* 30:758-767, 2002.
78. Gerber C, Ganz R: Clinical assessment of instability of the shoulder, *J Bone Joint Surg Br* 66:551-556, 1984.

79. Bigliani LU, Codd TP, Conner PM et al: Shoulder motion and laxity in the professional baseball player, *Am J Sports Med* 25:609-613, 1997.

80. McClusky GM: Classification and diagnosis of glenohumeral instability in athletes, *Sports Med Artho Rev* 8:158-169, 2000.

81. Bowen M, Warren R: Ligamentous control of shoulder stability based on selective cutting and static translation, *Clin Sports Med* 10:757-782, 1991.

82. Helmig P, Sojbjerg J, Kjaersgaard-Andersen P et al: Distal humeral migration as a component of multidirectional shoulder instability, *Clin Orthop* 252:139-143, 1990.

83. Neer CS: Anterior acromioplasty for the chronic impingement syndrome in the shoulder: a preliminary report, *J Bone Joint Surg Am* 54:41-50, 1972.

84. Dines DM, Warren RF, Inglis AE, Pavlov H: The coracoid impingement syndrome, *J Bone Joint Surg Br* 72:314-316, 1990.

85. Dorrestijn O, Stevens M, Winters JC et al: Conservative or surgical treatment for subacromial impingement syndrome? A systematic review, *J Shoulder Elbow Surg* 18:652-660, 2009.

86. Hawkins RJ, Mohtadi N: Rotator cuff problems in athletes. In DeLee J, Drez D, Stanitski CL (eds): *Orthopaedic sports medicine: principles and practice*, Philadelphia, 1994, Saunders.

87. Hawkins RJ, Kennedy JC: Impingement syndrome in athletes, *Am J Sports Med* 8:151-163, 1980.

88. Selkowitz DM, Chaney C, Stuckey SJ, Vlad G: The effects of scapular taping on the surface electromyographic signal amplitude of shoulder girdle muscles during upper extremity elevation in individuals with suspected shoulder impingement syndrome, *J Orthop Sports Phys Ther* 37:694-702, 2007.

89. Calis M, Akgun K, Birtane M et al: Diagnostic values of clinical diagnostic tests in subacromial impingement syndrome, *Ann Rheum Dis* 59:44-47, 2000.

90. Brossmann J, Preidler KW, Pedowitz KA et al: Shoulder impingement syndrome: influence of shoulder position on rotator cuff impingement—an anatomic study, *Am J Roentgenol* 167:1511-1515, 1992.

91. Valadic AL, Jobe CM, Pink MM et al: Anatomy of provocative tests for impingement syndrome of the shoulder, *J Shoulder Elbow Surg* 9:36-46, 2000.

92. Gerber C, Terrier F, Ganz R: The role of the coracoid process in the chronic impingement syndrome, *J Bone Joint Surg Br* 67:703-708, 1985.

93. Bigliani LU, Levine WN: Subacromial impingement syndrome, *J Bone Joint Surg Am* 79:1854-1868, 1997.

94. Connell DA, Potter HG, Wickiewicz TL et al: Noncontrast magnetic resonance imaging of superior labral lesions: 102 cases confirmed at arthroscopic surgery, *Am J Sports Med* 27:208-213, 1999.

95. MacDonald PB, Clark P, Sutherland K: An analysis of the diagnostic accuracy of the Hawkins and Neer subacromial impingement signs, *J Shoulder Elbow Surg* 9:299-301, 2000.

96. McFarland EG, Selhi HS, Keyurapan E: Clinical evaluation of impingement: what to do and what works, *J Bone Joint Surg Am* 88:432-441, 2006.

97. Priest JD, Nagel DA: Tennis shoulder, *Am J Sports Med* 4:28-42, 1976.

98. Leroux JL, Thomas E, Bonnel F et al: Diagnostic value of clinical tests for shoulder impingement, *Rev Rheum* 62:423-428, 1995.

99. Park HB, Yokota A, Gill HS et al: Diagnostic accuracy of clinical tests for the different degrees of subacromial impingement syndrome, *J Bone Joint Surg Am* 87:1446-1455, 2005.

100. Neer CS, Welsh RP: The shoulder in sports, *Orthop Clin North Am* 8:583-591, 1977.

101. Buchberger DJ: Introduction of a new physical examination procedure for the differentiation of acromioclavicular joint lesions and subacromial impingement, *J Manip Physiol Ther* 22:316-321, 1999.

102. Chronopoulus E, Kim TK, Park HB et al: Diagnostic value of physical tests for isolated chronic acromioclavicular lesions, *Am J Sports Med* 32:655-661, 2004.

103. Meister K: Injuries to the shoulder in the throwing athlete. II. Evaluation/treatment, *Am J Sports Med* 28:587-601, 2000.

104. Jobe CM: Posterior superior glenoid impingement: expanded spectrum, *Arthroscopy* 11:530-536, 1995.

105. Jobe CM: Superior glenoid impingement, *Clin Orthop Relat Res* 330:98-107, 1996.

106. Giombini A, Rossi F, Pettrone FA et al: Posterosuperior glenoid rim impingement as a cause of shoulder pain in top level water polo players, *J Sports Med Phys Fit* 37:273-278, 1997.

107. Parentis MA, Glousman RE, Mohr KS et al: An evaluation of the provocative tests for superior labral posterior lesions, *Am J Sports Med* 34:265-268, 2006.

108. Bankart ASB: The pathology and treatment of recurrent dislocations of the shoulder joint, *Br J Surg* 26:23-29, 1938.

109. Rathbun JB, Macnab I: The microvascular pattern of the rotator cuff, *J Bone Joint Surg Br* 52:540-553, 1970.

110. McFarland EG, Kim TK, Savino RM: Clinical assessment of three common tests for superior labral anterior-posterior lesions, *Am J Sports Med* 30:810-815, 2002.

111. Kibler WB: Specificity and sensitivity of the anterior slide test in throwing athletes with superior glenoid labral tears, *Arthroscopy* 11:296-300, 1995.

112. Kim SH, Ha KI, Ahn JH et al: Biceps load test II: a clinical test for SLAP lesions of the shoulder, *Arthroscopy* 17(2):160-164, 2001.

113. O'Brien SJ, Pagnoni MJ, Fealy S et al: The active compression test: a new and effective test for diagnosing labral tears and acromioclavicular joint abnormality, *Am J Sports Med* 26:610-613, 1998.

114. Zasler KR: Internal rotation resistance strength tests: a new diagnostic test to differentiate intra-articular pathology from outlet (Neer) impingement syndrome in the shoulder, *J Shoulder Elbow Surg* 10:23-27, 2001.

115. Kibler WB: Clinical examination of the shoulder. In Pettrone FA (ed): *Athletic injuries of the shoulder*, New York, 1995, McGraw Hill.

116. Andrews JR, Gillogly S: Physical examination of the shoulder in throwing athletes. In Zarins B, Andrews JR,

Carson WG (eds): *Injuries to the throwing arm,* Philadelphia, 1985, Saunders.

117. Walsh DA: Shoulder evaluation of the throwing athlete, *Sports Med Update* 4:24-27, 1989.

118. Kim SH, Ha KI, Han KY: Biceps load test: a clinical test for superior labrum anterior and posterior lesions in shoulder with recurrent anterior dislocations, *Am J Sports Med* 27:300-303, 1999.

119. Berg EE, Ciullo JV: A clinical test for superior glenoid labral or "SLAP" lesions, *Clin J Sports Med* 8:121-123, 1998.

120. Schultz JS, Leonard JA: Long thoracic neuropathy from athletic activity, *Arch Phys Med Rehabil* 73:87-90, 1992.

121. Fiddian NJ, King RJ: The winged scapula, *Clin Orthop* 185:228-236, 1984.

122. Sobush DC, Simoneau GG, Dietz KE et al: The Lennie test for measuring scapular position in healthy young adult females: a reliability and validity study, *J Orthop Sports Phys Ther* 23:39-50, 1996.

123. Kibler WB, Uhl TL, Maddux JW et al: Qualitative clinical evaluation of scapular dysfunction: a reliability study, *J Shoulder Elbow Surg* 11:550-556, 2002.

124. Kibler WB: Role of the scapula in the overhead throwing motion, *Contemp Orthop* 22:525-533, 1991.

125. Koslow PA, Prosser LA, Strony GA et al: Specificity of the lateral scapular slide test in asymptomatic competitive athletes, *J Orthop Sports Phys Ther* 33:331-336, 2003.

126. Odom CJ, Taylor AB, Hurd CE et al: Measurement of scapular asymmetry and assessment of shoulder dysfunction using the lateral scapular slide test: a reliability and validity study, *Phys Ther* 81:799-809, 2001.

127. Kibler WB: Scapular dyskinesis and its relation to shoulder pain, *J Am Acad Orthop Surg* 11:142-151, 2003.

128. Kibler WB: The role of the scapula in athletic shoulder function, *Am J Sports Med* 26:325-337, 1998.

129. Burkhart SS, Morgan CD, Kibler WB: Shoulder injuries in overhead athletes: the "dead arm" revisited, *Clin Sports Med* 19:125-158, 2000.

130. Goldbeck TG, Davies GJ: Test-retest reliability of the closed kinetic chain–upper extremity stability test: a clinical field test, *J Sports Rehab* 9:35-43, 2000.

131. Fraser-Moodie JA, Shortt NL, Robinson CM: Injuries to the acromioclavicular joint, *J Bone Joint Surg Br* 90:697-707, 2008.

132. Larsen E, Bjerg-Nielsen A, Christensen P: Conservative or surgical treatment of acromioclavicular dislocation: a prospective, controlled, randomized study, *J Bone Joint Surg Am* 68:552-555, 1986.

133. Macdonald PB, LaPointe P: Acromioclavicular and sternoclavicular joint injuries, *Orthop Clin North Am* 39:535-545, 2008.

134. Axe MJ: Acromioclavicular joint injuries in the athlete, *Sports Med Arthro Rev* 8:182-191, 2000.

135. Clark HD, McCann PD: Acromioclavicular joint injuries, *Orthop Clin North Am* 31:177-187, 2000.

136. Shaffer BS: Painful conditions of the acromioclavicular joint, *J Am Acad Orthop Surg* 7:176-188, 1999.

137. Holtby R, Razmjou H: Accuracy of the Speed's and Yergason's tests in detecting biceps pathology and SLAP lesions: comparison with arthroscopic findings, *Arthroscopy* 20:231-236, 2004.

138. Patrik GE, Kuhn JE: Validation of the lift-off test and analysis of subscapularis activity during maximal internal rotation, *Am J Sports Med* 24:589, 1996.

139. Holtby R, Razmjou H: Validity of the supraspinatus test as a single clinical test in diagnosing patients with rotator cuff pathology, *J Orthop Sports Phys Ther* 34:194-200, 2004.

140. Barth JR, Burkhart SS, DeBeer JF: The bear hug test: a new and sensitive test for diagnosing a subscapularis tear, *Arthroscopy* 222:1076-1084, 2006.

141. Greis PE, Kuhn JE, Schultheis J et al: Validation of the lift-off sign test and analysis of subscapularis activity during maximal internal rotation, *Am J Sports Med* 24: 589-593, 1996.

142. Hertel R, Ballmer FT, Lambert SM et al: Lag signs in the diagnosis of rotator cuff rupture, *J Shoulder Elbow Surg* 5:307-313, 1996.

143. Bell RH, Noble JB: Biceps disorders. In Hawkins RJ, Misamore GW (eds): *Shoulder injuries in the athlete,* New York, 1996, Churchill Livingstone.

144. Khan KM, Cook JL, Taunton JE et al: Overuse tendinosis, not tendinitis. Part 1. A new paradigm for a difficult clinical problem, *Phys Sportsmed* 28:38-48, 2000.

145. Yergason RM: Supination sign, *J Bone Joint Surg* 13:160, 1931.

146. Stefko JM, Jobe FW, Vanderwilde RS et al: Electromyographic and nerve block analysis of the subscapularis lift off test, *J Shoulder Elbow Surg* 6:347-355, 1997.

147. Jobe FW, Moynes DR: Delineation of diagnostic criteria and a rehabilitation program for rotator cuff injuries, *Am J Sports Med* 10:336-339, 1982.

148. Kelly BT, Kadrmas WR, Speer KP: The manual muscle examination for rotator cuff strength: an electromyographic investigation, *Am J Sports Med* 24:581-588, 1996.

149. Gerber C, Krushell RJ: Isolated ruptures of the tendon of the subscapularis muscle, *J Bone Joint Surg Br* 73: 389-394, 1991.

150. Lyons RP, Green A: Subscapularis tendon tears, *J Am Acad Orthop Surg* 13:353-363, 2005.

151. Williams GR: Complications of rotator cuff surgery. In Iannotti JP, Williams CR (eds): *Disorders of the shoulder,* Philadelphia, 1999, Lippincott Williams & Wilkins.

152. Burkhart SS, Lo IK, Brady PC: *A cowboy's guide to advanced shoulder arthroscopy,* Philadelphia, 2006, Lippincott, Williams & Wilkins.

153. Ticker JB, Warner JJ: Single-tendon tears of the rotator cuff: evaluation and treatment of subscapularis tears, *Orthop Clin North Am* 28:99-116, 1997.

154. Arroyo JS, Flatow EL: Management of rotator cuff disease: intact and repairable cuff. In Iannotti JP, Williams GR (eds): *Disorders of the shoulder,* Philadelphia, 1999, Lippincott Williams & Wilkins.

155. Walch G, Boulahia A, Calderone S et al: The "dropping" and "horn blower's" signs in evaluating rotator cuff tears, *J Bone Joint Surg Br* 80:624-628, 1998.

156. Cordasco FA, Bigliani LU: Large and massive tears: technique of open repair, *Orthop Clin North Am* 28: 179-193, 1997.

157. Brunnstrom S: Muscle testing around the shoulder girdle: a study of the function of shoulder blade fixators in 17 cases of shoulder paralysis, *J Bone Joint Surg Am* 23:263-272, 1941.

158. Kendall HO, Kendall FP: *Muscles: testing and function*, Baltimore, 1999, Williams & Wilkins.

159. Reese MB: *Muscle and sensory testing*, Philadelphia, 1999, Saunders.

160. Arcand MA, Reider B: Shoulder and upper arm. In Reider B (ed): *The orthopedic physical examination*, Philadelphia, 1999, Saunders.

161. Atasoy E: Thoracic outlet syndrome: anatomy, *Hand Clin* 20:7-14, 2004.

162. Ault J, Suutala K: Thoracic outlet syndrome, *J Man Manip Ther* 6:188-129, 1998.

163. Brantigan CO, Roos DB, David B: Etiology of neurogenic thoracic outlet syndrome, *Hand Clin* 20:17-22, 2004.

164. Dawson DM, Hallett M, Milender LH: *Entrapment neuropathies*, ed 2, Boston, 1990, Little, Brown.

165. Demondion X, Herbinet P, Van Sint Jan S et al: Imaging assessment of thoracic outlet syndrome, *RadioGraphics* 26:1735-1750, 2006.

166. Pecina MM, Krmpotic-Nemanic J, Markiewitz AP: *Tunnel syndromes: peripheral nerve compression syndromes*, ed 3, Boca Raton, 2001, CRC Press.

167. Wehbé MA: Thoracic outlet syndrome, *Hand Clin* 20:xi, 2004 [guest editorial].

168. Whitenack SH, Hunter JM, Read RL: Thoracic outlet syndrome: a brachial plexopathy. In Hunter JM, Mackin EJ, Callahan AD et al (eds): *Rehabilitation of the hand and upper extremity*, ed 5, St Louis, 2002, Mosby.

169. Roos DB: Congenital anomalies associated with thoracic outlet syndrome, *J Surg* 132:771-778, 1976.

170. Liebenson CS: Thoracic outlet syndrome: diagnosis and conservative management, *J Manip Physiol Ther* 11:493-499, 1988.

171. Ribbe EB, Lindgren SH, Norgren NE: Clinical diagnosis of thoracic outlet syndrome: evaluation of patients with cervicobrachial symptoms, *Man Med* 2:82-85, 1986.

172. Sallstrom J, Schmidt H: Cervicobrachial disorders in certain occupations, with special reference to compression in the thoracic outlet, *Am J Ind Med* 6:45-52, 1984.

173. Kaltenborn EM: *Mobilization of the extremity joints*, Oslo, 1980, Olaf Norlis Bokhandle.

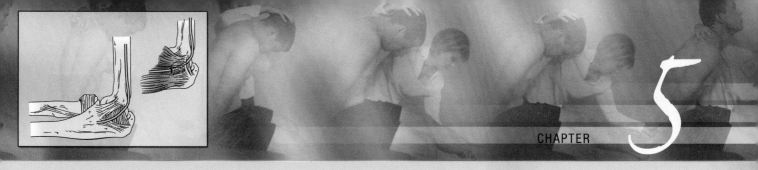

ELBOW

Précis of the Elbow Assessment*

History
Observation
Examination
Active movements
Elbow flexion
Elbow extension
Supination
Pronation
Combined movements (if necessary)
Repetitive movements (if necessary)
Sustained positions (if necessary)
Passive movements (as in active movements, if necessary)
Elbow flexion
Elbow extension
Supination
Pronation
Resisted isometric movements
Elbow flexion
Elbow extension
Supination
Pronation
Wrist flexion
Wrist extension
Reflexes and cutaneous distribution
Reflexes
Sensory scan
Peripheral nerves

Median nerve and branches
Ulnar nerve
Radial nerve and branches
Special tests
Ligamentous valgus instability test
Ligamentous varus instability test
Milking maneuver test
Moving valgus stress test
Lateral pivot-shift test
Posterolateral rotary drawer test
Posterolateral rotary apprehension test
Lateral epicondylitis (tennis elbow or Cozen's) test
Elbow flexion test
Pinch grip test
Joint play movements
Radial deviation of ulna and radius on humerus
Ulnar deviation of ulna and radius on humerus
Distraction of olecranon process on humerus in 90°
of flexion
Anterior-posterior glide of radius on humerus
Posterior-anterior glide of radius on humerus
Palpation
Diagnostic imaging

---

*The entire assessment may be done with the patient in the sitting position. After any examination, the patient should be warned that symptoms may be exacerbated as a result of the assessment.

SELECTED MOVEMENTS

ACTIVE MOVEMENTS[1]

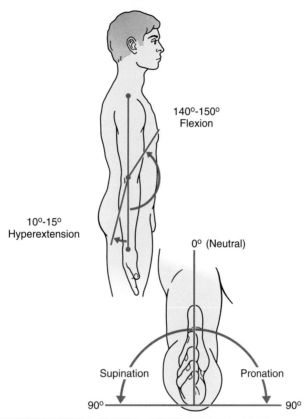

Figure 5–1
Range of motion at the elbow.

GENERAL INFORMATION If the patient has difficulty with or cannot complete a movement but the motion is pain free, the examiner must consider a severe injury to the contractile tissue (rupture) or a neurological injury. In such cases, further testing is necessary. It is important to remember that the most painful movements are done last. Structures outside the joint may affect range of motion (ROM). For example, with lateral epicondylitis, the long extensors of the forearm often are found to be tight or shortened. Therefore, the position of the wrist and fingers may affect the ROM at the elbow.

PATIENT POSITION The patient is sitting.

EXAMINER POSITION The examiner is positioned in front of the patient.

Flexion

TEST PROCEDURE The patient is asked to actively flex the elbow.

INDICATIONS OF A POSITIVE TEST Active elbow flexion is 140° to 150°. Movement usually is stopped by contact of the forearm with the muscles of the arm.

Continued

ACTIVE MOVEMENTS[1]—*cont'd*

CLINICAL NOTES	• The examiner should test active flexion in a neutral position as well as in the fully pronated and supinated positions. Differences in flexion ROM should be noted. • Terminal flexion loss is more disabling than the same degree of terminal extension loss, because flexion is needed for so many activities of daily living. Loss of either motion affects the reach of the hand, which in turn affects function.

Extension

TEST PROCEDURE	The patient is asked to actively extend the elbow.
INDICATIONS OF A POSITIVE TEST	Active elbow extension is 0°, although up to 10° of hyperextension may be seen, especially in women. This hyperextension is considered normal if it is equal on the two sides and the patient has no history of trauma.
CLINICAL NOTE	• Normally, the extension movement is arrested by the locking of the olecranon process of the ulna into the olecranon fossa of the humerus. Loss of elbow extension is a sensitive indicator of an intra-articular pathological condition. It is the first movement lost after injury to the elbow and the first regained with healing.

Pronation

TEST PROCEDURE	The patient is asked to flex the elbow to 90° and then to actively pronate the elbow.
INDICATIONS OF A POSITIVE TEST	Active pronation should be approximately 80° to 90°, so that the palm faces down. If the patient is unable to fully pronate the forearm while maintaining the elbow at the side of the body, pronation is restricted.
CLINICAL NOTES	• The examiner should make sure the patient does not abduct the shoulder in an attempt to increase the amount of pronation or to compensate for a lack of sufficient pronation. • For both supination and pronation, only about 75° of movement occurs in the forearm articulations; the remaining 15° is the result of wrist action.

Supination

TEST PROCEDURE	The patient is asked to flex the elbow to 90° and then to actively supinate the forearm.
INDICATIONS OF A POSITIVE TEST	Active supination should be 90°, so that the palm faces up. If the patient is unable to fully supinate the forearm while maintaining the elbow at the side of the body without adducting the shoulder, supination is restricted.
CLINICAL NOTES	• The examiner should make sure the patient's shoulder does not adduct further in an attempt to give the appearance of increased supination or to compensate for a lack of sufficient supination. • Loss of ROM with supination often is the result of wrist injuries or fracture. Therefore, loss of motion or symptom reproduction with supination does not always imply a pathological condition of the elbow. • If the patient history includes a complaint that combined movements, repetitive movements, or sustained positions cause pain, these specific movements should be included in the active movement assessment.

PASSIVE MOVEMENTS[1,2]

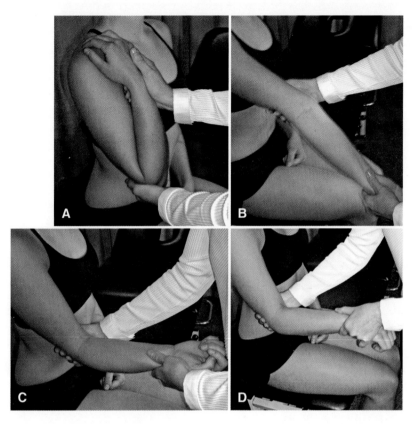

Figure 5–2

Testing passive movements of the elbow complex. **A,** Flexion. **B,** Extension. **C,** Supination **D,** Pronation.

PATIENT POSITION   The patient is either sitting or supine.

EXAMINER POSITION   The examiner is positioned directly in front of the patient.

TEST PROCEDURE   The examiner grasps the patient's distal wrist with one hand and uses the other hand to cup and stabilize the posterior aspect of the elbow. The elbow is passively guided into flexion, extension, supination, and pronation. If the motions are pain free, the examiner may choose to place additional overpressure on the joint to test the end feel in each direction. If the motion produces pain without overpressure, no overpressure should be applied.

INDICATIONS OF A POSITIVE TEST   ROM deficits and symptom reproduction both indicate a positive test result. The motion of the injured elbow should be compared with that of the contralateral side.

CLINICAL NOTES   • Passive movements should be carried out carefully to test the end feel and to test for a capsular pattern. Tissue approximation is the normal end feel of elbow flexion; in thin patients, the end feel may be bone to bone as a result of the coronoid process of the ulna hitting in the coronoid fossa of the humerus. Pronation also may be bone to bone in thin individuals. The examiner should note whether a capsular pattern is present.
• The capsular pattern for the elbow complex as a whole is more limitation of flexion than extension.

RESISTED ISOMETRIC MOVEMENTS[3,4]

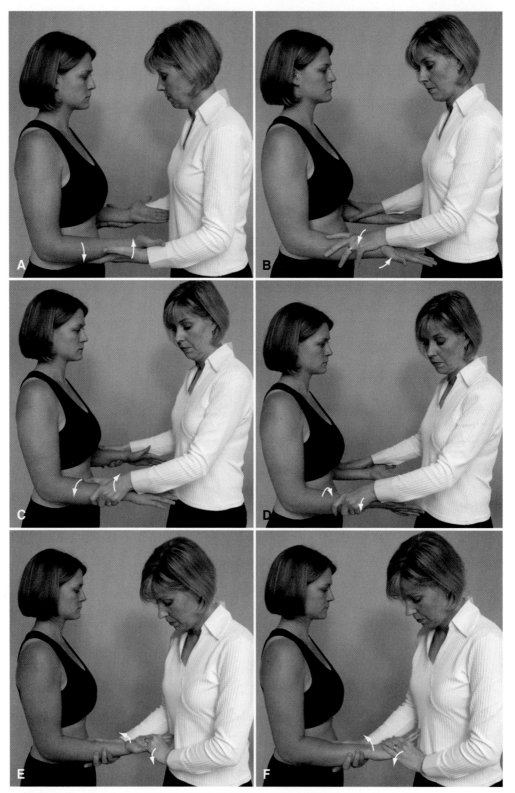

Figure 5–3
Positioning for resisted isometric movements. **A,** Elbow extension. **B,** Elbow flexion.
C, Forearm supination. **D,** Forearm pronation. **E,** Wrist flexion. **F,** Wrist extension.

RESISTED ISOMETRIC MOVEMENTS[3,4]—cont'd

PURPOSE

To assess the strength of the elbow musculature.

PATIENT POSITION

The patient is sitting.

EXAMINER POSITION

The examiner is positioned directly in front of the patient.

TEST PROCEDURE

The muscles of the elbow are tested isometrically, with the examiner positioning the patient and saying, "Don't let me move you." From this position, the examiner tests elbow flexion, extension, supination, and pronation. Wrist extension and flexion also must be tested, because a large number of muscles act over the wrist as well as the elbow. The examiner should slowly and steadily build up resistance when testing isometric muscle strength.

> **Elbow flexion.** The examiner places the palm of his or her hand on the superior aspect of the patient's forearm to provide resistance.
> **Elbow extension.** The examiner places the palm of his or her hand on the inferior aspect of the patient's forearm to provide resistance.
> **Pronation.** The examiner grasps the patient's forearm to provide resistance.
> **Supination.** The examiner grasps the patient's forearm to provide resistance.
> **Wrist flexion.** The examiner holds the patient's palm with one hand to provide resistance while stabilizing the forearm with the other.
> **Wrist extension.** The examiner holds the dorsum of the patient's hand with one hand to provide resistance while stabilizing the forearm with the other.

INDICATIONS OF A POSITIVE TEST

A positive test result is indicated by weakness or symptom reproduction (or both) compared with the contralateral, uninvolved side. If the resisted isometric contraction is weak and pain free, the examiner must consider a major injury to the contractile tissue (third-degree strain) or neurological injury.

CLINICAL NOTES

• If the patient has complained that combined movements under load, repetitive movements under load, or sustained positions under load cause pain, the examiner should carefully examine these resisted isometric movements and positions as well, but only after the basic movements have been tested isometrically.
• Muscle flexion power around the elbow is greatest in the range of 90° to 110° with the forearm supinated. At 45° and 135°, flexion power is only 75% of maximum.
• Research shows that men isometrically are two times stronger than women when testing elbow strength. In both men and women, extension is 60% of flexion and pronation is about 85% of supination.
• If the history indicates that concentric, eccentric, or econcentric movements have caused symptoms, these movements should also be tested with load or no load as required.

SPECIAL TESTS FOR LIGAMENTOUS INSTABILITY

Relevant Special Tests

Ligamentous valgus instability test
Ligamentous varus instability test
Milking maneuver
Moving valgus stress test
Lateral pivot-shift test
Posterolateral rotary drawer test
Posterolateral rotary apprehension test

Definition

The term *instability* can be used to describe a wide spectrum of clinical disorders ranging from traumatic elbow dislocation to ligament laxity secondary to repetitive strain. In any case, laxity and pain often are associated with the tissue damage.

Suspected Injury

Elbow dislocation
Elbow subluxation
Posterolateral instability
Medial collateral ligament sprain or tear
Lateral collateral ligament sprain or tear

Epidemiology and Demographics[5-12]

The elbow is the second most commonly dislocated joint in adults and the most commonly dislocated joint in children. Six in 100,000 people dislocate an elbow over a lifetime. Dislocations account for 10% to 25% of all injuries of the elbow.

The mean age for dislocation of the elbow is 30 years. About 40% of elbow dislocations occur during a sports activity, most often gymnastics, wrestling, basketball, or football. Dislocations occur 2 to 2.5 times more often in males than in females.

Medial collateral ligament injury is common with activities that require repetitive overuse. Young athletes who play overhead sports (e.g., baseball pitchers) often experience pain and injury to this ligament. The cause frequently is a combination of overuse and poor mechanics.

Relevant History

Patients may or may not have a prior history of damage to the elbow. Lateral instability occurs after elbow dislocation in 75% of cases.[13] Athletes who participate in overhead sports may have a history of lower extremity or back pain that does not allow normal throwing mechanics. This can lead to excessive stress in the elbow, especially on the medial collateral ligament.

Relevant Signs and Symptoms
Dislocation/Subluxation

With dislocation, the elbow is very painful and increased swelling is noted at the joint. The elbow is held in 90° of flexion, and the patient appears to closely guard the upper extremity. The forearm appears shorter than the upper extremity or contralateral side. All movements of the elbow are painful and limited. Even with reduction, ROM is limited, the joints are swollen, and muscle spasm and (at end range) pain are present.

Repetitive Stress Injuries

Patients with ligament laxity or overuse injuries complain of a vague pain and soreness with activity of the elbow. Intermittent episodes of snapping, popping, or clicking in the joint may be noted with activity. Episodes of apprehension or a feeling of slipping of the lateral structures, especially with loaded activities (i.e., weight on the arm), may be present with excessive joint laxity. The patient also may complain of episodes of the elbow giving way or the joint locking. The individual commonly has difficulty lifting with the forearm supinated, pushing, pulling, and pushing up out of a chair.

Mechanism of Injury
Dislocation/Subluxation

The definition of elbow dislocation implies a complete discontinuity of the ulnohumeral articulation with associated radiocapitellar disruption. This can occur with or without proximal radioulnar disruption, associated neurovascular injury, and/or residual elbow instability. Ligament damage can occur with or without a concomitant elbow dislocation, as in the case of elbow subluxation. A posterior elbow dislocation is caused by a fall on an outstretched arm with the elbow forced into hyperextension. Mechanically, the hand is supinated as the body rotates in a pronated direction in relation to the elbow; this produces a valgus force on the elbow. As the body continues in a forward motion, the elbow hyperextends and a posterior dislocation of the ulna in relation to the humerus occurs.

Repetitive Stress Injuries

The stability of the elbow relies on the stability and integrity of the ligaments. Ligaments are designed to resist primarily tensile loading. Activities that repetitively overstress the affected ligaments can lead to injury and eventual laxity. Damage to the medial collateral ligament occurs when a valgus force is applied to the elbow joint; damage to the lateral collateral ligament occurs when a varus force is applied. Such damage can be due to either trauma or repetitive overuse.

LIGAMENTOUS VALGUS INSTABILITY TEST[14,15]

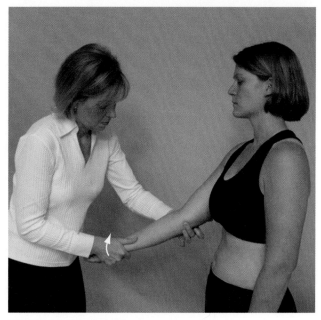

Figure 5–4
Testing the medial collateral ligament of the elbow.

PURPOSE	To assess the integrity of the medial (ulnar) collateral ligament of the elbow.
PATIENT POSITION	The patient may be tested while sitting, standing, or lying supine.
EXAMINER POSITION	The examiner stands immediately in front of the test elbow.
TEST PROCEDURE	To stabilize the patient's arm, the examiner uses one hand to stabilize the elbow and places the other hand above the wrist. While palpating the ligament with the fingers of the left hand as illustrated, the examiner applies an abduction or a valgus force at the distal forearm with the right hand to test the medial collateral ligament (valgus instability). The force is applied several times with increasing pressure, and the examiner notes any alteration in pain, stability, or ROM.
INDICATIONS OF A POSITIVE TEST	The examiner should note any laxity, decreased mobility, soft end feel, or altered pain compared with the uninvolved elbow.
CLINICAL NOTES	• Regan and Morrey[15] recommend doing the valgus stress test with the humerus in full lateral rotation. • Because the medial collateral ligament is multipennated and is designed to resist stress in multiple directions, the examiner should test the elbow in varying degrees of extension and flexion to test the various fibers of the ligament.
RELIABILITY/SPECIFICITY/ SENSITIVITY	Unknown

LIGAMENTOUS VARUS INSTABILITY TEST[16]

DVD

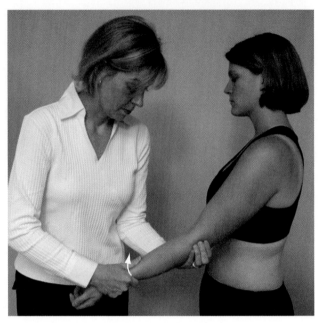

Figure 5–5
Testing the lateral collateral ligament of the elbow.

PURPOSE	To assess the integrity of the lateral (radial) collateral ligament of the elbow.
PATIENT POSITION	The patient may be tested while sitting, standing, or lying supine.
EXAMINER POSITION	The examiner stands immediately in front of the test elbow.
TEST PROCEDURE	To stabilize the patient's arm, the examiner uses the left hand as illustrated to stabilize the elbow and places the other hand above the wrist. With the patient's elbow slightly flexed (20° to 30°) and stabilized, and while palpating the ligament with the fingers of the left hand, the examiner applies an adduction or a varus force to the distal forearm to test the lateral collateral ligament (varus instability). The force is applied several times with increasing pressure, and the examiner notes any alteration in pain, stability, or ROM.
INDICATIONS OF A POSITIVE TEST	Normally, the examiner feels the ligament tense when stress is applied. Excessive laxity or a soft end feel indicates injury to the ligament (first-, second-, or third-degree sprain) and, especially with a third-degree sprain, may indicate posterolateral joint instability.
CLINICAL NOTES	• Regan and Morrey[15] recommend doing the varus stress test with the humerus in full medial rotation. • Posterolateral elbow instability is the most common pattern of elbow instability in which there is displacement of the ulna (accompanied by the radius) on the humerus so that the ulna supinates or laterally rotates away from or off the trochlea.
RELIABILITY/SPECIFICITY/ SENSITIVITY	Unknown

MILKING MANEUVER[14,17]

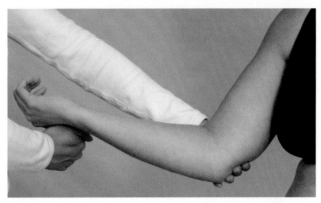

Figure 5–6
Milking maneuver to test the medial collateral ligament.

PURPOSE	To assess the integrity of the medial (ulnar) collateral ligament of the elbow.
PATIENT POSITION	The patient sits with the elbow flexed to 90° or more and the forearm supinated.
EXAMINER POSITION	The examiner stands immediately in front of the test elbow.
TEST PROCEDURE	The examiner uses the right hand as illustrated to grasp the patient's thumb by reaching underneath the patient's forearm; the other hand grasps and supports the distal humerus at the elbow with the other hand. The examiner then pulls on the patient's thumb, imparting a valgus stress to the elbow.
INDICATIONS OF A POSITIVE TEST	Reproduction of symptoms indicates a positive test result and a partial tear of the medial collateral ligament.
CLINICAL NOTE	• Pain indicates a positive test result. Laxity is seen if the ligament is torn (third-degree strain).
RELIABILITY/SPECIFICITY/ SENSITIVITY	Unknown

MOVING VALGUS STRESS TEST[14,17]

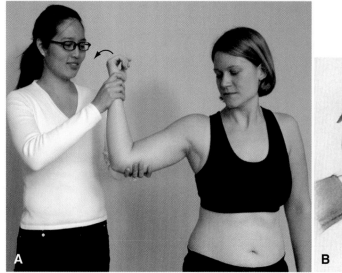
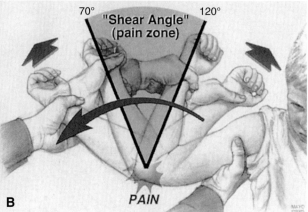

Figure 5–7
A, The moving valgus stress test. **B,** Schematic representation of the moving valgus stress test. The shear range refers to the range of motion that causes pain while the elbow is extended with valgus stress. The shear angle is the point that causes maximum pain.

PURPOSE	To assess the integrity of the medial (ulnar) collateral ligament of the elbow.
PATIENT POSITION	The patient lies supine or stands with the arm abducted and the elbow fully flexed.
EXAMINER POSITION	The examiner stands immediately adjacent to the test elbow.
TEST PROCEDURE	The examiner stabilizes the patient's arm by placing one hand at the elbow and the other hand around the wrist. While the fingers of the hand on the elbow palpate the medial collateral ligament, an abduction or a valgus force is applied at the distal forearm to test the medial collateral ligament (valgus instability). While maintaining the valgus stress, the examiner quickly extends the patient's elbow.
INDICATIONS OF A POSITIVE TEST	Reproduction of pain between 120° to 70° indicates a positive test result and a partial tear of the medial collateral ligament.
CLINICAL NOTE	• Pain indicates a positive test result, although laxity sometimes is felt.
RELIABILITY/SPECIFICITY/ SENSITIVITY	Unknown

LATERAL PIVOT-SHIFT TEST[14,16]

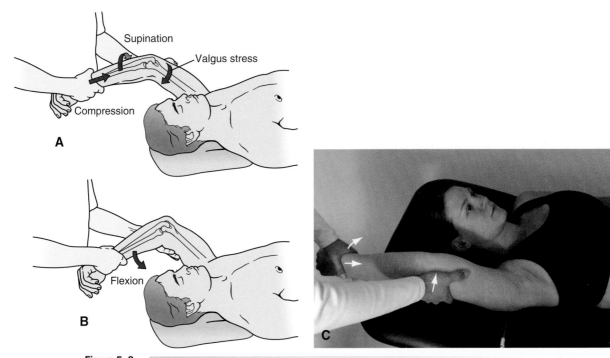

Figure 5–8

Posterolateral pivot-shift apprehension test of the elbow. **A,** The patient lies supine with the arm overhead. A mild supination force is applied to the forearm at the wrist. The elbow then is flexed while valgus stress and compression are applied to the elbow. **B,** If the examiner continues flexing the elbow at about 40° to 70°, subluxation and a clunk on reduction when the elbow is extended may occur, but usually only in an unconscious patient. **C,** Actual test with the elbow positioned to resemble the knee.

PURPOSE	To assess the integrity and stability of the posterolateral structures of the elbow.
PATIENT POSITION	The patient lies supine with the test arm overhead.
EXAMINER POSITION	The examiner stands immediately adjacent and cephalad to the test elbow.
TEST PROCEDURE	The examiner grasps the patient's wrist and forearm with one hand, with the patient's elbow extended and the forearm fully supinated. The examiner's other hand is placed on the lateral aspect of the distal humerus. The examiner flexes the patient's elbow and applies a valgus stress and axial compression to the elbow while maintaining supination. This causes the radius (and ulna) to sublux off the humerus, leading to a prominent radial head posterolaterally and a dimple between the radial head and capitellum if the posterolateral structures have been injured.
INDICATIONS OF A POSITIVE TEST	If the examiner continues flexing the elbow at about 40° to 70°, a sudden reduction (clunk) of the joint occurs, which can be palpated and seen.

Continued

LATERAL PIVOT-SHIFT TEST[14,16]—cont'd

CLINICAL NOTES

- If the patient is unconscious, subluxation and a clunk on reduction when the elbow is extended also may occur; however, these symptoms seldom are seen in a conscious patient.
- Care must be taken to ensure that the hand delivering the valgus force is on the humerus and not on the radius, which would block the radius' ability to sublux laterally.

RELIABILITY/SPECIFICITY/ SENSITIVITY

Unknown

POSTEROLATERAL ROTARY DRAWER TEST[14]   DVD

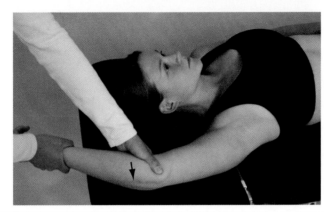

Figure 5–9
Posterolateral rotary drawer test.

PURPOSE	To assess the integrity and stability of the posterolateral structures of the elbow.
PATIENT POSITION	The patient lies supine with the test arm overhead and the elbow flexed 40° to 90°.
EXAMINER POSITION	The examiner stands immediately adjacent and cephalad to the test elbow.
TEST PROCEDURE	With one hand, the examiner grasps the patient's forearm with the patient's elbow extended and the forearm fully supinated. The examiner's left hand as illustrated is placed on the medial aspect of the distal humerus. The examiner holds the forearm and arm similar to the position for a drawer test of the knee. While stabilizing the humerus, the examiner pushes the radius and ulna posterolaterally.
INDICATIONS OF A POSITIVE TEST	A positive test result is produced if the radius and ulna rotate around an intact medial collateral ligament, indicating a tear of the lateral collateral ligament and posterolateral instability at the elbow.
CLINICAL NOTE	• The elbow is designed to resist stress in multiple directions. Therefore, the examiner should test the elbow in varying degrees of flexion to test the different structures.
RELIABILITY/SPECIFICITY/ SENSITIVITY	Unknown

POSTEROLATERAL ROTARY APPREHENSION TEST[7,10,14,16,18,19]

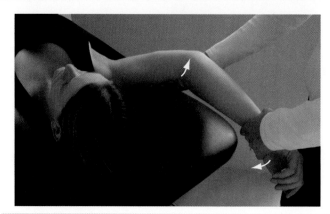

Figure 5–10

Posterolateral rotary apprehension test.

PURPOSE	To assess the integrity of the posterolateral structures of the elbow.
PATIENT POSITION	The patient lies supine with the test arm overhead.
EXAMINER POSITION	The examiner stands immediately adjacent and cephalad to the test elbow.
TEST PROCEDURE	With one hand, the examiner grasps the patient's wrist and forearm with the patient's elbow extended and the forearm fully supinated. The examiner's other hand is placed on the lateral aspect of the distal humerus. Maintaining the supination at the wrist, the examiner applies a valgus stress to the elbow while flexing the elbow.
INDICATIONS OF A POSITIVE TEST	If the joint is unstable, 20° to 30° of flexion, along with the valgus stress, will cause the patient to become apprehensive, and the patient's symptoms may be reproduced.
CLINICAL NOTES	• Actual subluxation is rare in a conscious patient. A positive test result indicates posterolateral rotary instability. • Care must be taken to ensure that the hand delivering the valgus force is on the humerus and not on the radius, which would block the radius' ability to sublux laterally.
RELIABILITY/SPECIFICITY/ SENSITIVITY	Unknown

SPECIAL TEST FOR EPICONDYLITIS

Relevant Special Test

Lateral epicondylitis test (tennis elbow or Cozen's test)

Definition

Epicondylitis is an injury to the extensor tendons (tennis elbow, or lateral epicondylitis) or the flexor tendons (golfer's elbow, or medial epicondylitis). Epicondylosis is a chronic overuse injury to the same elbow structures affected by epicondylitis. Both of these conditions result from repeated microtrauma to the tendon, leading to disruption and degeneration of the tendon's internal structure (tendinosus). Epicondylosis appears to be a degenerative condition in which the tendon fails to heal properly after repetitive microtrauma.

Suspected Injury

Lateral epicondylitis
Lateral epicondylosis
Medial epicondylitis
Medial epicondylosis

Epidemiology and Demographics[20-25]

About 1% to 2% of the overall population is affected by either epicondylitis or epicondylosis. About 5% to 10% of patients diagnosed with lateral epicondylitis are tennis players. The incidence of lateral epicondylitis is five to nine times greater than that of medial epicondylitis, and lateral epicondylitis occurs in the dominant arm in 75% of cases. Lateral epicondylitis/epicondylosis occurs most frequently between the age of 35 and 50, with the median age being 41 years old. The incidence is 2 to 3.5 times higher in those over age 40. Males and females are equally affected.

About 64% of cases of medial epicondylitis occur because of work-related activities that require heavy load and repetitive hand functions.

Relevant History

The patient often complains of an insidious, gradually worsening pain that sometimes radiates down the forearm. The subjective history includes reports of engaging in activities that require repetitive wrist extension or flexion or activities that require wrist stabilization. The patient may report progressive loss of grip strength. Improper form or technique (or both) may cause microtrauma, especially in novice athletes.

Relevant Signs and Symptoms

Medial Epicondylitis/Epicondylosis

- Grasp/grip strength is weak, and pain occurs with repetitive wrist flexion and pronation.
- Elbow flexion contracture is uncommon but can occur in a throwing athlete.
- Pain may be described as a dull ache immediately after activity and at rest or as a sharp or achy pain that radiates down the medial forearm.

Lateral Epicondylitis/Epicondylosis

- Local tenderness is present directly over the lateral epicondyle, and occasional forearm referral symptoms occur.
- Pain is aggravated by strong gripping.
- Grip strength is diminished because extensor muscles stabilize the wrist during grip.
- Pain occurs with passive stretching of the palmar forearm muscles.
- Radiography reveals tendon calcification in 20% of patients.

Mechanism of Injury

The mechanism of injury for epicondylitis/epicondylosis generally is insidious and involves repetitive microtrauma caused by eccentric and concentric overloading of the extensor carpi radialis brevis and other wrist extensors (lateral epicondylitis/epicondylosis) or wrist flexors (medial epicondylitis/epicondylosis). Acute trauma to the lateral or medial epicondyle can cause epicondylitis.

Generally, overload of the muscle-tendon unit results in the initial inflammatory process, and continued use results in the tendon breakdown seen in epicondylosis.

The term *epicondylitis* suggests an inflammatory process. However, acute inflammation occurs only in the early stages of the disease. Scientists and physicians have accepted the fact that the term *tendonitis* refers to the clinical syndrome and not the actual histopathology of the disorder. The actual histopathology of the disorder is called tendinopathy. With tendinopathy, collagen becomes disorganized, with a loss of parallel orientation, asymmetrical crimping and loosening, and microtears. Because of the hypovascularity of the tendons, the collagen fibers tend to break down during attempts to repair them after excessive load and trauma.

Specificity/Sensitivity Comparison

Unknown

LATERAL EPICONDYLITIS TEST (TENNIS ELBOW OR COZEN'S TEST)[26]

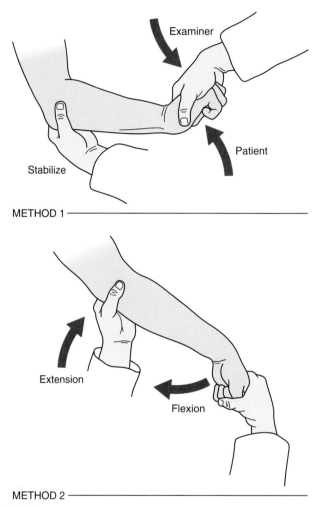

Figure 5–11
Test for tennis elbow.

PURPOSE	To assess for lateral epicondylopathy of the elbow.
PATIENT POSITION	The patient may be standing, sitting, or lying supine.
EXAMINER POSITION	The examiner stands immediately in front of the test elbow.
TEST PROCEDURE	**Method 1:** One of the examiner's hands supports the patient's elbow. The thumb of this hand rests on the lateral epicondyle. The examiner's other hand grasps the dorsal aspect of the patient's hand. The patient is asked to actively make a fist, pronate the forearm, and radially deviate and extend the wrist while the examiner resists the motion.
	Method 2: The test may also be done passively by the examiner. While palpating the lateral epicondyle, the examiner passively pronates the forearm and flexes the wrist fully; then, while holding these two positions, the examiner extends the elbow. The symptoms would be the same as for the active test.

LATERAL EPICONDYLITIS TEST (TENNIS ELBOW OR COZEN'S TEST)[26]—cont'd

INDICATIONS OF A POSITIVE TEST A positive test result is indicated by a sudden, severe pain in the area of the lateral epicondyle of the humerus. The epicondyle may be palpated to determine the origin of the pain.

CLINICAL NOTES
- Although classically designed to test for lateral epicondylitis, this technique can be used to test for any pathological condition of the lateral epicondyle.
- The examiner should be aware that the passive test stretches the radial nerve, which may lead to symptoms that may be similar to those seen with tennis elbow.

RELIABILITY/SPECIFICITY/ SENSITIVITY Unknown

SPECIAL TESTS FOR NEUROLOGICAL SYMPTOMS

Relevant Special Tests

Elbow flexion test
Pinch grip test

Definition

Nerves are sensitized structures designed to propagate electrical impulses along their axons. The axon of the nerve also transmits nutrients and chemicals down its lumen. Any pathological condition that prevents the nerve from completing these activities results in varying degrees of neurological symptoms. Tests for neurological symptoms in the elbow fall into two categories: tests designed to identify patients with changes in nerve function, and tests designed to identify patients with limits in the mobility of the upper extremity nerves. This section focuses on tests that identify patients with changes in nerve function. Upper extremity nerve mobility tests were described as upper limb tension tests in the cervical spine.

Suspected Injury

Cubital tunnel syndrome (ulnar nerve entrapment in the cubital tunnel at the elbow)
Pronator teres syndrome (anterior interosseous nerve entrapment at the pronator teres muscle)

Epidemiology and Demographics[27-34]

Cubital Tunnel Syndrome

Cubital tunnel syndrome is the second most common nerve compression injury in the upper extremity (the most common one is carpal tunnel syndrome). Historically, cubital tunnel syndrome has been more common in men and manifests between the ages of 13 and 20 years. The incidence is higher in men largely because more men than women participate in repetitive and high velocity throwing activities, which have a high reported incidence compared with other sports-related activities. However, the incidence of ulnar neuritis in the workplace is on the rise, especially in occupations requiring repetitive and prolonged compressive forces on the elbow. Examples of this are truck drivers who place their arm on the truck window still while driving or computer programmers who rest upon their elbows while using the computer. This type of neuritis is not age determined, but rather activity and time correlated.

Pronator Teres Syndrome

Pronator teres syndrome tends to be linked to a specific activity, trauma, disease, or anatomical makeup rather than a particular age group. Nerve entrapment occurs more frequently among office workers, manual workers, and individuals who engage in repetitive movement pattern activities, such as musicians, artists, and sports participants. Pronator teres syndrome usually manifests in the fifth decade of life and is four times more common in females than in males.

Relevant History

Patients with cubital tunnel syndrome and pronator teres syndrome commonly have a past history of trauma or a space-occupying lesion that compresses the nerve. However, the trauma also can be the result of prolonged positions or repetitive overuse from occupational and recreational hazards. A history of recent fracture, dislocation, or a traumatic incident with injury to the nerve is common. Other factors include systemic disease (e.g., rheumatoid arthritis) and space-occupying lesions such as gout, ganglions, lipomas, osteophytes, hematomas, and anomalous muscles.

Relevant Signs and Symptoms
Cubital Tunnel Syndrome

Initially the patient complains of pain, point tenderness, and swelling of the medial aspect of the elbow, primarily in the cubital tunnel. This progresses to numbness, tingling, and a cold feeling in the medial distal third of the forearm and the little and ring fingers. The numbness increases over time, and the individual often complains of waking up at night with numbness and tingling in the same area (especially those who habitually sleep with the elbows fully flexed) or increased symptoms during work or an aggravating activity. As the symptoms worsen, the muscles supplied by the ulnar nerve begin to atrophy, but more significantly, the patient complains of having difficulty gripping, clumsiness, and frequently dropping objects because of hand weakness.

Pronator Teres Syndrome

Pronator teres syndrome commonly presents with weakness of and difficulty moving the index and middle fingers (flexor digitorum profundus) combined with weakness in the thumb (flexor pollicis longus), which make the pinch grip difficult. The numbness worsens, and the patient often complains of waking up at night with numbness and tingling into the lateral three fingers. As the symptoms worsen, the muscles supplied by the median nerve in the forearm and hand atrophy, but more significantly, the patient complains of having difficulty gripping, clumsiness, and frequently dropping objects because of hand weakness. Patients may also complain of numbness in the palm consistent with the distribution of the palmar cutaneous branch of the median nerve.

Mechanism of Injury

Cubital Tunnel Syndrome

Several different mechanisms of injury have been identified for cubital tunnel syndrome. It can be caused by trauma (e.g., hitting the "funny bone"), prolonged compressive or stretching forces, secondary trauma, or joint disfigurement or dysfunction. Joint disfigurement occurs secondary to osteophyte formation or changes in bony composition from previous fractures or trauma. Prolonged compression or stretching forces are seen in patients with a history of sleeping in a position of prolonged elbow flexion, occupational positions requiring prolonged elbow flexion, or students or workers who spend a prolonged time working at a computer or desk while leaning on the elbows or the proximal forearms.

Pronator Teres Syndrome

Pronator teres syndrome may occur when the nerve is compressed at the tendinous origin of the deep head of pronator teres (the most common presentation) or as it passes between the two heads of pronator teres. The term "pronator syndrome" refers to median nerve compression between the two pronator teres heads before it branches to form the anterior interosseous nerve. Entrapment also can occur under the bicipital aponeurosis at the elbow or under the flexor digitorum superficialis tendon. The pain is aggravated by activities that require repetitive pronation and supination. Examples of such activities are assembly workers who are required to repetitively pronate and supinate their hands, construction workers who use screwdrivers or wrenches, or grocery clerks as they scan products for purchase. The syndrome also has been associated with repetitive exertional grasping activities, such as are performed by carpenters or tennis players.

ELBOW FLEXION TEST[35,36]

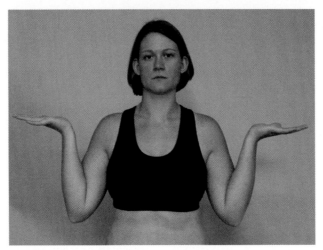

Figure 5–12
Elbow flexion test for a pathological condition of the ulnar nerve.

PURPOSE	To assess for ulnar nerve entrapment in the cubital tunnel.
PATIENT POSITION	The patient is sitting or standing.
EXAMINER POSITION	The examiner stands in front of the patient to observe and communicate with the patient. No patient contact is required for this test.
TEST PROCEDURE	The patient is asked to fully flex the elbows with extension of the wrists and abduction and depression of the shoulder girdle. The patient is asked to hold this position for 3 to 5 minutes.
INDICATIONS OF A POSITIVE TEST	Tingling or paresthesia in the ulnar nerve distribution of the forearm and hand indicate a positive test result.
RELIABILITY/SPECIFICITY/ SENSITIVITY	Unknown

PINCH GRIP TEST[37]

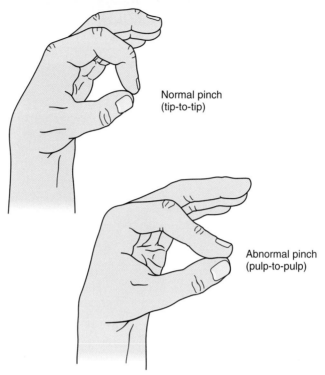

Normal pinch
(tip-to-tip)

Abnormal pinch
(pulp-to-pulp)

Figure 5–13

Normal tip-to-tip pinch compared with the abnormal pulp-to-pulp pinch seen in anterior interosseous nerve syndrome.

PURPOSE	To assess for entrapment of the anterior interosseous nerve (a branch of the median nerve) at the pronator teres muscle.
PATIENT POSITION	Generally, the patient is tested while seated.
EXAMINER POSITION	The examiner stands in front of the patient to observe and to communicate with the patient. No patient contact is required for this test.
TEST PROCEDURE	The patient is asked to pinch the tips of the index finger and thumb together (tip-to-tip pinch).
INDICATIONS OF A POSITIVE TEST	Normally, the patient should be able to achieve and maintain a tip-to-tip pinch. A positive test result for a pathological condition of the anterior interosseous nerve is indicated if the patient is unable to pinch tip to tip and instead goes into a pulp-to-pulp pinch of the index finger and thumb.
CLINICAL NOTE	• A pulp-to-pulp pinch also may indicate entrapment of the anterior interosseous nerve as it passes between the two heads of the pronator teres muscle.
RELIABILITY/SPECIFICITY/ SENSITIVITY	Unknown

JOINT PLAY MOVEMENTS

RADIAL DEVIATION OF THE ULNA AND RADIUS ON THE HUMERUS

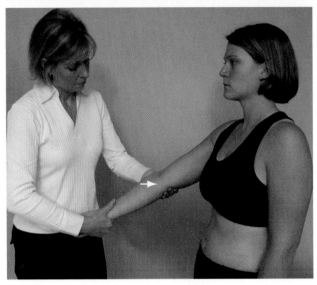

Figure 5–14
Radial deviation of the ulna on the humerus.

PATIENT POSITION	The patient may be standing, sitting, or lying supine, depending on which position is most comfortable and most likely to allow the patient to relax the arm for the test.
EXAMINER POSITION	The examiner stands adjacent to the patient's elbow.
TEST PROCEDURE	The examiner stabilizes the patient's elbow by holding the posterior lateral aspect of the humerus firmly with one hand while grasping above the wrist with the other hand. The examiner then applies a medially directed force to the elbow and a lateral counterforce at the wrist while maintaining the elbow extended.
INDICATIONS OF A POSITIVE TEST	The examiner compares the amount of available joint play and end feel on the affected side with the movement on the unaffected side and notes whether the movements affect the patient's symptoms. As the joint play movements are performed, the examiner should note any decreased ROM, pain, or difference in end feel.
CLINICAL NOTES	• Radial deviation of the ulna and radius on the humerus is performed in a fashion similar to that used for the radial collateral ligament test but with less elbow flexion. • When examining the joint play movements, the examiner must compare the injured side with the unaffected side. • When the patient's elbow is almost straight (extended) during the movement, the end feel should be bone to bone.

ULNAR DEVIATION OF THE ULNA AND RADIUS ON THE HUMERUS   DVD

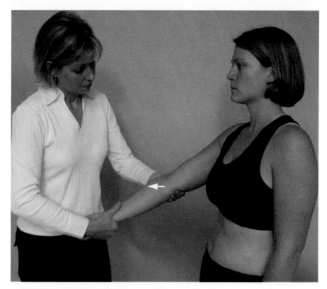

Figure 5–15
Ulnar deviation of the ulna on the humerus.

PATIENT POSITION	The patient may be standing, sitting, or lying supine, depending on which position is most comfortable and most likely to allow the patient to relax the arm for the test.
EXAMINER POSITION	The examiner stands adjacent to the patient's elbow.
TEST PROCEDURE	The examiner stabilizes the patient's elbow by holding the posterior medial aspect of the humerus firmly and using the other hand to grasp above the wrist. The examiner then applies a laterally directed force onto the elbow and a medial counterforce at the wrist to the extended elbow.
INDICATIONS OF A POSITIVE TEST	The examiner compares the amount of available joint play and end feel on the affected side with the movement on the unaffected side and notes whether the movements affect the patient's symptoms. As the joint play movements are performed, the examiner should note any decreased ROM, pain, or difference in end feel.
CLINICAL NOTES	• Ulnar deviation of the ulna and radius on the humerus is performed in a fashion similar to that used for the ulnar collateral ligament test but with less elbow flexion. • When examining the joint play movements, the examiner must compare the injured side with the unaffected side. • When the patient's elbow is almost straight (extended) during the movement, the end feel should be bone to bone.

ELBOW DISTRACTION

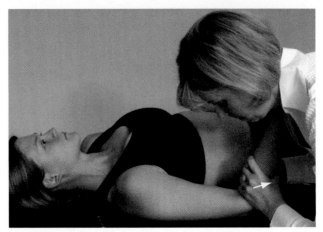

Figure 5–16
Distraction of the olecranon process from the humerus.

PATIENT POSITION	The patient is supine.
EXAMINER POSITION	The examiner kneels or stands adjacent to the patient's elbow.
TEST PROCEDURE	The examiner flexes the patient's elbow to 90° and wraps both hands around the forearm, close to the elbow. The patient's hand rests comfortably on the examiner's shoulder. The examiner then applies a distractive force at the elbow, ensuring that no rotation torque is applied to the elbow.
INDICATIONS OF A POSITIVE TEST	The examiner compares the amount of available joint play and end feel on the affected side with the movement on the unaffected side and notes whether the movements affect the patient's symptoms. As the joint play movements are performed, the examiner should note any decreased ROM, pain, or difference in end feel.
CLINICAL NOTES	• If the patient has a sore shoulder, counterforce should be applied with one hand around the humerus. • Because of the shape of the olecranon, the distraction force often is a scooping motion in a direction distal (toward the patient's feet) and anterior (away from the table).

ANTERIOR-POSTERIOR GLIDE OF THE RADIUS ON THE HUMERUS

DVD

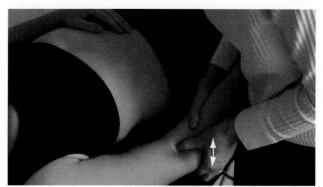

Figure 5–17
Anterior-posterior glide of the radius.

PATIENT POSITION	The patient is supine.
EXAMINER POSITION	The examiner stands adjacent to and facing the patient's elbow.
TEST PROCEDURE	The examiner stabilizes the patient's forearm. The patient's arm is held between the examiner's body and upper arm. The examiner places the thumb of his or her hand over the anterior radial head and then pushes the radial head posteriorly with the thumb.
INDICATIONS OF A POSITIVE TEST	The examiner compares the amount of available joint play and end feel on the affected side with the movement on the unaffected side and notes whether the movements affect the patient's symptoms. As the joint play movements are performed, the examiner should note any decreased ROM, pain, or difference in end feel.
CLINICAL NOTES/CAUTIONS	• Commonly, posterior gliding movement is easier to obtain than anterior glide (see the next test). • This movement must be performed with care, because it can be very painful as a result of pinching of the skin between the examiner's digits and the bone. • Pain may result from application of the force even in the normal arm; therefore, the two sides must be compared for differences in symptoms.

POSTERIOR-ANTERIOR GLIDE OF THE RADIUS ON THE HUMERUS

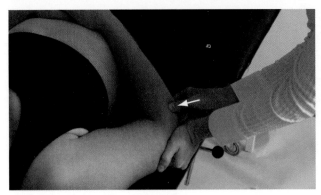

Figure 5–18
Posterior-anterior glide of the radius.

PATIENT POSITION	The patient is lying supine with the arm at the side and the hand resting on the stomach.
EXAMINER POSITION	The examiner stands adjacent to the patient's elbow.
TEST PROCEDURE	The examiner places the thumbs over the posterior aspect of the radial head and then carefully pushes the radial head anteriorly with the thumbs.
INDICATIONS OF A POSITIVE TEST	The examiner compares the amount of available movement and end feel on the affected side with the movement on the unaffected side and notes whether the movements affect the patient's symptoms. As the joint play movements are performed, the examiner should note any decreased ROM, pain, or difference in end feel.
CLINICAL NOTES/CAUTIONS	• This movement must be performed with care, because it can be very painful as a result of pinching of the skin between the examiner's thumbs and the bone. • Pain may result from application of the force even in the normal arm; therefore, the two sides must be compared for differences in symptoms.

References

1. Tarr RR, Garfinkel AI, Sarmiento A: The effects of angular and rotational deformities of both bones of the forearm, *J Bone Joint Surg Am* 66:65-70, 1984.
2. Clarkson HM: *Musculoskeletal assessment: joint range of motion and manual muscle strength*, Philadelphia, 2000, Lippincott Williams & Wilkins.
3. Kapandji AI: *The physiology of the joints*, vol 1, *Upper limb*, New York, 1970, Churchill Livingstone.
4. Askew LJ, An KN, Morrey BF et al: Isometric elbow strength in normal individuals, *Clin Orthop* 222:261-266, 1987.
5. Cheung EV: Chronic lateral elbow instability, *Orthop Clin North Am* 39:221-228, 2008.
6. Kuhn MA, Ross G: Acute elbow dislocations, *Orthop Clin North Am* 39:155-161, 2008.
7. Mehta JA, Bain GI: Elbow dislocations in adults and children, *Clin Sports Med* 23:609-627, 2004.
8. Mehlhoff TL, Noble PC, Bennett JB et al: Simple dislocation of the elbow in the adult, *J Bone Joint Surg Am* 70A:244, 1988.
9. O'Driscoll SW, Morrey BF, Korninek S et al: Elbow subluxation and dislocation: a spectrum of instability, *Clin Orthop* 280:186-280, 1992.
10. O'Driscoll SW, Bell DF, Morrey BF: Posterolateral rotary instability of the elbow, *J Bone Joint Surg Am* 73:440-446, 1991.
11. Protzman RR: Dislocation of the elbow joint, *J Bone Joint Surg* 60:539, 1978.
12. Smith III JP, Savoie FH, Field LD: Posterolateral rotatory instability of the elbow, *Clin Sports Med* 20:47-57, 2001.
13. Moore L: Elbow subluxations. In Sueki D, Brechter J (eds): *Orthopedic rehabilitation clinical advisor*, St Louis, 2010, Mosby.
14. O'Driscoll SW: Acute, recurrent and chronic elbow instabilities. In Norris TR (ed): *Orthopedic knowledge update 2: shoulder and elbow*, Rosemont, Ill, 2002, American Academy of Orthopedic Surgeons.
15. Regan WD, Morrey BF: The physical examination of the elbow. In Morrey BF (ed): *The elbow and its disorders*, Philadelphia, 1993, Saunders.
16. O'Driscoll SW: Classification and evaluation of recurrent instability of the elbow, *Clin Orthop Relat Res* 370:34-43, 2000.
17. O'Driscoll SW, Lawton RM, Smith AM: The "moving valgus stress test" for medial collateral ligament tears of the elbow, *Am J Sports Med* 33:231-239, 2005.
18. Lee ML, Rosenwasser MP: Chronic elbow instability, *Orthop Clin North Am* 30:81-89, 1999.
19. Kalainov DM, Cohen MS: The posterolateral rotary instability of the elbow in association with lateral epicondylitis: a report on three cases, *J Bone Joint Surg Am* 87:1120-1125, 2005.
20. Ciccotti MC, Schwartz MA, Cicotti MG: Diagnosis and treatment of medial epicondylitis of the elbow, *Clin Sports Med* 23:693-705, 2004.
21. Maffulli N, Wong J, Almekinders LC: Types and epidemiology of tendinopathy, *Clin Sports Med* 23:675-692, 2003.
22. Nirschl PR, Ashman ES: Elbow tendinopathy: tennis elbow, *Clin Sports Med* 22:813-836, 2003.
23. Pimentel L: Orthopedic trauma: office management of major joint injury, *Med Clin North Am* 90:355-382, 2006.
24. Whaley AL, Baker CL: Lateral epicondylitis, *Clin Sports Med* 23:677-691, 2004.
25. Wilson JJ, Best TM: Common overuse tendon problems: a review and recommendations for treatment, *Am Family Physician* 72:811-818, 2005.
26. Roles NC, Maudsley RH: Radial tunnel syndrome: resistant tennis elbow as a nerve entrapment, *J Bone Joint Surg Br* 54:499-508, 1972.
27. Bencardino JT, Rosenberg ZS: Entrapment neuropathies of the shoulder and elbow in the athlete, *Clin Sports Med* 25:465-487, 2006.
28. Chin DH, Meals R: Anterior interosseous nerve syndrome, *J Hand Surg* 1:249-257, 2001.
29. Gomes I, Becker J, Ehlers JA, Nora DB: Prediction of the neurophysiological diagnosis of carpal tunnel syndrome from the demographic and clinical data, *Clin Neurophysiol* 117:964-971, 2006.
30. Izzi J, Dennison D, Noerdlinger M et al: Nerve injuries of the elbow, wrist, and hand in athletes, *Clin Sports Med* 20:203-217, 2001.
31. Koo JT, Szabo RM: Compression neuropathies of the median nerve, *J Hand Surg* 4:156-175, 2004.
32. Latinovic R, Gulliford MC, Hughes RA: Incidence of common compressive neuropathies in primary care, *J Neurol Neurosurg Psychiatry* 77:263-265, 2006.
33. Nithi K: Physiology of the peripheral nervous system, *Surgery* 21:264a-264e, 2003.
34. Pratt N: Anatomy of nerve entrapment sites in the upper quarter, *J Hand Ther* 18:216-229, 2005.
35. Buehler MJ, Thayer DT: The elbow flexion test: a clinical test for the cubital tunnel syndrome, *Clin Orthop* 233:213-216, 1988.
36. Butler DS: *Mobilisation of the nervous system*, Melbourne, 1991, Churchill Livingstone.
37. Bigg-Wither G, Kelly P: Diagnostic imaging in musculoskeletal physiotherapy. In Refshauge K, Gass E (eds): *Musculoskeletal physiotherapy: clinical science and practice*, Oxford, 1995, Butterworth-Heinemann.

FOREARM, WRIST, AND HAND

Précis of the Forearm, Wrist, and Hand Assessment*

History (sitting)
Observation (sitting)
Examination (sitting)
Active movements
   Pronation of the forearm
   Supination of the forearm
   Wrist flexion
   Wrist extension
   Radial deviation of wrist
   Ulnar deviation of wrist
   Finger flexion (at MCP, PIP, and DIP joints)
   Finger extension (at MCP, PIP, and DIP joints)
   Finger abduction
   Finger adduction
   Thumb flexion
   Thumb extension
   Thumb abduction
   Thumb adduction
   Opposition of the thumb and little finger
Passive movements (as in active movements)
   Fanning and folding of the hand
Resisted isometric movements (as in active movements, in the neutral position)
Functional testing
   Functional grip tests
   Pinch tests
   Coordination tests
Special tests (sitting)
   Ligamentous finger instability
   Thumb ulnar collateral ligamentous laxity
   Lunotriquetral ballottement (Reagan's) test
   Lunotriquetral shear test
   Watson (scaphoid shift) test
   Triangular fibrocartilage complex load test

   Finkelstein test
   Tinel's sign
   Phalen's test
   Reverse Phalen's test
   Allen test
   Digit blood flow test
Reflexes and cutaneous distribution (sitting)
   Reflexes
   Sensory scan
   Nerve injuries
   Median nerve
   Ulnar nerve
   Radial nerve
Joint play movements (sitting)
   Long axis extension of the wrist
   Anterior-posterior glide of the wrist
   Side glide of the wrist
   Shear test of the individual carpal bones
   Anterior-posterior glide of the intermetacarpal joints
   Long axis extension of the joints of the fingers
   Anterior-posterior glide of the joints of the fingers
   Rotation of the joints of the fingers
   Side glide of the joints of the fingers
Palpation (sitting)
Diagnostic imaging

---

*After any examination, the patient should be warned of the possibility of exacerbation of symptoms as a result of the assessment. *DIP,* Distal interphalangeal; *MCP,* metacarpophalangeal; *PIP,* proximal interphalangeal.

SELECTED MOVEMENTS

ACTIVE MOVEMENTS

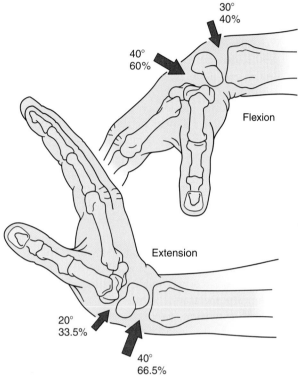

30°
40%

40°
60%

Flexion

Extension

20°
33.5%

40°
66.5%

Figure 6–1
During flexion of the wrist, the motion is more midcarpal and less radiocarpal. During extension of the wrist, the motion is more radiocarpal and less midcarpal. (Modified from Sarrafian SK, Melamed JL, Goshgarian GM: Study of wrist motion in flexion and extension, *Clin Orthop* 126:156, 1977.)

GENERAL INFORMATION   Active movements sometimes are referred to as *physiological movements*. If a pathological condition affects only one area of the hand or wrist, only that area needs to be assessed, provided the examiner is satisfied that the condition does not affect or has not affected the function of the other areas of the forearm, wrist, and hand. For example, if the patient has suffered a fall on the outstretched hand (FOOSH) injury to the wrist, the examiner spends most of the examination looking at the wrist. However, because positioning of the wrist can affect the function of the rest of the hand and forearm, the examiner must determine the functional effect of the injury on these other areas. Also, if the injury is chronic, adaptive changes may have occurred in adjacent joints.

PATIENT POSITION   The patient is sitting.

EXAMINER POSITION   The examiner faces the patient.

TEST PROCEDURE   The patient is asked to actively flex, extend, ulnarly deviate, and radially deviate the wrist. The patient next is asked to flex, extend, and ulnarly and radially deviate the joints of the digits. The most painful movements are done last. If active movement is pain free, overpressure can be added at the end of each movement. If active movement is painful, no overpressure should be added. The tests are most commonly assessed with the forearm in a pronated position, but it can be valuable for the examiner to test the patient's active range of motion (ROM) with the forearm in neutral and in a supinated position. In some cases, the position of the elbow could affect the active movements of the wrist and hand.

Continued

ACTIVE MOVEMENTS—*cont'd*

INDICATIONS OF A POSITIVE TEST

Pronation and supination. Active pronation and supination of the forearm and wrist are approximately 85° to 90°, although this varies from individual to individual. It is more important to compare the movement with that of the normal side. Approximately 75° of supination or pronation occurs in the forearm articulations. The remaining 15° is the result of wrist action.

Wrist flexion and extension. Wrist flexion is 80° to 90°; wrist extension is 70° to 90°. The end feel of each movement is tissue stretch.

Radial and ulnar deviation. Radial and ulnar deviations of the wrist are 15° and 30° to 45°, respectively. The normal end feel of these movements is bone to bone.

Finger flexion. Flexion of the fingers occurs at the metacarpophalangeal joints (85° to 90°), followed by the proximal interphalangeal joints (100° to 115°) and the distal interphalangeal joints (80° to 90°).

Finger extension. Extension occurs at the metacarpophalangeal joints (30° to 45°), the proximal interphalangeal joints (0°), and the distal interphalangeal joints (20°). The end feel of finger flexion and extension is tissue stretch.

Finger abduction and adduction. Finger abduction occurs at the metacarpophalangeal joints (20° to 30°); the end feel is tissue stretch. Finger adduction (0°) occurs at the same joint.

Thumb flexion. Thumb flexion occurs at the carpometacarpal joint (45° to 50°), the metacarpophalangeal joint (50° to 55°), and the interphalangeal joint (80° to 90°). It is associated with medial rotation of the thumb as a result of the saddle shape of the carpometacarpal joint.

Thumb extension. Extension of the thumb occurs at the interphalangeal joint (0° to 5°); it is associated with lateral rotation. Flexion and extension take place in a plane parallel to the palm of the hand.

Thumb abduction and adduction. Thumb abduction is 60° to 70°; thumb adduction is 30°. These movements occur in a plane at right angles to the flexion-extension plane.

CLINICAL NOTES/CAUTIONS

- Pathological conditions in structures other than the joint may restrict ROM (e.g., muscle spasm, tight ligaments/capsules). If the examiner suspects a problem with these structures, passive movement end feels will help differentiate the problem.
- Most functional activities of the hand require the fingers and thumb to open at least 5 cm (2 inches), and the fingers should be able to flex within 1 to 2 cm (0.4 to 0.8 inches) of the distal palmar crease.
- If the patient complains of pain on supination, the examiner can differentiate between the distal radioulnar joint and the radiocarpal joints by passively supinating the ulna on the radius with no stress on the radiocarpal joint. If this passive movement is painful, the problem is in the distal radioulnar joint, not the radiocarpal joints. The normal end feel of both movements is tissue stretch, although in thin patients, the end feel of pronation may be bone to bone.
- Wrist flexion decreases as the fingers are flexed, just as finger flexion decreases as the wrist flexes, and movements of flexion and extension are limited, usually by the antagonistic muscles and ligaments.
- The digits are medially deviated slightly in relation to the metacarpal bones. When the fingers are flexed, they should point toward the scaphoid tubercle. In addition, the metacarpals are at an angle to each other.

FANNING AND FOLDING OF THE HAND[1]

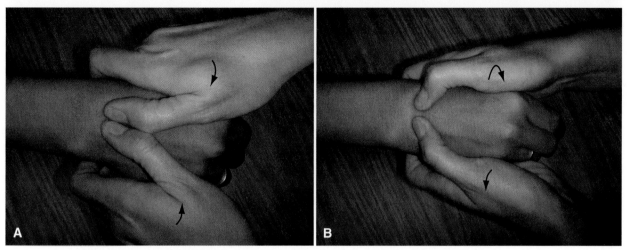

DVD

Figure 6–2
Fanning (**A**) and folding (**B**) of the hand.

PURPOSE	To assess conjunction rotation of the hand
PATIENT POSITION	The patient is sitting.
EXAMINER POSITION	The examiner sits facing the patient.
TEST PROCEDURE	The examiner holds the scaphoid and trapezium with the index and middle finger of one hand and the pisiform and hamate of the other hand while the capitate is held with the thumbs on the dorsum of the hand.
INDICATIONS OF A POSITIVE TEST	The examiner folds and fans the hand, feeling the movement while monitoring motion and feeling for crepitus and joint motion. Reproduction of symptoms also is assessed. Symptom reproduction or abnormal movement or shifting of joints is an indication of a positive test result.
CLINICAL NOTE	• The test is used as a general screening examination. It is difficult to identify specific structures as the source of a pathological condition with this test, because it tests multiple structures and joints. There is also a wrist and hand scan that may be done.
RELIABILITY/SPECIFICITY/ SENSITIVITY	Unknown

SPECIAL TESTS FOR LIGAMENT, CAPSULE, AND JONT INSTABILITY[2-5]

Relevant Special Tests

Ligamentous instability test for the fingers
Thumb ulnar collateral ligament laxity or instability test
Lunotriquetral ballottement (Reagan's) test
Lunotriquetral shear test
Watson (scaphoid shift) test
Triangular fibrocartilage complex (TFCC) load test

Definition

Stability within the hand and wrist are critical for optimal upper extremity function. Instability can occur at any of the joints of the forearm, wrist, or hand. Typically, the stability of a joint depends on the coordinated interaction between the passive elements of the region (i.e., bone, cartilage, and ligaments) and the active elements (i.e., muscle, tendon, and neuromuscular control). Instability occurs when injury or a pathological condition alters this balance.

Suspected Injury

Collateral ligament of the finger sprain or tear (3° sprain)
Instability of the lunotriquetral joint
Lunotriquetral ligament sprain or tear
Ulnar collateral ligament of the thumb sprain or tear
Instability of the triangular fibrocartilage complex
Instability of the scapholunate joint
Scapholunate ligament sprain or tear

Epidemiology and Demographics

Dobyns et al.[4] estimated that 10% of all carpal injuries result in carpal instability. This number increases when distal radius fractures occur. Tang[5] reported that 30% of patients with distal radius fractures also have carpal instability.

Degeneration of the TFCC begins in the third decade of life and progressively increases in frequency and severity in subsequent decades. Studies have found no normal-appearing TFCCs after the fifth decade of life.

Ulnar collateral ligament injuries to the thumb occur nine times more frequently than radial collateral ligament injuries. Individuals active in sports such as skiing and mountain bike riding are prone to this injury.

Relevant History

If instability and laxity are the result of injury or trauma, no prior history of pathology needs to be present in the region. If the instability or laxity is the result of disease processes, the patient may have a past history of diseases that affect soft tissues. A prime example of this is rheumatoid arthritis, which significantly affects the laxity of the joints of the hand and wrist.

Relevant Signs and Symptoms

• Localized pain may occur over the injured tissue, especially when the individual is gripping, using the hand, or weight bearing on the hand.
• Generalized pain may be present.
• Swelling may or may not be present.
• Clicking or catching may be noted with functional use.
• The patient may complain of weakness in the hand and wrist.

Mechanism of Injury

The most common mechanism of injury is trauma, such as a fall onto the hand (FOOSH) or wrist. Injury also can occur whenever the ligaments are subjected to tensile forces that exceed their physiological capacities. Because the ligaments are damaged, passive stability is lost and active stability is needed. The muscles, tendons, and nerves of the wrist and forearm provide the active stability to the region. However, in the wrist and hand, most joints have no direct muscle or tendon attachment. Instead, the tendons of the muscle overlie the affected joint and have no direct control over the wrist motion or stability. As a result, instability is common after trauma and persists without the neuromuscular system contribution. Although the initial mechanism is different when ligament damage is the result of disease processes, the reason for the lack of stability in the joint is similar.

LIGAMENTOUS INSTABILITY TEST FOR THE FINGERS

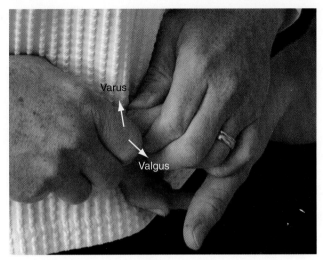

Figure 6-3
Position for testing ligamentous instability of the fingers.

PURPOSE	To assess the integrity of the collateral ligaments of the metacarpophalangeal and interphalangeal joints of the fingers.
SUSPECTED INJURY	Collateral ligament sprain or tear Rheumatoid arthritis
PATIENT POSITION	The patient is sitting.
EXAMINER POSITION	The examiner sits directly in front of the patient.
TEST PROCEDURE	The uninvolved hand is tested first. The examiner stabilizes the finger with one hand proximal to the joint to be tested. With the other hand, the examiner grasps the finger distal to the test joint and places the joint in the resting position. The examiner's distal hand then is used to apply a varus or valgus stress to the joint (proximal or distal phalanx) to test the integrity of the collateral ligaments.
INDICATIONS OF A POSITIVE TEST	The results for the uninvolved hand are compared for laxity with those of the affected hand.
CLINICAL NOTE	• The finger joints should be tested in varying degrees of flexion to assess the integrity of the different fibers of the ligament.
RELIABILITY/SPECIFICITY/SENSITIVITY	Unknown

THUMB ULNAR COLLATERAL LIGAMENT LAXITY OR INSTABILITY TEST[6,7]

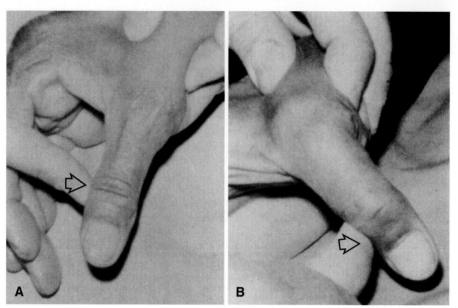

Figure 6–4

A and **B,** Testing the stability of the ulnar collateral ligament in the thumb of a normal individual. In extension, the thumb was stable, but in flexion, it appeared to be unstable. This was caused by the laxity of the dorsal capsule at the metacarpophalangeal joint. (From Nicholas JA, Hershman EB (eds): *Upper extremity in sports medicine,* p 580, St. Louis, 1989, Mosby.)

PURPOSE	To assess the integrity of the ulnar collateral ligament of the thumb.
SUSPECTED INJURY	Ulnar collateral ligament sprain or tear Gamekeeper's thumb Skier's thumb
PATIENT POSITION	The patient is sitting.
EXAMINER POSITION	The examiner sits directly in front of the patient.
TEST PROCEDURE	The examiner stabilizes the patient's hand with one hand and takes the patient's thumb into extension with the other hand. While holding the thumb in extension, the examiner applies a valgus stress to the metacarpophalangeal joint of the thumb, stressing the ulnar collateral ligament and accessory collateral ligament.
INDICATIONS OF A POSITIVE TEST	Valgus movement greater than 30° to 35° indicates a complete tear of the ulnar collateral and accessory collateral ligaments. Laxity of less than 30° to 35° indicates a partial tear, which is still greater than would be seen on the unaffected side (normal laxity in extension is about 15°).
CLINICAL NOTE	• To test the collateral ligament in isolation, the carpometacarpal joint is flexed to 30° and a valgus stress is applied.
RELIABILITY/SPECIFICITY/ SENSITIVITY	Unknown

LUNOTRIQUETRAL BALLOTTEMENT (REAGAN'S) TEST[8-10]

DVD

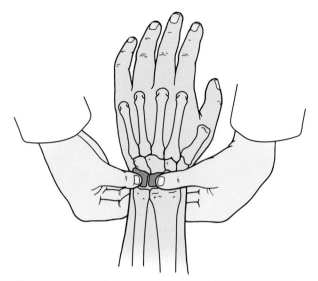

Figure 6-5
Lunotriquetral ballottement test for lunatotriquetral interosseous membrane dissociations.

PURPOSE	To assess the integrity and stability of the lunotriquetral ligament and lunotriquetral joint in the wrist.
SUSPECTED INJURY	Lunotriquetral ligament sprain or tear Lunotriquetral joint instability Lunotriquetral joint subluxation
PATIENT POSITION	The patient is sitting.
EXAMINER POSITION	The examiner sits directly in front of the patient.
TEST PROCEDURE	The examiner grasps the triquetrum between the thumb and second finger of one hand and the lunate with the thumb and second finger of the other hand. The examiner then stabilizes the triquetrum with a finger and the thumb of one hand and moves the lunate up and down (anteriorly and posteriorly) with the finger and thumb of the other hand.
INDICATIONS OF A POSITIVE TEST	Joint laxity, crepitus, or pain all are indicators of a positive test result for lunotriquetral instability.
CLINICAL NOTE/CAUTION	• Because this test focuses on small bones, the examiner must take care to grasp only the triquetrum and lunate. If the force is placed over other bones, the results may not be true indications of the status of the lunotriquetral joint.
RELIABILITY/SPECIFICITY/SENSITIVITY	Unknown

LUNOTRIQUETRAL SHEAR TEST[8,11]

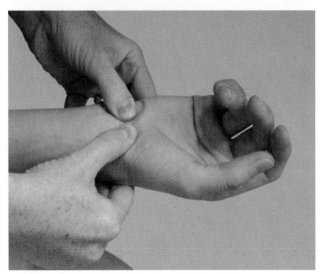

Figure 6-6
Lunotriquetral shear test.

PURPOSE	To assess the integrity and the stability of the lunotriquetral ligament and lunotriquetral joint at the wrist.
SUSPECTED INJURY	Lunotriquetral ligament sprain or tear Lunotriquetral joint instability Lunotriquetral joint subluxation
PATIENT POSITION	The patient sits with the elbow flexed in neutral rotation and resting on the examining table.
EXAMINER POSITION	The examiner faces the patient.
TEST PROCEDURE	With one hand the examiner grasps the patient's wrist so that the examiner's thumb rests in the patient's palm and the examiner's fingers are placed over the dorsum of the proximal row of carpals to support the lunate. The thumb of the examiner's other hand loads the pisotriquetral joint on the palmar aspect, applying a shearing force to the lunotriquetral joint.
INDICATIONS OF A POSITIVE TEST	Pain, crepitus, or abnormal movements are considered a positive test result.
CLINICAL NOTE/CAUTION	• Because this test focuses on small bones, the examiner must take care to grasp only the appropriate bones. If the force is placed over other bones, the results may not be a true indication of the status of the lunotriquetral joint.
RELIABILITY/SPECIFICITY/ SENSITIVITY	Unknown

WATSON (SCAPHOID SHIFT) TEST[10,12-15]

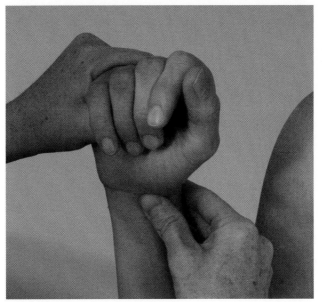

Figure 6-7
Watson (scaphoid shift) test.

PURPOSE	To assess the integrity and the stability of the scapholunate ligament and scapholunate joint in the wrist.
SUSPECTED INJURY	Scapholunate ligament sprain or tear Scapholunate joint instability Scapholunate joint subluxation
PATIENT POSITION	The patient sits with the elbow resting on the table and the forearm pronated.
EXAMINER POSITION	The examiner faces the patient.
TEST PROCEDURE	With the right hand the examiner takes the patient's wrist into full ulnar deviation and slight extension while holding the metacarpals with left hand, as illustrated. The examiner presses the thumb of the other hand against the distal pole of the scaphoid on the palmar side to prevent it from moving toward the palm while the fingers provide a counterpressure on the dorsum of the forearm. With the first hand the examiner radially deviates and slightly flexes the patient's hand while maintaining pressure on the scaphoid.
INDICATIONS OF A POSITIVE TEST	This test creates a subluxation stress if the scaphoid is unstable. If the scaphoid (and lunate) are unstable, the dorsal pole of the scaphoid subluxes, or "shifts," over the dorsal rim of the radius and the patient will complain of pain, indicating a positive test result.
CLINICAL NOTE	• If the scaphoid subluxes with the thumb pressure, it commonly returns to its normal position with a "thunk" when the thumb is removed. If the ligamentous tissue is intact, the scaphoid normally moves forward, pushing the thumb forward with it.
RELIABILITY/SPECIFICITY/ SENSITIVITY	Unknown

TRIANGULAR FIBROCARTILAGE COMPLEX (TFCC) LOAD TEST[16]

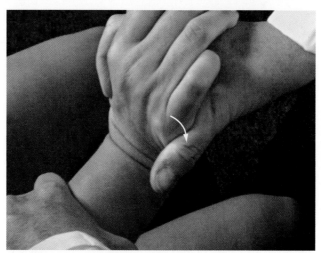

Figure 6-8
Triangular fibrocartilage complex (TFCC) load test.

PURPOSE	To assess the integrity and the stability of the triangular fibrocartilage complex in the wrist.
SUSPECTED INJURY	Triangular fibrocartilage complex injury
PATIENT POSITION	The patient sits with the elbow flexed in neutral rotation and resting on the examining table.
EXAMINER POSITION	The examiner faces the patient.
TEST PROCEDURE	The examiner holds the patient's forearm with the left hand and the patient's hand with the right hand as illustrated. The examiner then proceeds to axially load and ulnarly deviate the wrist, which compresses the TFCC. While maintaining the compressive load, the examiner "grinds" or "scours" the ulnar aspect of the wrist by moving the wrist dorsally and palmarly or by rotating the forearm.
INDICATIONS OF A POSITIVE TEST	Pain, clicking, or crepitus in the area of the TFCC indicates a positive test result.
CLINICAL NOTES	• Degeneration of the TFCC begins in the third decade of life and progressively increases in frequency and severity in subsequent decades. Studies have observed no normal-appearing triangular fibrocartilage complexes after the fifth decade of life. • Gymnasts (males more than females) incur TFCC injuries as a result of using the wrist as a weight-bearing joint. • The patient may complain of pain when putting weight on the hand (wrist extended) and then pronating the forearm.
RELIABILITY/SPECIFICITY/ SENSITIVITY	Unknown

SPECIAL TEST FOR MUSCLE OR TENDON PATHOLOGY[17-19]

Relevant Special Test

Finkelstein test

Definition

Pathologically, de Quervain's tenosynovitis is a chronic irritation of the extensor pollicis brevis (EPB) and abductor pollicis longus (APL) tendons as they pass deep to the extensor retinaculum in the first dorsal compartment. Stenosing tenosynovitis of the first dorsal compartment may occur and usually involves irritation of the EPB and APL tendons on the radiodorsal aspect of the wrist

Suspected Injury

De Quervain's tenosynovitis

Epidemiology and Demographics

De Quervain's tenosynovitis is a relatively common problem that occurs with equal frequency in people of all races. It is somewhat more common in women than in men.

Relevant History

• Recurrent episodes are common.
• Work requiring repetitive wrist motion often is cited as a factor.

• The condition may appear in women after giving birth, probably because of altered hand use in lifting the infant and positioning the baby for breast-feeding. Research also has demonstrated laxity in the wrist joint postpartum, which may contribute to the development of pain in the region.

Relevant Signs and Symptoms

• Pain is felt in the radial aspect of the wrist, especially over the involved tendons.
• Symptoms may refer into the thumb and up the radial side of the forearm.

Mechanism of Injury

The pathological condition occurs secondary to overuse or misuse, often as a result of a change in the customary use patterns for the wrist and thumb, leading to inflammation. It may be precipitated by discrete trauma, such as a blow to the wrist, but the onset usually is gradual. Initially, physical irritation results in acute inflammation of the tendon sheath. Over time, chronic degenerative changes develop as a result of the inflammation, resulting in tendinosis. Repeated wrist radial deviation and/or thumb palmar or radial abduction, especially under load, is the most common mechanism of injury.

FINKELSTEIN TEST[20,21]

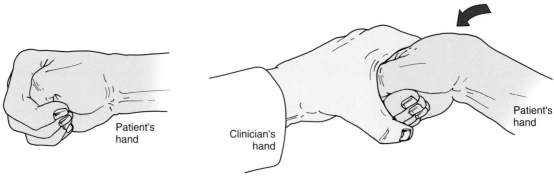

Figure 6-9
Finkelstein test.

PURPOSE	To assess for irritation of the extensor pollicis brevis and abductor pollicis longus tendons as they pass deep to the extensor retinaculum in the first dorsal compartment in the wrist.
PATIENT POSITION	Usually the patient sits with the elbow flexed in neutral rotation and resting on the examining table.
EXAMINER POSITION	The examiner faces the patient.
TEST PROCEDURE	The patient makes a fist with the thumb inside the fingers. The examiner stabilizes the forearm with one hand and then passively deviates the wrist toward the ulnar side with the other hand while keeping the patient's thumb enclosed in the patient's fist.
INDICATIONS OF A POSITIVE TEST	Pain or reproduction of symptoms over the abductor pollicis longus and extensor pollicis brevis tendons at the wrist is a positive test result and indicates a paratenonitis or tendinosus of these two tendons.
CLINICAL NOTE/CAUTION	• Because the test can cause some discomfort even in normal individuals, the examiner should compare the pain caused on the test side with that on the unaffected side. The test result is considered positive only if greater pain or symptom reproduction is noted on the affected side.
RELIABILITY/SPECIFICITY/ SENSITIVITY	Unknown

SPECIAL TESTS FOR NEUROLOGICAL SYMPTOMS[22-32]

Relevant Special Tests

Tinel's sign (at the wrist)
Phalen's (wrist flexion) test
Reverse Phalen's (prayer) test

Definition

A pathological condition of the nerves is a common source of symptoms and dysfunction in the forearm, wrist, and hand. The term *carpal tunnel syndrome* refers to compression of the median nerve as it passes through the channel created by the trapezoid, the capitate, and the flexor retinaculum (transverse carpal ligament) and its attachments to the scaphoid tubercle, trapezium, hook of hamate, and pisiform.

Suspected Injury

Carpal tunnel syndrome

Epidemiology and Demographics

Carpal tunnel syndrome is among the most commonly reported nerve entrapments. It is seen more than twice as often in women as in men and usually occurs between 45 and 54 years of age. It also is frequently seen during pregnancy. Median nerve entrapments are more common in office workers, manual workers, and individuals who engage in repetitive movement pattern activities, such as musicians, artists, and sports participants.

Relevant History

Median nerve entrapment can occur as a result of a broad spectrum of associated causative factors; consequently, the past history for the pathological condition may vary widely from individual to individual. Anatomical anomalies involving bony structures, vascular structures, and connective tissue (fascia) may predispose a person to a pathological condition, together with underlying disease and medical issues such as diabetes mellitus, osteoarthritis, obesity, pregnancy, menopause, and space-occupying lesions. The patient may have a history of trauma (e.g., fractures of the wrist or forearm) or may pursue work or leisure activities that involve repetitive movement patterns or vibration exposure.

Relevant Signs and Symptoms

Carpal tunnel syndrome commonly presents with progressively worsening pain (classically described as aching and burning) and paraesthesia in the thumb, forefinger, middle finger, hand, and wrist that may extend to the forearm, elbow, shoulder, and neck. Symptoms frequently are worse nocturnally. The patient also may complain of problems with grip and weakness in the wrist and hand. With median nerve involvement, fine motor skills (precision grip) are affected more than power grip.

Variations in the innervation of the hand, particularly the Martin Gruber anastomosis, where the motor nerve crosses over from the median nerve to the ulnar nerve (seen in 10% to 15% of the population), can cause the presentation of entrapment to vary significantly. The condition may involve the flexor pollicis brevis, adductor pollicis, abductor pollicis brevis, lumbricals, and abductor digiti minimi, or even the entire hand.

Mechanism of Injury

In general, nerve injury is classified according to the severity of the injury and the potential for reversibility. Nerve injury may be classified according to the amount of nerve damage and the nerve structure involved. Five categories of nerve injury are frequently used (Sunderland classification).

- *First-degree neuropraxia* involves distortion of myelin about the nodes of Ranvier caused by ischemia, mechanical compression, or electrolyte imbalance, resulting in temporary loss of nerve conduction.
- *Second-degree axonotmesis* involves interruption of the axon with secondary wallerian degeneration but preservation of the supporting tissue around the axon. Recovery may be complete but takes longer and depends on the distance between the site of injury and the end structure (denervated muscle).
- *Third-degree neurotmesis* involves extensive disruption of the nerve and its supporting structures; however, although the endoneurium is disrupted, the perineurium and epineurium remain intact.
- *Fourth-degree neurotmesis* involves disruption of all neural components except the epineurium.
- *Fifth-degree neurotmesis* involves complete transection and discontinuity of the nerve, with no capacity for regeneration. Neurotmesis rarely occurs as a result of entrapment. However, when continuity has been disrupted, complete recovery is not possible, even with surgical techniques, and the eventual outcome depends on the individual circumstances.

Reliability/Specificity/Sensitivity Comparison[30-32]

	Validity	Interrater Reliability	Intrarater Reliability	Specificity	Sensitivity
Tinel's Sign	No association with the severity of carpal tunnel syndrome and test results $p > 0.11$	0.77	0.80	87%	23%
Phalen's Test	Patients with more severe carpal tunnel syndrome are more likely to have a positive test result $p < 0.05$	0.65	0.53	76%	51%
Reverse Phalen's Test	Unknown	Unknown	Unknown	Unknown	Unknown

TINEL'S SIGN (AT THE WRIST)[20]

DVD

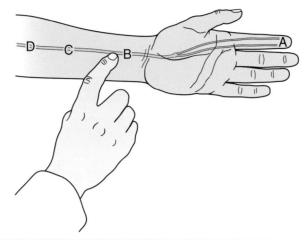

Figure 6-10

Tinel's sign at the wrist. Light percussion is applied along the nerve, starting at "A," and progresses proximally. The point where paresthesia is elicited is the level of axonal regrowth.

PURPOSE	To assess for median nerve involvement through the carpal tunnel of the wrist.
PATIENT POSITION	The patient sits with the elbow flexed in neutral rotation and resting on the examining table.
EXAMINER POSITION	The examiner sits directly in front of the test wrist.
TEST PROCEDURE	The examiner supinates the patient's hand and wrist and stabilizes the forearm with one hand. The other hand is used to test along the median nerve pathway. The examiner taps over the carpal tunnel at the wrist with the index and/or middle finger, working up the arm and following the path of the median nerve.
INDICATIONS OF A POSITIVE TEST	A positive test result is indicated by tingling or paresthesias into the thumb, index finger (forefinger), and middle and lateral half of the ring finger (median nerve distribution). For a positive test result, the tingling or paresthesia must be felt distal to the point of tapping.
CLINICAL NOTES/CAUTIONS	• This test gives an indication of the rate of regeneration of sensory fibers of the median nerve. The most distal point at which the abnormal sensation is felt represents the limit of nerve regeneration. • Tinel's sign can be used to test any superficial nerve along its pathway. • Tests for neurological dysfunction are highly suggestive of a particular nerve lesion if they produce a positive result, but they do not rule out the problem if the result is negative. In fact, test results may be negative 50% of the time or more often even when the condition actually exists. Electrodiagnostic tests are more conclusive.
RELIABILITY/SPECIFICITY/ SENSITIVITY[30-36]	Reliability range: 0.51-0.80 Specificity range: 63% to 100% Sensitivity range: 23% to 64%

PHALEN'S (WRIST FLEXION) TEST[37]

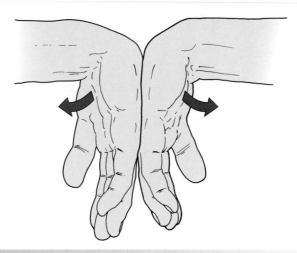

Figure 6-11
Phalen's test.

PURPOSE	To assess for median nerve involvement through the carpal tunnel of the wrist.
PATIENT POSITION	The patient sits with the dorsal aspect of one hand in contact with the dorsum of the other hand.
EXAMINER POSITION	The examiner is seated in front of the patient to observe the patient. The examiner should have a clock to monitor time. No manual contact is required for this test.
TEST PROCEDURE	The patient flexes the wrists maximally and holds the wrists in the test position. The patient then pushes the wrists together and holds this position for 1 minute.
INDICATIONS OF A POSITIVE TEST	A positive test result is indicated by tingling in the thumb, index finger, and middle and lateral half of the ring finger. A positive result is indicative of carpal tunnel syndrome caused by pressure (compression) on the median nerve.
CLINICAL NOTE/CAUTION	• Tests for neurological dysfunction are highly suggestive of a particular nerve lesion if they produce a positive result, but they do not rule out the problem if the result is negative. In fact, test results may be negative 50% of the time or more often even when the condition actually exists. Electrodiagnostic tests are more conclusive.
RELIABILITY/SPECIFICITY/ SENSITIVITY[30-36]	Reliability range: 0.53-0.58 Specificity range: 54% to 100% Sensitivity range: 51% to 87%

REVERSE PHALEN'S (PRAYER) TEST[9]

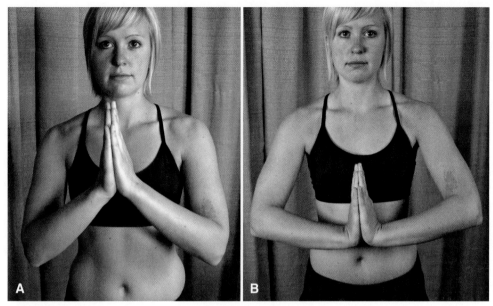

Figure 6-12
Reverse Phalen's (prayer) test (alternative method). **A,** Start position. **B,** End position.

PURPOSE	To assess for median nerve involvement through the carpal tunnel of the wrist.
PATIENT POSITION	The patient is sitting.
EXAMINER POSITION	The examiner is seated in front of the patient.
TEST PROCEDURE	The examiner extends the patient's wrist with one hand while asking the patient to grip the examiner's hand. The thumb or index finger of the examiner's other hand is placed directly over the patient's carpal tunnel. The examiner then applies direct pressure over the carpal tunnel for 1 minute. As an alternative method, the patient can be asked to put the palms of the two hands together and bring the hands down toward the waist while keeping the palms in full contact ("prayer" test), thus causing extension of the wrist.
INDICATIONS OF A POSITIVE TEST	A positive test result is indicated by production of the same symptoms seen in Phalen's test (i.e., tingling in the thumb, index finger, and middle and lateral half of the ring finger). A positive result is indicative of carpal tunnel syndrome caused by stretching of the median nerve.
CLINICAL NOTE	• See Phalen's test.
RELIABILITY/SPECIFICITY/ SENSITIVITY	Unknown

SPECIAL TESTS FOR CIRCULATION AND SWELLING IN THE WRIST AND HAND

Relevant Special Tests

Allen test
Digit blood flow test

Definition

An understanding of the inflammatory process plays an important role in the clinical diagnosis and treatment of musculoskeletal pathological conditions. Inflammation is a normal and natural process. It is a critical part of the body's process of healing. Swelling is a natural byproduct of this inflammatory process. Both swelling and inflammation are influenced by circulation. Measurement of blood flow and swelling allows the examiner to quantify improvement or deficits in both of these processes.

Suspected Injury

Any injury to a region results in an inflammatory response in the body. Highly vascularized structures generally produce a faster inflammatory response. Conversely, regions that are poorly vascularized have a slower inflammatory response, but the swelling and inflammation remain in the region longer if circulation and lymphatic drainage in the area are poor.

Epidemiology and Demographics

Pathological conditions that affect circulation or lymphatic drainage can impede the process and resolution of swelling. Disease processes such as diabetes can greatly affect the body's ability to heal. Cancer and the associated surgery that removes lymphatic tissue often result in the accumulation of interstitial fluid in the hand and wrist. Diet, medications, cardiovascular conditions, and hypertension likewise can have a positive or negative effect on swelling and circulation in the hand and wrist.

In addition to injury, complex regional pain syndromes and sympathetic responses into the upper extremity can result in altered circulatory patterns and edema in the wrist and hand.

Relevant History

The patient may have a history of trauma, cancer and lymph node removal, diabetes, cardiovascular disorders, and kidney or liver dysfunction. Diet, medications, and stress also can affect circulation and swelling in the wrist and hand region.

Relevant Signs and Symptoms

- Swelling is more obvious on the dorsum of the hand, where the skin is looser.
- Tightness and stiffness in the hand joints often are seen.
- Rings and jewelry on the hands and fingers may fit tightly.
- Coldness or weakness in the hands and arms may be noted.
- Color changes may be seen in the upper extremity.
- Wounds or injuries of the hand may heal poorly.
- Changes may occur in the skin and nail beds.

Mechanism of Injury

No single specific mechanism of injury is consistent with every instance of swelling or altered circulation in the upper extremity. Injury may or may not have been a trigger. Both vascular edema and neurological edema can result in altered circulation or the accumulation of fluid and other products of inflammation.

ALLEN TEST[37,38]

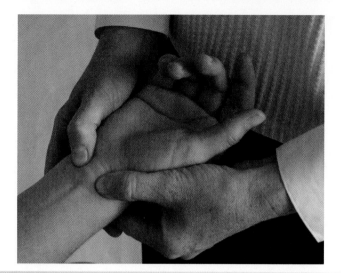

Figure 6-13
Allen test.

PURPOSE	To assess the patency of the radial and ulnar arteries and determine which artery provides the major blood supply to the hand.
PATIENT POSITION	The patient is sitting.
EXAMINER POSITION	The examiner is seated in front of the patient to observe the circulatory response to the test.
TEST PROCEDURE	The patient is asked to open and close the test hand several times as quickly as possible and then squeeze the hand tightly. The examiner then compresses both the radial and ulnar arteries, using both hands. The patient opens the hand while the examiner maintains pressure over the arteries. One artery is tested by releasing the pressure over that artery to see how quickly the hand flushes. The other artery then is tested in a similar fashion.
INDICATIONS OF A POSITIVE TEST	A positive test result is indicated by a slow return of normal color in the hand; the test also indicates which artery is the major vessel of the hand.
CLINICAL NOTE	• Both hands should be tested for comparison.
RELIABILITY/SPECIFICITY/ SENSITIVITY/ODDS RATIO	Unknown

DIGIT BLOOD FLOW TEST

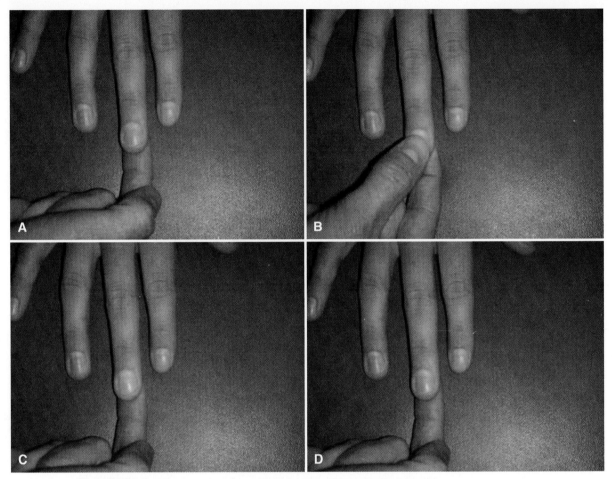

Figure 6-14
Checking digital blood flow. **A,** Starting position. **B,** Compression on finger. **C,** Immediately after pressure released. **D,** Three seconds after pressure released.

PURPOSE	To determine the patency of the digital arteries to the fingers of the hand.
PATIENT POSITION	The patient sits with the hands and wrists pronated and resting on the table.
EXAMINER POSITION	The examiner is seated in front of the patient to observe the circulatory response to the test.
TEST PROCEDURE	The examiner compresses the nail bed and then releases it, noting the time required for color to return to the nail.
INDICATIONS OF A POSITIVE TEST	Normally, color returns to the nail bed within 3 seconds after the release of pressure. If the return takes longer, arterial insufficiency to the fingers should be suspected.
CLINICAL NOTE	• Comparison with the unaffected side gives some indication of restricted flow.
RELIABILITY/SPECIFICITY/ SENSITIVITY	Unknown

JOINT PLAY MOVEMENTS

LONG AXIS EXTENSION OF THE WRIST

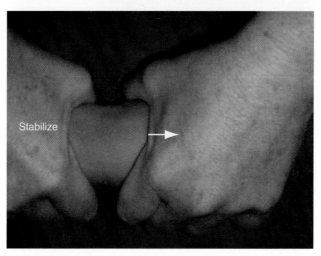

Stabilize

Figure 6-15
Long axis extension (traction) of the wrist.

PATIENT POSITION	The patient may be sitting or supine.
EXAMINER POSITION	The examiner is adjacent to the patient's hand.
TEST PROCEDURE	The examiner stabilizes the radius and ulna with one hand and places the other hand just distal to the wrist over the proximal carpal bone. The examiner then applies a longitudinal traction movement with the distal hand.
INDICATIONS OF A POSITIVE TEST	The amount of movement obtained by the joint play is compared with that on the unaffected side. The test result is considered significant only if a difference is seen between the two sides. Reproduction of the patient's symptoms also indicates the joints at fault.
CLINICAL NOTE	• The patient's elbow may be flexed to 90°, and stabilization may be applied at the elbow if no pathological condition is present at the elbow.

ANTERIOR-POSTERIOR GLIDE OF THE WRIST

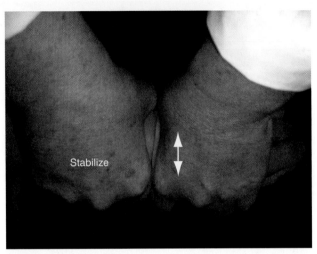

Figure 6-16
Anterior-posterior glide of the wrist.

PATIENT POSITION	The patient may be sitting or supine.
EXAMINER POSITION	The examiner usually is adjacent to the patient's hand.
TEST PROCEDURE	*Step 1: Radiocarpal joint.* The examiner first places the forearm in a supinated or pronated position. The examiner's stabilizing hand then is placed around the distal end of the radius and ulna, just proximal to the radiocarpal joint, and the other hand is placed around the proximal row of carpal bones. If the examiner's hands are positioned properly, they should touch. The examiner applies an anteroposterior gliding movement of the proximal row of carpal bones on the radius and ulna, testing the amount of movement and end feel.
	Step 2: Midcarpal joint. The examiner moves the stabilizing hand slightly distally (less than 1 cm [0.4 inch]) so that it is around the proximal row of carpal bones and places the mobilizing hand around the distal row of carpal bones. An anteroposterior gliding movement is applied to the distal row of carpal bones on the proximal row to test the amount of movement and end feel (midcarpal joint).
	Step 3: Carpometacarpal joint. The examiner then moves the stabilizing hand slightly distally again (less than 1 cm [0.4 inch]); the hand will be around the distal carpal bones. The mobilizing hand is placed around the metacarpals. An anteroposterior gliding movement is applied to the base of the metacarpals to test the amount of joint play and end feel.
INDICATIONS OF A POSITIVE TEST	The amount of movement obtained by the joint play is compared with that on the unaffected side. The test result is considered significant only if a difference is seen between the two sides. Reproduction of the patient's symptoms also indicates the joints at fault.
CLINICAL NOTE	• These movements sometimes are called the *anteroposterior drawer tests of the wrist.*

SIDE GLIDE OF THE WRIST

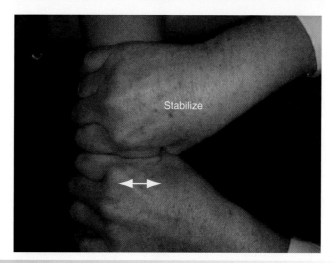

Stabilize

Figure 6-17
Wrist side glide.

PATIENT POSITION   The patient may be sitting or supine.

EXAMINER POSITION   The examiner is adjacent to the patient's hand.

TEST PROCEDURE   The examiner positions the patient's forearm in supination or pronation. The examiner stabilizes the radius and ulna by placing the stabilizing hand around the distal radius and ulna just proximal to the radiocarpal joint at the side of the wrist (usually the ulnar side) and the mobilizing hand around the patient's hand at the side of the wrist (usually the ulnar side). The examiner then glides the proximal carpals radially or ulnarly on the radius and ulna. Similar to the anterior to posterior glide at the wrist, the examiner can also do side glide at the midcarpal and carpometacarpal joints.

INDICATIONS OF A POSITIVE TEST   The amount of movement obtained by the joint play is compared with that on the unaffected side. The test result is considered significant only if a difference is seen between the two sides. Reproduction of the patient's symptoms also indicates the joints at fault.

CLINICAL NOTE   • The forearm can be positioned in varying degrees of pronation, neutral, or supination to assess how forearm and wrist positions affect side gliding and other motions of the wrist joint.

SHEAR TEST OF THE INDIVIDUAL CARPAL BONES

DVD

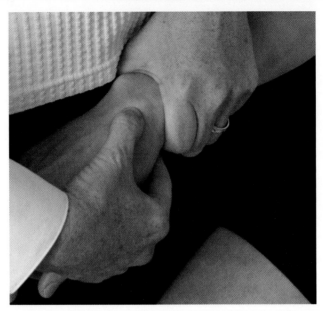

Figure 6-18
Shear test of the individual carpal bones.

PATIENT POSITION	The patient may be sitting or supine.
EXAMINER POSITION	The examiner usually is adjacent to the patient's hand.
TEST PROCEDURE	The examiner grasps the dorsal and palmar aspects of one carpal bone between the thumb and index finger to stabilize the bone. The finger and thumb of the other hand grasp the adjacent carpal bone to be mobilized in a similar fashion. The examiner then glides (mobilizes) the one bone on the other in a dorsal or palmar direction. All carpals may be tested in this fashion.
INDICATIONS OF A POSITIVE TEST	The amount of movement obtained by the joint play is compared with that on the unaffected side. The test result is considered significant only if a difference is seen between the two sides. Pain on any of these joint play movements done in neutral, flexion, or extension may indicate a pathological condition in the joint between the two bones.
CLINICAL NOTES/CAUTIONS	• Because the carpal bones are small, correct hand position is critical for the success of this test. • A firm grasp of anatomy is required for success when doing these movements. Carpal joint locations are difficult to palpate; therefore, an understanding of the anatomical location of the individual bones helps the examiner identify their position and facilitates testing of the joint. • Reagan's test, Watson's test, and the lunotriquetral test are done in a similar fashion.

ANTERIOR-POSTERIOR GLIDE OF THE INTERMETACARPAL JOINTS

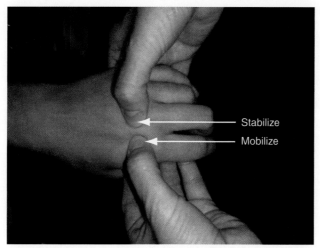

Stabilize
Mobilize

Figure 6-19
Anterior-posterior glide of the intermetacarpal joints.

PATIENT POSITION	The patient may be sitting or supine.
EXAMINER POSITION	The examiner is adjacent to the patient's hand.
TEST PROCEDURE	The examiner grasps the dorsal and palmar aspects of one metacarpal bone between the thumb and index finger to stabilize it. The other hand grasps the adjacent metacarpal bone in a similar fashion to mobilize it. The examiner stabilizes one metacarpal bone and moves the adjacent metacarpal anteriorly or posteriorly in relation to the fixed bone. The process is repeated for each joint.
INDICATIONS OF A POSITIVE TEST	The amount of movement obtained by the joint play is compared with that on the unaffected side. The test result is considered significant only if a difference is seen between the two sides. Pain on any of these joint play movements done in neutral, flexion, or extension may indicate a pathological condition in the joint between the two bones.
CLINICAL NOTE/CAUTION	• Minimal movement is felt during the test.

LONG AXIS EXTENSION OF THE JOINTS OF THE FINGERS

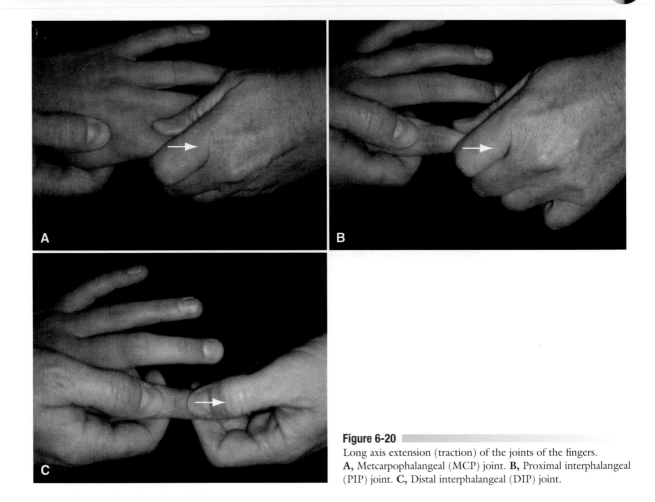

Figure 6-20
Long axis extension (traction) of the joints of the fingers.
A, Metcarpophalangeal (MCP) joint. **B,** Proximal interphalangeal
(PIP) joint. **C,** Distal interphalangeal (DIP) joint.

PATIENT POSITION	The patient may be sitting or supine.
EXAMINER POSITION	The examiner is adjacent to the patient's hand.
TEST PROCEDURE	The examiner stabilizes the proximal segment or bone using the fingers of one hand while placing the fingers of the other hand around the distal segment or bone of the particular test joint (metacarpophalangeal, proximal interphalangeal, or distal interphalangeal joint). With the mobilizing (usually distal) hand, the examiner applies a longitudinal traction to the joint.
INDICATIONS OF A POSITIVE TEST	The amount of movement obtained by the joint play is compared with that on the unaffected side. The test result is considered significant only if a difference is seen between the two sides. Pain on any of these joint play movements done in neutral, flexion, or extension may indicate a pathological condition in the joint between the two bones.
CLINICAL NOTE	• The joint play movements for the fingers are the same for the metacarpophalangeal, proximal interphalangeal, and distal interphalangeal joints; the hand position of the examiner simply moves farther distally.

ANTERIOR-POSTERIOR GLIDE OF THE JOINTS OF THE FINGERS

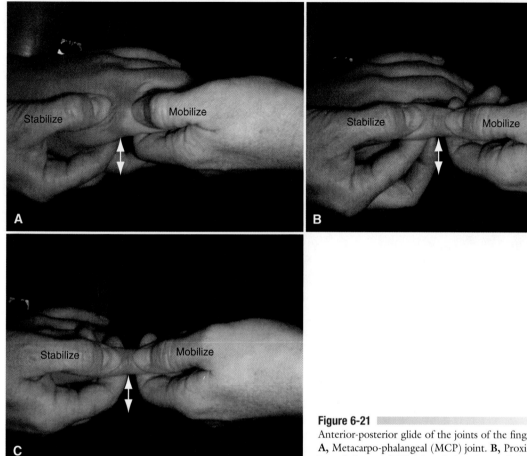

Figure 6-21
Anterior-posterior glide of the joints of the fingers.
A, Metacarpo-phalangeal (MCP) joint. **B,** Proximal interphalangeal (PIP) joint. **C,** Distal interphalangeal (DIP) joint.

PATIENT POSITION	The patient may be sitting or supine.
EXAMINER POSITION	The examiner is adjacent to the patient's hand.
TEST PROCEDURE	The examiner stabilizes the proximal bone with the fingers of one hand. The fingers of the mobilizing hand are placed around the distal segment of the joint. The examiner applies an anterior and/or posterior movement to the distal segment of the desired joint (metacarpophalangeal, proximal interphalangeal, or distal interphalangeal joint), making sure to maintain the joint surfaces parallel to one another while determining the amount of movement and end feel.
INDICATIONS OF A POSITIVE TEST	The amount of movement obtained by the joint play is compared with that on the unaffected side. The test result is considered significant only if a difference is seen between the two sides. Pain on any of these joint play movements done in neutral, flexion, or extension may indicate a pathological condition in the joint between the two bones.
CLINICAL NOTES	• A minimal amount of traction may be applied to bring about slight separation of the joint surfaces before the anterior or posterior movement is done. • The examiner must position both hands close to the joint line so that the motion tested reflects true joint play and not finger flexion or extension.

ROTATION OF THE JOINTS OF THE FINGERS

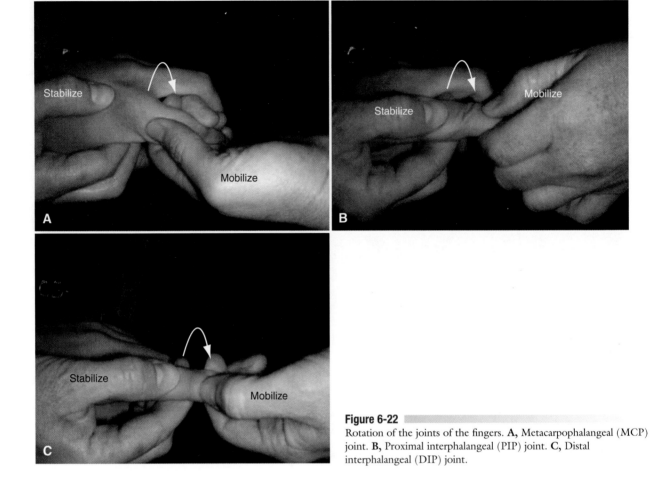

Figure 6-22
Rotation of the joints of the fingers. **A,** Metacarpophalangeal (MCP) joint. **B,** Proximal interphalangeal (PIP) joint. **C,** Distal interphalangeal (DIP) joint.

PATIENT POSITION	The patient may be sitting or supine.
EXAMINER POSITION	The examiner is adjacent to the patient's hand.
TEST PROCEDURE	The examiner grasps the proximal bone between the index finger and thumb of one hand. The fingers of the other hand are placed around the distal segment of the joint. Rotation of the joints of the fingers is accomplished by slightly distracting the joint surfaces and then rotating the distal segment of the desired joint (metacarpophalangeal, proximal interphalangeal, or distal interphalangeal joint) on the proximal segment to determine the end feel and joint play.
INDICATIONS OF A POSITIVE TEST	The amount of movement obtained by the joint play is compared with that on the unaffected side. The test result is considered significant only if a difference is seen between the two sides. Pain on any of these joint play movements done in neutral, flexion, or extension may indicate a pathological condition in the joint between the two bones.
CLINICAL NOTE	• Excessive joint distraction affects the amount of rotation achieved.

SIDE GLIDE OF THE JOINTS OF THE FINGERS

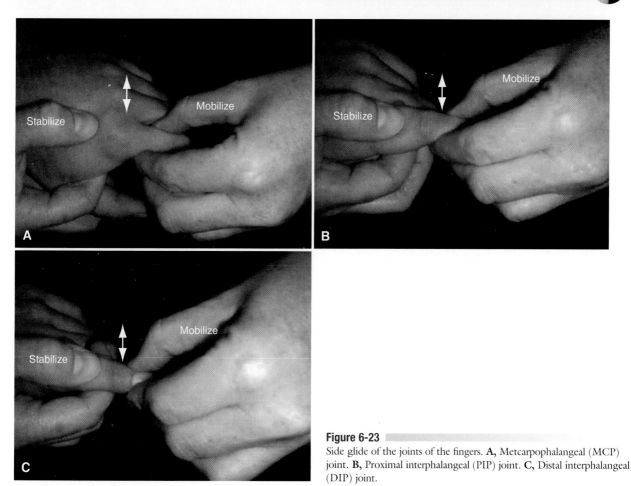

Figure 6-23
Side glide of the joints of the fingers. **A,** Metcarpophalangeal (MCP) joint. **B,** Proximal interphalangeal (PIP) joint. **C,** Distal interphalangeal (DIP) joint.

PATIENT POSITION	The patient may be sitting or supine.
EXAMINER POSITION	The examiner is adjacent to the patient's hand.
TEST PROCEDURE	The examiner positions the patient's forearm in supination or pronation. The examiner grasps the proximal bone between the index finger and thumb of one hand to stabilize it. The fingers of the other hand are placed around the distal segment of the joint to mobilize or move it. The examiner applies slight traction to the joint with the mobilizing hand to distract the joint surfaces and then moves the distal segment of the desired joint (metacarpophalangeal, proximal interphalangeal, or distal interphalangeal joint) sideways, keeping the joint surfaces parallel to one another to determine joint play and end feel.
INDICATIONS OF A POSITIVE TEST	The amount of movement obtained by the joint play is compared with that on the unaffected side. The test result is considered significant only if a difference is seen between the two sides. Pain on any of these joint play movements done in neutral, flexion, or extension may indicate a pathological condition in the joint between the two bones.
CLINICAL NOTES	• Excessive joint distraction affects the amount of side glide achieved. • The examiner must position both hands close to the joint line so that the motion tested reflects true joint play and not finger abduction or adduction.

References

1. Dutton M: *Orthopedic examination, evaluation and intervention,* New York, 2004, McGraw Hill.
2. Cooney WP: Tears of the triangular fibrocartilage of the wrist. In Cooney WP, Linscheid RL, Dobyns J (eds): *The wrist: diagnosis and operative treatment,* St Louis, 1998, Mosby.
3. Newland CC: Gamekeeper's thumb, *Orthop Clin North Am* 23:41-48, 1992.
4. Dobyns JH, Linschid RL, Chao EYS: Traumatic instability of the wrist, *American Academy of the Orthopaedic Surgeons Instructional Course Lectures,* 1975.
5. Tang JB: Carpal instability associated with fracture of the distal radius: incidence, influencing factors and pathomechanics, *Chin Med J (Engl)* 105:758-765, 1992.
6. Heyman P, Gelberman RH, Duncan K, Hipp JA: Injuries of the ulnar collateral ligament of the thumb metacarpophalangeal joint, *Clin Orthop* 292:165-171, 1993.
7. Heyman P: Injuries to the ulnar collateral ligament of the thumb metacarpophalangeal joint, *J Am Acad Orthop Surg* 5:224-229, 1997.
8. Shin AY, Battaglia MJ, Bishop AT: Lunotriquetral instability: diagnosis and treatment, *J Am Acad Orthop Surg* 8:170-179, 2000.
9. Post M: *Physical examination of the musculoskeletal system,* Chicago, 1987, Year Book Medical.
10. Taliesnik J: Soft tissue injuries of the wrist. In Strickland JW, Rettig AC (eds): *Hand injuries in athletes,* Philadelphia, 1992, Saunders.
11. Kleinman WB: The lunotriquetral shuck test, *Am Soc Surg Hand Corr News* 51, 1985.
12. Watson HK, Ballet FL: The SLAC wrist: scapulolunate advanced collapse pattern of degenerative arthritis, *J Hand Surg Am* 9:358-365, 1984.
13. Burton RI, Eaton RG: Common hand injuries in the athlete, *Orthop Clin North Am* 4:309-338, 1975.
14. Taleisnik J: Carpal instability, *J Bone Joint Surg Am* 70:1262-1268, 1988.
15. Watson HK, Ashmead D, Makhlouf MV: Examination of the scaphoid, *J Hand Surg Am* 13:657-660, 1988.
16. Skirven T: Clinical examination of the wrist, *J Hand Surg* 9:96-107, 1996.
17. Ilyas AM, Ast M, Schaffer AA et al: De Quervain tenosynovitis of the wrist, *J Am Acad Orthop Surg* 15:757-764, 2007.
18. Marnach ML, Ramin KD, Masey PS et al: Characterization of the relationship between joint laxity and maternal hormones in pregnancy, *Obstet Gynecol* 101:331-335, 2003.
19. Burks R: De Quervain's syndrome. In Sueki D, Brechter J (eds): *Orthopedic rehabilitation clinical advisor,* St Louis, 2010, Mosby.
20. Finkelstein H: Stenosing tendovaginitis at the radial styloid process, *J Bone Joint Surg* 12:509, 1930.
21. Johnstone AJ: Tennis elbow and upper limb tendinopathies, *Sports Med Arthro Rev* 8:69-79, 2000.
22. Atoshi I, Gummesson C, Johnsson R et al: Prevalence of carpal tunnel syndrome in a general population, *JAMA* 282:153-158, 1999.
23. de Krom MC, Kester AD, Knipschild PG et al: Risk factors for carpal tunnel syndrome, *Am J Epidemiol* 132:1102-1110, 1990.
24. Palmer KT, Harris EC, Coggon D: Carpal tunnel syndrome and its relation to occupation: a systematic literature review, *Occup Med (Lond)* 57:57-66, 2007.
25. Pratt N: Anatomy of nerve entrapment sites in the upper quarter, *J Hand Ther* 18:216-219, 2005.
26. Seitz WH, Matsuoka H, McAdoo J et al: Acute compression of the median nerve at the elbow by the lacertus fibrosis, *J Shoulder Elbow Surg* 16:91-94, 2007.
27. Leibovic SJ, Hasting H: Martin-Gruber revisited, *J Hand Surg* 17:47-53, 1992.
28. Rodriguez-Niedenfuhr M, Vazquez T, Parkin I et al: Martin-Gruber anastomosis revisited, *Clin Anat* 15:129-134, 2002.
29. Graham S: Median nerve entrapments. In Sueki D, Brechter J (eds): *Orthopedic rehabilitation clinical advisor,* St Louis, 2010, Mosby.
30. Prignac VW, Henry SM: The relationship among five common carpal tunnel syndrome tests and the severity of carpal tunnel syndrome, *J Hand Ther* 16:225-236, 2003.
31. Marx RG, Hudak PL, Bombarier C et al: The reliability of physical examination for carpal tunnel syndrome, *J Hand Surg Br* 23(4):499-502, 1998.
32. Kuhlman KA, Hennessey WJ: Sensitivity and specificity of carpal tunnel syndrome signs, *Am J Phys Med Rehabil* 76(6):451-457, 1997.
33. MacDermid JC, Kramer JF, McFarlane RM, Roth JH: Inter-rater agreement and accuracy of clinical tests used in diagnosis of carpal tunnel syndrome, *Work* 8:37-44, 1997.
34. Szabo RM, Slater RR, Farver TB et al: The value of diagnostic testing in carpal tunnel syndrome, *J Hand Surg Am* 24(4):704-714, 1999.
35. Buch-Jaeger N, Foucher G: Correlation of clinical signs with nerve conduction tests in the diagnosis of carpal tunnel syndrome, *J Hand Surg Br* 19(6):720-724, 1994.
36. Wiederien RC, Feldman TD, Heusel LD, et al: The effect of the median nerve compression test on median nerve conduction across the carpal tunnel, *Electromyogr Clin Neurophysiol* 42(7):413-421, 2002.
37. American Society for Surgery of the Hand: *The hand: examination and diagnosis,* Aurora, Colorado, 1978, The Society.
38. Allen EV: Thromboangiitis obliterans: methods of diagnosis of chronic occlusive arterial lesions distal to the wrist with illustrative cases, *Am J Med Sci* 178:237-244, 1929.

Thoracic Spine

Selected Movements
Active Movements
Costovertebral Expansion
Rib Motion
Passive Movements

Special Test for Neurological Dysfunction
Slump Test (Sitting Dural Stretch Test)

Précis of the Thoracic Spine Assessment*

History
Observation (standing)
Examination
    Active movements (standing or sitting)
        Forward flexion
        Extension
        Side flexion (left and right)
        Rotation (left and right)
        Costovertebral expansion
        Rib motion
        Combined movements (if necessary)
        Repetitive movements (if necessary)
        Sustained postures (if necessary)
    Passive movements (sitting)
        Forward flexion
        Extension
        Side flexion (left and right)
        Rotation (left and right)
    Resisted isometric movements (sitting)
        Forward flexion
        Extension
        Side flexion (left and right)
        Rotation (left and right)

Special test (sitting)
    Slump test
Reflexes and cutaneous distribution (sitting)
    Sensation scan
Special test (prone lying)
    Rib motion
Joint play movements (prone lying)
    Posteroanterior central vertebral pressure
    Posteroanterior unilateral vertebral pressure
    Transverse vertebral pressure
    Rib springing
Palpation (prone lying)
Palpation (supine lying)
Diagnostic imaging

*The précis is shown in an order that limits the amount of movement the patient must do but ensures that all necessary structures are tested. After any assessment, the patient should be warned that symptoms may be exacerbated by the assessment.

SELECTED MOVEMENTS

ACTIVE MOVEMENTS[1-3]

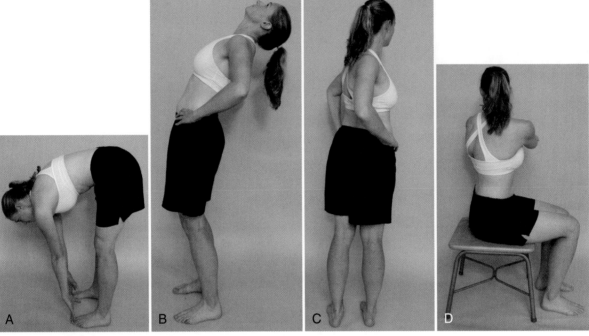

Figure 7–1

Active movement. **A,** Forward flexion. **B,** Extension. **C,** Rotation (standing). **D,** Rotation (sitting).

GENERAL INFORMATION   Movement in the thoracic spine is limited by the rib cage and the long spinous processes of the thoracic spine. When assessing the thoracic spine, the examiner should be sure to note whether the movement occurs in the spine (thoracic or lumbar) or in the hips. A patient can touch the toes with a completely rigid spine if the hip joints have sufficient range of motion (ROM). Likewise, tight hamstrings may alter the results. The thoracic movements may be done with the patient sitting to reduce or eliminate the effect of hip movement.

  If the patient history indicates that repetitive motion, sustained postures, or combined movements aggravate the symptoms, these movements also should be tested; however, this should be done only after the original movements of flexion, extension, side flexion, and rotation have been tested. Repetitive motion testing depends partly on the patient's *irritability* (i.e., the ease with which symptoms are aggravated). If the patient's symptoms are highly irritable (easily aggravated), repetitive motion testing is not advisable. Combined movements that may be tested in the thoracic spine include forward flexion and side bending, backward bending and side flexion, and lateral bending with flexion and lateral bending with extension. Any restriction of motion, excessive movement (hypermobility) or curve abnormality should be noted. Shoulder motion may be restricted if the upper thoracic segments or ribs are hypomobile.

ACTIVE MOVEMENTS[1-3]—cont'd

PATIENT POSITION The patient is standing or sitting.

EXAMINER POSITION The examiner is positioned directly in front or in back of the patient so as to instruct the patient and observe motion.

Forward Flexion

TEST PROCEDURE **Method 1.** Because the ROM at each vertebra is difficult to measure, the examiner can use a tape measure to derive an indication of overall movement. The examiner first measures the length of the spine from the C7 spinous process to the T12 spinous process with the patient in the normal standing posture. The patient then is asked to bend forward, and the spine is again measured.

Method 2. If the examiner wishes, the spine may be measured from the C7 to the S1 spinous processes with the patient in the normal standing position. The patient then is asked to bend forward, and the spine is again measured. In this case, the examiner is measuring movement in the lumbar spine as well as in the thoracic spine.

INDICATIONS OF A POSITIVE TEST The normal ROM of forward flexion (forward bending) in the thoracic spine is 20° to 45°.

Method 1: A difference of 2.7 cm (1.1 inch) in tape measure length (C7-T12) is considered normal.

Method 2: A difference of 10 cm (4 inches) in tape measure length (C7-S1) is considered normal, with most movement occurring between T12 and L1.

CLINICAL NOTES
- An alternative test method involves having the patient bend forward and try to touch the toes while keeping the knees straight. The examiner then measures from the fingertips to the floor and records the distance. With this method, the examiner must keep in mind that, in addition to the thoracic spine movement, movement also may occur in the lumbar spine and hips; in fact, movement could occur totally in the hips.
- Each of the methods described is indirect. Measurement of the ROM at each vertebral segment requires a series of radiographs. The examiner can decide which method to use. It is of primary importance, however, to note on the patient's chart how the measuring was done and which reference points were used.
- While the patient is flexed forward, the examiner can observe the spine from the "skyline" view. With nonstructural scoliosis, the scoliotic curve disappears on forward flexion; with structural scoliosis, it remains. With the skyline view, the examiner is looking for a hump on one side (convex side of the curve) and a hollow on the other side (concave side of the curve). This "hump and hollow" sequence is caused by vertebral rotation in idiopathic scoliosis, which pushes the ribs and muscles out on one side and causes the paravertebral valley on the opposite side. The vertebral rotation is most evident in the flexed position.
- When the patient flexes forward, the thoracic spine should curve forward in a smooth, even manner with no rotation or side flexion. The examiner should look for any apparent tightness or sharp angulation, such as a gibbus (hump) when the movement is performed. If the patient has an excessive kyphosis to begin with, very little forward flexion movement occurs in the thoracic spine.
- McKenzie[1] advocates testing flexion while the patient is sitting to reduce pelvic and hip movements. While sitting, the patient slouches forward, flexing the thoracic spine. The patient can put the hands around the neck to apply overpressure at the end of flexion. If symptoms arise from forward flexion on the spine with the neck flexed by the hands, the examiner should repeat the movement with the neck slightly extended and the hands removed. This can help differentiate between cervical and thoracic pain.

Continued

ACTIVE MOVEMENTS[1-3]—cont'd

Extension

TEST PROCEDURE

The examiner first measures the length of the spine from the C7 spinous process to the T12 spinous process with the patient in the normal standing posture. The patient then is asked to bend backward, and the spine is again measured. The examiner can use a tape measure and obtain the distance between the same two points (the C7 and T12 spinous processes).

INDICATIONS OF A POSITIVE TEST

Extension (backward bending) in the thoracic spine is normally 25° to 45°. A difference of 2.5 cm (1 inch) in tape measure length between standing and extension is considered normal.

CLINICAL NOTES

- Because extension occurs over 12 vertebrae, the movement between the individual vertebrae is difficult to detect visually.
- McKenzie[1] advocates having the patient place the hands in the small of the back to add stability while performing the backward movement or to do extension while the patient is sitting or in the prone-lying (sphinx) position.
- As the patient extends, the thoracic curve should curve backward or at least straighten in a smooth, even manner with no rotation or side flexion.
- Lee[2] advocates asking the patient to fully forward-flex the arms during extension to facilitate extension.
- The examiner should look for any apparent tightness or angulation when the movement is performed.
- If the patient shows excessive kyphosis, the kyphotic curvature remains on extension; that is, the thoracic spine remains flexed, whether the movement is tested while the patient is standing or lying prone.
- The test also may be done with the patient in the prone-lying position. If this position is used, the normal kyphotic posture should flatten. If it does not, the patient has a structural kyphosis.

Rotation

TEST PROCEDURE

The patient is asked to cross the arms in front or place the hands on opposite shoulders and then rotate to the right and left while the examiner looks at the amount of rotation, comparing the two directions.

INDICATIONS OF A POSITIVE TEST

Rotation in the thoracic spine is approximately 35° to 50°.

CLINICAL NOTE

- The examiner must remember that movement occurs in the lumbar spine and hips as well as in the thoracic spine.

Side Flexion

TEST PROCEDURE

The patient is asked to run a hand down the side of the leg as far as possible without bending forward or backward. The examiner then can estimate the angle of side flexion or use a tape measure to determine the distance from the fingertips to the floor and compare it with the findings on the other side.

ACTIVE MOVEMENTS[1-3]—cont'd

INDICATIONS OF A POSITIVE TEST   Side (lateral) flexion is approximately 20° to 40° to the right and left in the thoracic spine. Normally, the distances should be equal.

CLINICAL NOTES
- The examiner must remember that movement in the lumbar spine, as well as in the thoracic spine, is being measured with these movements.
- As the patient bends sideways, the spine should curve sideways in a smooth, even, sequential manner. The examiner should look for any tightness or abnormal angulation, which may indicate hypomobility or hypermobility at a specific segment when the movement is performed. On side flexion, if the ipsilateral paraspinal muscles tighten or their contracture is evident (Forestier's bowstring sign), ankylosing spondylitis or a pathological condition causing muscle spasm should be considered.

COSTOVERTEBRAL EXPANSION

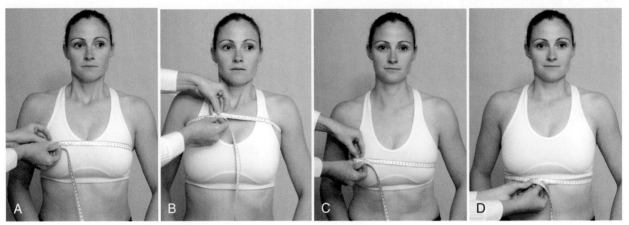

Figure 7–2
Costovertebral joint movement usually is determined by measuring chest expansion. **A,** Fourth lateral intercostal space. **B,** Axilla. **C,** Nipple line. **D,** Tenth rib.

TEST PROCEDURE   **Method 1.** Costovertebral joint movement usually is determined by measuring chest expansion. The examiner places the tape measure around the chest at the level of the fourth intercostal space. The patient is asked to exhale as much as possible, and the examiner takes a measurement. The patient then is asked to inhale as much as possible and to hold the breath while the second measurement is taken.

Method 2. Chest expansion also can be measured at three different levels. If this method is used, the examiner must take care to ensure that the levels of measurement are noted for consistency. The levels are (1) under the axillae for apical expansion, (2) at the nipple line or xiphisternal junction for midthoracic expansion, and (3) at the T10 rib level for lower thoracic expansion. The measurements are taken after expiration and inspiration.

INDICATIONS OF A POSITIVE TEST   The normal difference between inspiration and expiration is 3 to 7.5 cm (1 to 3 inches).

CLINICAL NOTES/CAUTIONS
- After chest expansion has been measured, it is worthwhile to have the patient take a deep breath and cough so that the examiner can determine whether this action causes or alters any pain. If it does, the examiner may suspect a respiratory-related problem or a condition that is increasing intrathecal pressure in the spine.
- Evjenth and Gloeck[3] have noted a way to differentiate thoracic spine and rib pain during movement. If pain is present on flexion, the patient is returned to neutral and asked to take a deep breath and hold it. While holding the breath, the patient flexes until pain is felt. At this point, the patient stops flexing and exhales. If further flexion can be accomplished after the exhale, the problem is more likely to be the ribs than the thoracic spine. Extension can be tested in a similar fashion.

RIB MOTION[4,5]

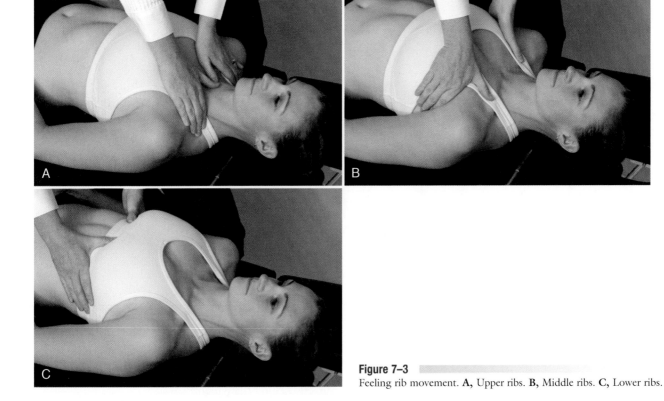

Figure 7–3
Feeling rib movement. **A,** Upper ribs. **B,** Middle ribs. **C,** Lower ribs.

PURPOSE	To assess rib mobility in the thoracic spine.

Rib Movement During Respiration

PATIENT POSITION	The patient is supine.
EXAMINER POSITION	The examiner stands adjacent to the patient's thoracic region.
TEST PROCEDURE	The examiner's hands are placed in a relaxed fashion over the upper chest. In this position, the examiner is feeling anteroposterior movement of the ribs. To test lateral movement of the ribs, the examiner's hands are placed around the sides of the rib cage approximately 45° to the vertical axis of the patient's body. The patient is instructed to inhale and exhale normally. As the patient inhales and exhales, the examiner should compare the two sides to see whether the movement is equal. Any restriction or difference in motion should be noted. The examiner then moves the hands down the patient's chest, testing the movement in the middle and lower ribs in a similar fashion.
INDICATIONS OF A POSITIVE TEST	If a rib stops moving relative to the other ribs on inhalation, it is classified as a depressed rib. If a rib stops moving relative to the other ribs on exhalation, it is classified as an elevated rib. The examiner must keep in mind that restriction of one rib affects the adjacent ribs.
CLINICAL NOTES/CAUTIONS	• If a depressed rib is implicated, the highest restricted rib usually is the one that causes the greatest problem. If an elevated rib is present, the lowest restricted rib usually is the one that causes the greatest problem. • Rib dysfunctions may be categorized as structural, torsional, or respiratory.

Continued

RIB MOTION[4,5]—*cont'd*

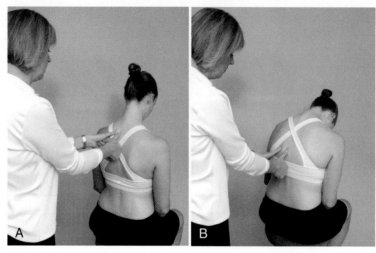

Figure 7–4

Testing the mobility of the rib relative to the thoracic vertebra. Note that one thumb is on the transverse process of the vertebra, and the other thumb is on the rib. **A,** Upper ribs. **B,** Lower ribs.

Rib Movement Relative to the Thoracic Spine

PATIENT POSITION	The patient is sitting.
EXAMINER POSITION	The examiner sits or kneels directly behind the patient.
TEST PROCEDURE	The examiner places one thumb or finger on the transverse process and the thumb of the other hand just lateral to the tubercle of the rib. The goal is to palpate and test the rib and transverse process of the same spinal segment. The patient is asked to forward-flex the head (for the upper thoracic spine) and the thorax (for the lower thoracic spine) while the examiner feels the movement of the rib.
INDICATIONS OF A POSITIVE TEST	Normally, on forward movement, the rib rotates anteriorly and the rib tubercle stays at the same level as the transverse process. If the rib is hypermobile, it elevates relative to the transverse process. If the rib is hypomobile, its motion stops before the thoracic spine.
CLINICAL NOTES	• Extension may be tested in a similar fashion, but the rib rotates posteriorly.
	• To test lateral movement of the ribs, the examiner begins at the level of the axilla and works down the lateral aspect of the ribs, feeling the movement of the ribs during inspiration and expiration and noting any restriction.

PASSIVE MOVEMENTS

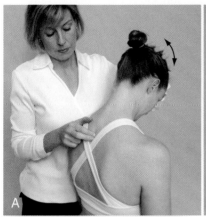

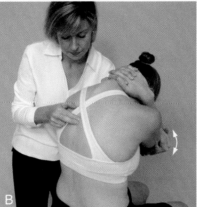

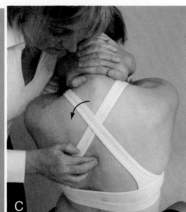

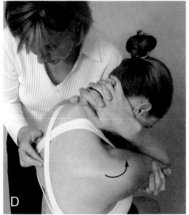

Figure 7–5

Passive movements of the thoracic spine. **A,** Upper thoracic spine. **B,** Middle and lower thoracic spine. **C,** Passive side flexion of the thoracic spine. **D,** Passive rotation of the thoracic spine.

PATIENT POSITION	**Upper thoracic spine (C5-T3):** The patient is seated with the arms by the side.
	Lower thoracic spine (T3 and T11): The patient is seated with the fingers clasped behind the neck and the elbows together in front.
EXAMINER POSITION	The examiner stands beside or behind the patient.
TEST PROCEDURE	**Upper thoracic spine (C5-T3).** The examiner places one hand on the patient's forehead or on top of the head. With the other hand, the examiner palpates over and between the spinous processes of the lower cervical and upper thoracic spines, feeling for movement between the spinous processes. To test the movement properly, the examiner places the middle finger in the space (interspace) between two spinous processes. The index and ring fingers are placed over two adjacent spinous processes. The examiner then flexes, extends, side-flexes, and rotates the patient's head while palpating for movement in the interspace. The examiner should feel the movement occurring, assess its quality, and note whether the movement is hypomobile or hypermobile relative to the adjacent vertebrae.
	Lower thoracic spine (T3 and T11). The examiner places one hand and arm around the patient's elbows while palpating over and between the spinous processes, as previously described. The examiner then flexes and extends the spine by

Continued

lifting and lowering the patient's elbows. Side flexion and rotation of the trunk may be performed in a similar fashion to test these movements. The patient sits with the hands clasped behind the head. The examiner uses the thumb on one side of the spinous process and/or the index finger and/or the middle finger on the other side to palpate just lateral to the interspinous space. For side flexion, the examiner moves the patient into right side flexion and then left side flexion and by palpation compares the amount and quality of right and left movement, including adjacent segments. For rotation, the examiner rotates the patient's shoulders to the right or left, comparing by palpation the amount and quality of movement of each segment and that of adjacent segments.

INDICATIONS OF A POSITIVE TEST

Hypomobility or hypermobility of the tested motion segment, compared with adjacent spinal segments, indicates a positive test result.

CLINICAL NOTES

- Because passive movements in the thoracic spine are difficult to perform in a gross fashion, the movement between each pair of vertebrae may be assessed.
- When the spinous processes are palpated, if one process appears to be out of alignment, the examiner can palpate the transverse processes on each side and compare them with the levels above and below to determine whether the vertebra is truly rotated or side-flexed. For example, if the spinous process of T5 is shifted to the right and if rotation has occurred at that level, the left transverse process would be more superficial posteriorly, whereas the right one would appear deeper. Spinous processes commonly are structurally abnormal, and as a result, the process may be deformed to the right or to the left. In this case the spinal segment would appear rotated, but in reality, the spinous process is structurally deformed. If the spinous process rotation is an anomaly, the transverse processes would be equal, as would the ribs.
- Palpating the transverse processes while the patient does passive or active movement of the spine helps indicate abnormal movement when the two sides are compared or when one level is compared with another. If the alignment is normal to begin with and becomes abnormal with movement or if it is abnormal to begin with and becomes normal with movement, this indicates a functional asymmetry rather than a structural one. Generally, a structural asymmetry remains through all movements.

SPECIAL TEST FOR NEUROLOGICAL DYSFUNCTION

Relevant Special Test

Slump test (sitting dural stretch test)

Definition

Classically, neurological testing has been divided into two categories: tests that assess the function of the nerve and its ability to conduct neural impulses, and tests that assess the mobility of the nerve. Tests of nerve function in the thoracic spine are not commonplace. Tests that assess the patency of thoracic spinal nerve roots are not part of a normal spine examination. Entrapment of the spinal cord in the thoracic spine can be assessed through reflex testing, assessment of spasticity and clonus, or Babinski testing of the lower extremity. The mobility of the spinal cord, the associated thoracic nerve roots, and the sympathetic nervous system as it travels through the thoracic spine can be assessed through neural mobility testing.

Suspected Injury

Thoracic disc herniation
Thoracic compression fracture
T4 syndrome
Thoracic spine hypomobility or hypermobility

Epidemiology and Demographics

Thoracic disc herniation. The thoracic spine is reported to be the spinal region least likely to experience a disc herniation. The thoracic spine has been reported to account for 0.25% to 5% of intervertebral disc herniations. One in 1 million patients experiences symptoms of thoracic disc herniation every year. Of these patients, 2% have herniation at the lower thoracic spine (T11-T12), and 70% have herniation in a posterolateral direction. The age range for thoracic disc herniation has been reported to be 11 to 82 years, with a peak age of 40 to 50 years. The condition appears to occur more often in men than in women.[6-9]

Thoracic compression fracture. Spinal compression fractures occur in more than 750,000 people a year in the United States. About two thirds of spinal compression fractures are never diagnosed, because many patients and families think that back pain is merely a sign of aging and arthritis. Compression fractures are more prevalent in two groups of patients: the elderly, because of osteoporosis and an increased risk of falls; and young adults, as a result of trauma, such as motor vehicle accidents or a fall from a great height.[10,11]

T4 syndrome. The prevalence of this pathological condition is unknown. Those most prone to development of the syndrome are individuals over 35 years of age. The gender and cultural prevalence also are unknown.[12-14]

Relevant History

The patient history varies, depending on the associated pathological condition. Patients may have a prior history of trauma to the thoracic spine. Trauma such as a fall onto the buttock also may be reported. Many patients with thoracic compression fractures or disc herniations report that their symptoms began after lifting a heavy object while in flexion. Other precipitating activities include coughing or sneezing. Patients with a history of osteoporosis, asthma, pulmonary dysfunction, or respiratory illness may be predisposed to injury in the thoracic region.

Relevant Signs and Symptoms

Thoracic disc herniation. Disc herniations in the thoracic spine may be asymptomatic. However, patients may complain of intermittent backache, thoracic root pain and paresthesia, and/or spinal cord compression symptoms.

Thoracic compression fracture. A patient with a thoracic compression fracture may complain of pain in the thoracic region over the affected vertebra. The symptoms may be described as severe, sharp, and exacerbated by motion. Pain is noted when the person lifts and carries objects or with breathing. The patient may or may not have signs of cord compression, depending on the magnitude of injury.

T4 syndrome. Patients with T4 syndrome complain of unilateral or bilateral paresthesia in all five hand digits, or in the whole hand, or in the forearm and hand (i.e., glove type [long/short]). The hands may feel hot or cold, swelling may be present, and the patient may complain that the arms feel heavy. Aches and pains may be present in a nondermatomal pattern. The patient may complain that the pain feels like a tight band around the arms. The person also may complain of a combination of neck, upper thoracic, and cranial pain, without abnormal neurological signs.

Mechanism of Injury

Injury to the thoracic spine can be varied and diverse. Several factors make the thoracic spine susceptible to neural entrapment. First, it is considered the "watershed" area of the spine; that is, it has a very poor blood supply. From a clinical perspective, this means that injured tissue in this region takes longer to heal and recover. The second factor that makes the thoracic spine an area for injury and neural entrapment is the fact that the spinal canal of the thoracic spine is smaller in diameter then that of the cervical or lumbar region. Therefore, a lesion in the spine that protrudes into the thoracic canal has a greater impact on spinal cord mobility than a lesion of equal size in the cervical or lumbar spine. It also has been hypothesized that the impact of the thoracic spine on nerve mobility extends beyond the mobility of the spinal cord or the thoracic spinal nerve roots. Preliminary evidence suggests that the sympathetic nervous system may play a role in limiting nerve mobility. The bulk of the sympathetic nervous system runs within the thoracic spine. Some have hypothesized that limited mobility of the sympathetic nervous system also could affect nerve movement and mobility.

SLUMP TEST (SITTING DURAL STRETCH TEST)[15-17]

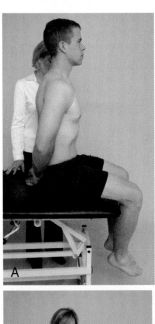
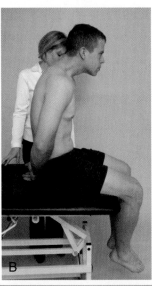
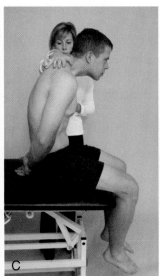
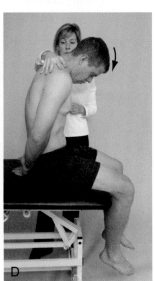

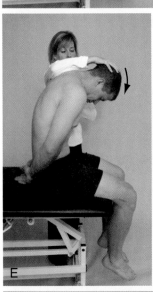
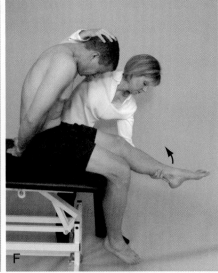

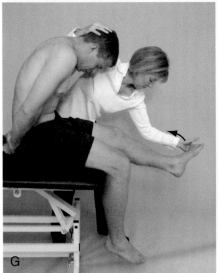
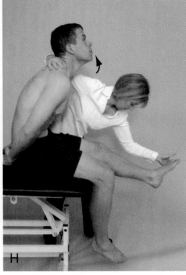

Figure 7–6

Sequence of subject postures in the slump test. **A,** The patient sits erect with the hands behind the back. **B,** The patient slumps the lumbar and thoracic spine while either the patient or the examiner keeps the head in neutral. **C,** The examiner pushes down on the shoulders while the patient holds the head in neutral. **D,** The patient flexes the head. **E,** The examiner carefully applies overpressure to the cervical spine. **F,** The examiner extends the patient's knee while holding the cervical spine flexed. **G,** While holding the knee extended and the cervical spine flexed, the examiner dorsiflexes the foot. **H,** The patient extends the head, which should relieve any symptoms. If symptoms are reproduced at any stage, further sequential movements are not attempted.

SLUMP TEST (SITTING DURAL STRETCH TEST)[15,17]—cont'd

PURPOSE	To assess for impingement of the dura and spinal cord or nerve roots.
PATIENT POSITION	The patient sits on the edge of the examining table with the legs supported, the hips in neutral position (i.e., no rotation, abduction, or adduction), and the hands behind the back. In this position, the patient should have no symptoms.
EXAMINER POSITION	The examiner sits or stands directly adjacent to the patient so as to control head and lower extremity motion.
TEST PROCEDURE	The examination is performed in sequential steps. First, the patient is asked to "slump" the back into thoracic and lumbar flexion. The examiner maintains the patient's chin in the neutral position to prevent neck and head flexion. If no symptoms are produced, the examiner places one hand on the patient's head and neck to control cervical and upper thoracic motion. The examiner then uses the same arm that has the hand resting on the head to apply overpressure across the shoulders to maintain flexion of the thoracic and lumbar spines. While this position is held, the patient is asked to actively flex the cervical spine and head as far as possible (i.e., chin to chest). The examiner then applies overpressure to maintain the cervical flexion of all three parts of the spine (cervical, thoracic, and lumbar) using the hand of the same arm to maintain overpressure in the cervical spine. Provided there are no symptoms, starting with the normal leg, the examiner's other hand is placed on the patient's foot or lower extremity to control lower extremity motion. The examiner then extends the patient's knee. If that does not produce symptoms, the examiner takes the patient's foot into maximum dorsiflexion. The test is repeated with the affected leg and then with both legs at the same time.
INDICATIONS OF A POSITIVE TEST	Symptoms of sciatic pain or reproduction of the patient's symptoms indicates a positive test result, implicating impingement of the dura and spinal cord or nerve roots.
CLINICAL NOTES	• The uninvolved leg is always tested before the involved leg. • Butler[16] suggested that when the thoracic spine is tested with the patient in the slump position, trunk rotation left and right should be added to increase the stress on the intercostal nerves. • With a positive test result, pain usually is produced at the site of the lesion. • If bilateral symptoms are produced, the examiner must consider a myelopathy.
RELIABILITY/SPECIFICITY/ SENSITIVITY[17]	Reliability (interrater) range: k = 0.83-0.89

References

1. McKenzie RA: *The cervical and thoracic spine: mechanical diagnosis and therapy,* Waikanae, New Zealand, 1981, Spinal Publications.

2. Lee D: *Manual therapy for the thorax: a biomechanical approach,* Delta, BC, 1994, DOPC.

3. Evjenth O, Gloeck C: *Symptoms localization in the spine and the extremity joints,* Minneapolis, 2000, OPTP.

4. Stoddard A: *Manual of osteopathic technique,* London, 1959, Hutchinson Medical Publications.

5. Bookhout MR: Evaluation of the thoracic spine and rib cage. In Flynn TW (ed): *The thoracic spine and rib cage,* Boston, 1996, Butterworth-Heinemann.

6. Arce CA, Dohrmann GJ: Herniated thoracic discs, *Neurosurg Clin* 3:392, 1985.

7. Levi N, Gjerris F, Dons K: Thoracic disc herniation, *J Neurosurg* 88:148-150, 1998.

8. Mellion LR, Ladeira CE: The herniated thoracic disc: a review of the literature, *J Man Manip Ther* 9:154-163, 2001.

9. Whitcomb DC, Martin SP, Schoen RE, Jho HD: Chronic abdominal pain caused by thoracic disk herniation, *Am J Gastroenterol* 90:835-837, 1995.

10. Cooper C, Atkinson EJ, O'Fallon WM, Melton LJ: Incidence of clinically diagnosed vertebral fractures: a population-based study in Rochester, Minnesota, 1985-1989, *J Bone Miner Res* 7:221-227, 1992.

11. Melton LJ, Kan SH, Frye MA et al: Epidemiology of vertebral fractures in women, *Am J Epidemiol* 129: 1000-1011, 1989.

12. Conroy J, Schneiders A: The T4 syndrome, *Man Ther* 10:292-296, 2005.

13. DeFranca GG, Levine LJ: The T4 syndrome, *J Manip Physiol Ther* 18:34-37, 1995.

14. Evans P: The T4 syndrome: some basic science aspects, *Physiotherapy* 83:186-189, 1997.

15. Maitland GD: The slump test: examination and treatment, *Aust J Physiother* 31:215-219, 1985.

16. Butler DS: *Mobilization of the nervous system,* Melbourne, 1991, Churchill Livingstone.

17. Philip K, Lew P, Matyas TA: The inter-therapist reliability of the slump test, *Austr J Phys Ther* 35(2): 89-94, 1989.

LUMBAR SPINE

Précis of the Lumbar Spine Assessment*

History (sitting)
Observation (standing)
Examination
Active movements (standing)
　　Forward flexion
　　Extension
　　Side flexion (left and right)
　　Rotation (left and right)
　　Quick test (if possible)
　　Trendelenburg's test and S1 nerve root test (modified Trendelenburg's test)
Passive movements (only with care and caution)
Peripheral joint scan (standing)
　　Sacroiliac joints
Special tests (standing)
　　H and I stability test
　　Quadrant test
　　One leg standing lumbar extension test
Resisted isometric movements (sitting)
　　Forward flexion
　　Extension
　　Side flexion (left and right)
　　Rotation (left and right)
Special tests (sitting)
　　Slump test
　　Test of posterior lumbar spine instability
　　Sitting root test
Resisted isometric movements (supine lying)
　　Isometric abdominal test
　　Dynamic abdominal endurance test
　　Internal/external abdominal obliques test
　　Double straight leg lowering
　　Dynamic horizontal side support (side bridge or side plank) test
Peripheral joint scan (supine lying)
　　Hip joints (flexion, abduction, adduction, and medial and lateral rotation)
　　Knee joints (flexion and extension)
　　Ankle joints (dorsiflexion and plantar flexion)
　　Foot joints (supination, pronation)
　　Toe joints (flexion, extension)
Myotomes (supine lying)
　　Hip flexion (L2)
　　Knee extension (L3)
　　Ankle dorsiflexion (L4)

　　Toe extension (L5)
　　Ankle eversion or plantar flexion (S1)
Special tests (supine lying)
　　Straight leg raise test and its variants
　　Bowstring test (Cram test or popliteal pressure sign)
　　Sign of the buttock
Reflexes and cutaneous distribution (anterior and side aspects)
Palpation (supine lying)
Resisted isometric movements (side lying)
　　Horizontal side support
Special tests (side lying)
　　Femoral nerve traction test
　　Test of anterior lumbar spine stability
　　Specific lumbar spine torsion test
Joint play movements (side lying)
　　Flexion
Peripheral joint scan (prone lying)
　　Hip joints (extension, medial and lateral rotation)
Myotomes (prone lying)
　　Hip extension (S1)
　　Knee flexion (S1-S2)
Resisted isometric movements (prone lying)
　　Dynamic extensor test
　　Isometric extensor test
Special tests (prone lying)
　　Prone knee bending test
Reflexes and cutaneous distribution (prone lying)
Reflexes and cutaneous distribution (posterior aspect)
Joint play movements (prone lying)
　　Posterior-anterior central vertebral pressure (PACVP)
　　Posterior-anterior unilateral vertebral pressure (PAUVP)
　　Transverse vertebral pressure (TVP)
Palpation (prone lying)
Resisted isometric movements (quadriped position)
　　Back rotators/multifidus test
Diagnostic imaging

---

*The assessment is shown in an order that limits the amount of movement the patient must do but ensures that all necessary structures are tested. After any assessment, the patient should be warned that symptoms may be exacerbated by the assessment.

SELECTED MOVEMENTS

ACTIVE MOVEMENTS

DVD

GENERAL INFORMATION

The range of motion (ROM) that occurs during active movement is the summation of the movements of the entire lumbar spine, not just movement at one level, along with hip movement. If the problem is mechanical, one or more of the movements will be painful.

While the patient is doing the active movements, the examiner looks for limitation of movement and possible causes, such as pain, spasm, stiffness, or blocking. If the patient reports that a sustained position increases the symptoms, the examiner should consider having the patient maintain the position (e.g., flexion) at the end of the ROM for 10 to 20 seconds to see whether the symptoms increase. Likewise, if the patient history indicates that repetitive motion or combined movements cause symptoms, these movements should be performed, but only after the patient has completed the basic movements.

The greatest motion in the lumbar spine occurs between the L4 and L5 vertebrae and between L5 and S1. Considerable individual variability is seen in the ROM of the lumbar spine. In fact, little obvious movement occurs in the lumbar spine, especially in the individual segments, because of the shape of the facet joints, the tightness of the ligaments, the presence of the intervertebral discs, and the size of the vertebral bodies.

McKenzie[1] recommended repeating the active movements, especially flexion and extension, 10 times to see whether the movement increases or decreases the symptoms.

If the examiner finds that side flexion and rotation are equally limited and extension is limited to a lesser extent, a capsular pattern may be suspected. A capsular pattern in one lumbar segment, however, is difficult to detect.

Because back injuries rarely occur during a "pure" movement, such as flexion, extension, side flexion, or rotation, some have suggested that combined movements of the spine should be included in the examination. The examiner may want to test the more habitual combined movements, such as lateral flexion in flexion, lateral flexion in extension, flexion and rotation, and extension and rotation. These combined movements may cause signs and symptoms different from those produced by single-plane movements, and they definitely are indicated if the patient has shown that symptoms are caused by a combined movement. For example, if the patient has a facet syndrome, combined extension and rotation is the movement most likely to exacerbate symptoms. Other symptoms that indicate facet involvement include absence of radicular signs or neurological deficit, hip and buttock pain, and sometimes leg pain above the knee, no paresthesia, and low back stiffness.

Testing of active ROM depends on the irritability of the patient. Full motion testing and combined or repetitive motion testing can be performed on patients who are not irritable. Patients whose pain is easily produced and who remain in pain for some time once the pain is produced should undergo a limited ROM test. Motion should be tested just until the onset of symptoms, and the painful directions of motion should be tested last.

PATIENT POSITION

The patient is standing.

EXAMINER POSITION

The examiner is positioned directly in front or in back of the patient so as to instruct the patient and observe motion.

Continued

ACTIVE MOVEMENTS—*cont'd*

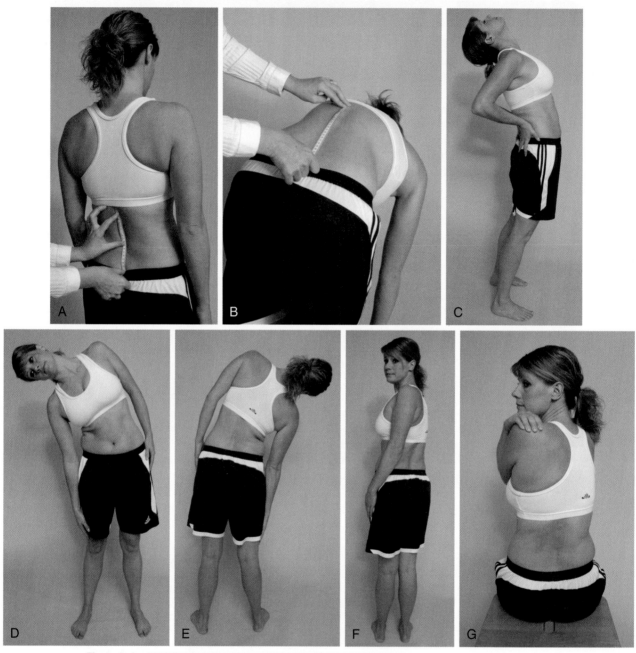

Figure 8–1
Active movements of the lumbar spine. **A** and **B,** Measuring forward flexion with a tape measure.
C, Extension. **D,** Side flexion (anterior view). **E,** Side flexion (posterior view). **F,** Rotation (standing).
G, Rotation (sitting).

ACTIVE MOVEMENTS—cont'd

Forward Flexion

TEST PROCEDURE

The patient is asked to bend forward and to try to touch the toes while keeping the knees straight. The examiner may use a tape measure to measure the increase in the distance between L1 spinous process and S1 on forward flexion. The examiner should note how far forward the patient is able to bend (i.e., to the midthigh, knees, midtibia, or floor).

INDICATIONS OF A POSITIVE TEST

For flexion (forward bending), the maximum ROM in the lumbar spine normally is 40° to 60°. If a tape measure is used, the measurement should increase about 7.5 cm (3 inches) if taken between the T12 spinous process and S1.

CLINICAL NOTES/CAUTIONS

- On forward flexion, the lumbar spine should move from its normal lordotic curvature to at least a straight or slightly flexed curve. If this change does not occur, some hypomobility probably is present in the lumbar spine either from tight structures or muscle spasm.
- In a patient with no back pain, when returning to the upright posture from forward flexion, the person first rotates the hips and pelvis to about 45° of flexion; during the last 45° of extension, the low back resumes its lordosis.
- In a patient with back pain, most movement usually occurs in the hips, accompanied by knee flexion; in some cases, the patient also uses hand support, working up the thighs.
- The examiner must differentiate the movement that occurs in the lumbar spine from that occurring in the hips or thoracic spine. Some patients can touch their toes by flexing the hips, even if no movement occurs in the spine. The degree of injury also has an effect. For example, the more severely a disc is injured (e.g., if sequestration has occurred rather than a protrusion), the greater is the limitation of movement.
- Often, an "instability jog" may be seen during one or more movements, especially flexion, returning to neutral from flexion, or side flexion. An instability jog is a sudden movement shift or rippling of the muscles during active movement, which indicates an unstable segment.
- Similarly, muscle twitching during movement or complaints of something "slipping out" during lumbar spine movement may indicate instability.
- If the patient bends one or both knees on forward flexion, the examiner should watch for nerve root symptoms or tight hamstrings, especially if spinal flexion is decreased when the knees are straight.

Extension

TEST PROCEDURE

The patient is asked to bend backward. While performing the movement, the patient should place the hands in the small of the back to help stabilize it.

INDICATIONS OF A POSITIVE TEST

Extension (backward bending) normally is limited to 20° to 35° in the lumbar spine.

CLINICAL NOTE

- Bourdillon and Day[2] recommend having the patient do this movement in the prone-lying position to hyperextend the spine. They called the resulting position the "sphinx position." The patient hyperextends the spine by resting on the elbows with the hands holding the chin and allows the abdominal wall to relax. The position is held for 10 to 20 seconds to see whether symptoms occur or worsen if already present.

Continued

ACTIVE MOVEMENTS—*cont'd*

Rotation

TEST PROCEDURE	The patient is instructed to rotate, or turn, to the left and then to the right, or vice versa, depending on which is the painful side (the painful side is tested last).
INDICATIONS OF A POSITIVE TEST	Rotation in the lumbar spine normally is 3° to 18° to the left or right is accomplished by a shearing movement of the lumbar vertebrae on each other.
CLINICAL NOTE	• Although the patient usually is in the standing position, rotation may be performed while the patient is sitting to eliminate or decrease pelvic and hip movement. If the patient stands, the examiner must take care to watch for this accessory movement and try to eliminate it by stabilizing the pelvis.

Side Flexion

TEST PROCEDURE	The patient is asked to run a hand down the side of the leg and not to bend forward or backward while performing the movement. The examiner can eyeball the movement and compare it with that on the other side. The distance from the fingertips to the floor also may be measured on both sides, and any difference should be noted.
INDICATIONS OF A POSITIVE TEST	Side (lateral) flexion, or side bending, is approximately 15° to 20° in the lumbar spine. As the patient side-flexes, the examiner should watch the lumbar curve. Normally, the lumbar curve forms a smooth curve on side flexion, and there should be no obvious sharp angulation at only one level. If angulation does occur, it may indicate hypomobility below the level or hypermobility above the level in the lumbar spine.
CLINICAL NOTES/CAUTIONS	• If a movement (e.g., side flexion) toward the painful side increases the symptoms, the lesion is probably intra-articular, because the muscles and ligaments on that side are relaxed.
	• If a disc protrusion is present and lateral to the nerve root, side flexion to the painful side increases the pain and radicular symptoms on that side.
	• If a movement (e.g., side flexion) away from the painful side alters the symptoms, the lesion may be articular or muscular in origin, or it may be a disc protrusion medial to the nerve root.
	• In the spine, the movement of side flexion is a coupled movement with rotation. Because of the position of the lumbar facet joints, side flexion and rotation occur together, although the amount and direction of movement may not be the same.
	• Patients often deviate into forward flexion instead of remaining in true side flexion. To prevent this, the patient can be cued to run the hand down the back of the thigh instead of the side of the thigh.

TRENDELENBURG'S TEST (MODIFIED)

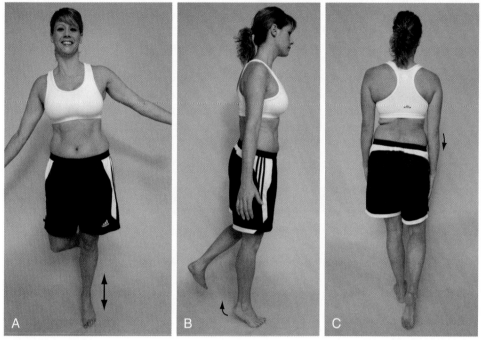

Figure 8–2

Trendelenburg's/S1 nerve root test. **A,** Anterior view, negative test result. **B,** Side view, negative test result. **C,** Posterior view, positive test result for a weak right gluteus medius.

PURPOSE	To assess for gluteus medius weakness or coxa vara; this test also may be used to assess for S1 nerve root lesions.
PATIENT POSITION	The patient stands, unsupported.
EXAMINER POSITION	The examiner is positioned so as to view the patient's pelvic position.
TEST PROCEDURE	The patient is asked to balance on one leg and to go up and down on the toes four or five times.
INDICATIONS OF A POSITIVE TEST	While the patient balances on one leg, the examiner watches for Trendelenburg's sign. A positive Trendelenburg sign is indicated if the ilium on the nonstance side drops instead of elevating, as it normally would when a person is standing on one leg. If the nonstance side drops, it is a positive test for a weak gluteus medius on the stance side. Both legs are tested. If the patient is unable to go up and down on the toes four or five times, the examiner should suspect an S1 nerve root lesion.
CLINICAL NOTES	• This is, in effect, a modified Trendelenburg's test. A weak gluteus medius muscle or a coxa vara (abnormal shaft-neck angle of the femur) on the stance leg side may produce a positive sign on the nonstance side.
	• The examiner should look for patient compensations when completing the test. The most common compensation is trunk side flexion toward the stance leg. The patient side flexes to move his or her center of gravity over the stance leg, thus decreasing the demand on the gluteus medius. Therefore, the test may appear normal because the ilium responds normally, but if the side flexion is corrected, the positive response occurs.

ADVANCED RESISTED MOVEMENTS OF THE LUMBAR SPINE

GENERAL INFORMATION Provided neutral resisted isometric testing in sitting is normal or causes only a small amount of pain, the examiner can go on to other tests that place greater stress on the muscles. These tests often are dynamic and provide both concentric and eccentric work for the muscles supporting the spine. With all of the following tests, the examiner should make sure the patient can hold a neutral pelvis before doing that test. If excessive movement of the anterior superior iliac spines (ASISs) (supine) or posterior superior iliac spines (PSISs) (prone) is noted when the patient does any of the movements, the tests should be stopped. In normal individuals, the ASIS or PSIS does not move during these tests. Motivation may also affect the results.[3]

ISOMETRIC ABDOMINAL TEST[4-7]

DVD

PURPOSE To assess the endurance of the abdominal muscles.

PATIENT POSITION The patient is supine with the hips at 45°, the knees at 90°, and the hands at the sides. Both feet rest flat on the table.

EXAMINER POSITION The examiner is positioned so as to observe for altered mechanics.

TEST PROCEDURE The patient starts the test in the patient position noted above. The examiner then sequentially asks the patient to move to the end position of each level of testing. The patient is instructed to hold the end position for as long as possible. Testing begins with the Trace Grade and progresses sequentially to the Normal Grade (see Table 8-1).

INDICATIONS OF A POSITIVE TEST The number of seconds the patient holds the contraction before cheating (e.g., holding the breath, altered mechanics) or the onset of fatigue is recorded as the manual muscle test (MMT) score. The grading for this isometric abdominal test is described in Table 8-1.

RELIABILITY/SPECIFICITY/ SENSITIVITY[5] Reliability (interrater) ICC = 0.25

Table 8-1
Isometric Abdominal Test Grading

Grade	MMT Score	Patient Position
Normal	5	With the hands clasped behind the neck, able to raise the upper body until the scapulae clear the table (20- to 30-second hold)
Good	4	With the arms crossed over the chest, able to raise the upper body until the scapulae clear the table (15- to 20-second hold)
Fair	3	With the arms straight, able to raise the upper body until the scapulae clear the table (10- to 15-second hold)
Poor	2	With the arms extended toward the knees, able to raise the upper body until the top of the scapulae lift from the table (1- to 10-second hold)
Trace	1	Unable to raise more than the head off the table

MMT, Manual muscle test.

ISOMETRIC ABDOMINAL TEST[4-7]—cont'd

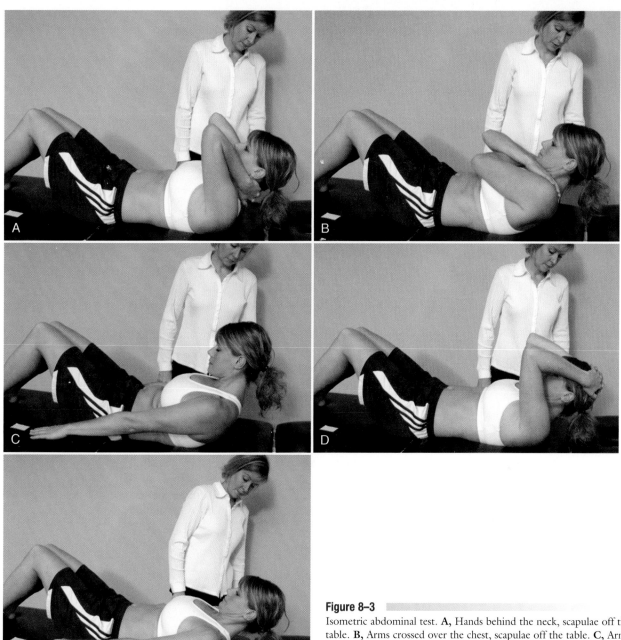

Figure 8–3

Isometric abdominal test. **A,** Hands behind the neck, scapulae off the table. **B,** Arms crossed over the chest, scapulae off the table. **C,** Arms straight, scapulae off the table. **D,** Hands behind the head, only the head off the table. **E,** Arms straight, only the head off the table.

DYNAMIC ABDOMINAL ENDURANCE TEST[5,8]

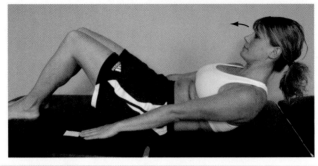

Figure 8–4
Dynamic abdominal endurance test. The patient tucks in the chin and curls up the trunk, lifting the trunk off the bed. Ideally, the scapulae should clear the bed.

PURPOSE	To assess the endurance of the abdominal muscles.
PATIENT POSITION	The patient lies supine with the hips at 45°, the knees at 90°, and the hands at the sides. The feet are flat on the table.
EXAMINER POSITION	The examiner is positioned so as to observe for altered mechanics.
TEST PROCEDURE	A line is drawn 8 cm (patients over age 40) or 12 cm (patients under age 40) distal to the fingers. The patient tucks in the chin and curls (flexes) the trunk to touch the line with the fingers and repeats as many curls as possible using a cadence of 25 repetitions per minute.
INDICATIONS OF A POSITIVE TEST	The number of repetitions possible before cheating (e.g., holding the breath, altered mechanics) or the onset of fatigue is recorded as the score.
CLINICAL NOTE/CAUTION	• This test places significant stress upon the lumbar discs, so if disc pathology is suspected, the examiner should consider whether it is advisable to do the test.
RELIABILITY/SPECIFICITY/ SENSITIVITY[5]	Interrater ICC = 0.78

ISOMETRIC EXTENSOR TEST[5,9,10]

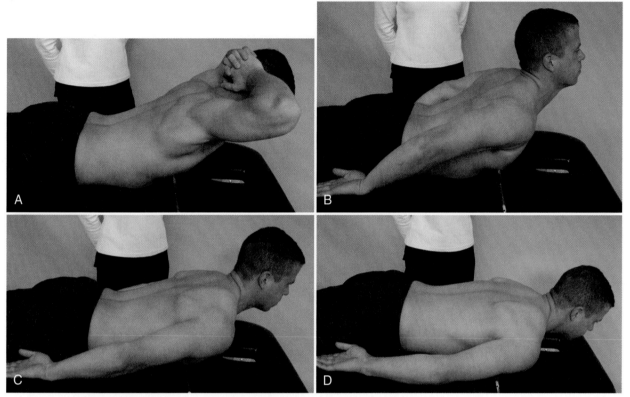

Figure 8–5

Isometric extensor test. **A,** With the hands behind the head, the patient lifts the head, chest, and ribs off the bed. **B,** With the hands at the side, the patient lifts the head, chest, and ribs off the bed. **C,** With the hands at the side, the patient lifts the sternum off the bed. **D,** With the hands at the side, the patient lifts the head off the bed.

PURPOSE	To test the strength of the iliocostalis lumborum (erector spinae) and multifidus.
PATIENT POSITION	The patient is prone lying.
EXAMINER POSITION	The examiner is positioned so as to observe for altered mechanics.
TEST PROCEDURE	The patient attempts to extend the spine as far as possible by lifting up the head and trunk. Depending on how the patient does the test (the aim is to get the highest score possible) and how long the position is held (see Table 8-2), the examiner records the MMT score. The patient holds the end position as long as possible.

Continued

ISOMETRIC EXTENSOR TEST[5,9,10]—cont'd

INDICATIONS OF A POSITIVE TEST The examiner times how long the patient can hold the extended position. The test is graded as described in Table 8-2.

RELIABILITY/SPECIFICITY/ SENSITIVITY[5] Interrater reliability: ICC = 0.24

Table 8-2

Isometric Extensor Test Grading

Grade	MMT Score	Patient Position
Normal	5	With the hands clasped behind the head, extends the lumbar spine, lifting the head, chest, and ribs from the bed/floor (20- to 30-second hold)
Good	4	With the hands at the side, extends the lumbar spine, lifting the head, chest, and ribs from the bed/floor (15- to 20-second hold)
Fair	3	With the hands at the side, extends the lumbar spine, lifting the sternum off the bed/floor (10- to 15-second hold)
Poor	2	With the hands at the side, extends the lumbar spine, lifting the head off the bed/floor (1- to 10-second hold)
Trace	1	Only slight contraction of the muscle with no movement

MMT, Manual muscle test.

INTERNAL/EXTERNAL ABDOMINAL OBLIQUE TEST[6,11] DVD

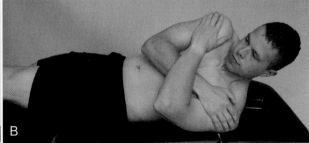

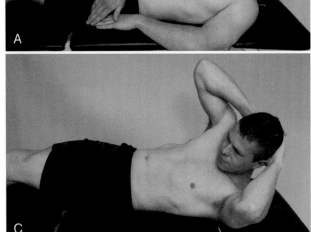

Figure 8–6

Internal/external abdominal oblique test. **A,** Test position with the hands at the side. **B,** Test position with the hands on the shoulders. **C,** Test position with the hands behind the head.

INTERNAL/EXTERNAL ABDOMINAL OBLIQUE TEST[6,11]—cont'd

PURPOSE To check the combined action of the internal oblique muscle of one side and the external oblique muscle on the opposite side.

PATIENT POSITION The patient is supine lying with the hands by the side.

EXAMINER POSITION The examiner is positioned so as to observe for altered mechanics.

TEST PROCEDURE The patient is asked to lift the head and the shoulder on one side and reach over and touch the fingernails of the other hand or to flex and rotate the trunk. Depending on how the patient does the test (the aim is to get the highest score possible) and how long the position is held (see Table 8-3), the examiner records the MMT score. The patient holds the end position as long as possible. The patient's feet should not be supported, and the patient should breathe normally.

INDICATIONS OF A POSITIVE TEST The number of seconds the contraction is held before cheating (e.g., holding the breath, altered mechanics) or the onset of fatigue is recorded as the score. The test is graded as described in Table 8-3.

CLINICAL NOTE • This test also can be done dynamically, to test endurance, by counting the number of repetitions to each side the patient is able to do before cheating.

RELIABILITY/SPECIFICITY/ SENSITIVITY Unknown

Table 8-3

Internal/External Abdominal Oblique Test Grading

Grade	MMT Score	Patient Position
Normal	5	Flexes and rotates the lumbar spine fully with the hands behind the head (20- to 30-second hold)
Good	4	Flexes and rotates the lumbar spine fully with the hands across the chest (15- to 20-second hold)
Fair	3	Flexes and rotates the lumbar spine fully with the arms reaching forward (10- to 15-second hold)
Poor	2	Unable to flex and rotate fully
Trace	1	Only slight contraction of the muscle with no movement
None	0	No contraction of the muscle

MMT, Manual muscle test.

DOUBLE STRAIGHT LEG LOWERING TEST[6,11-13]

DVD

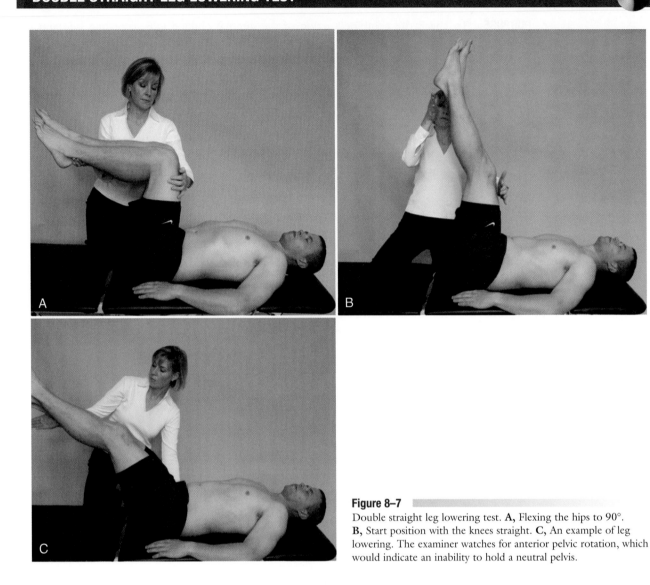

Figure 8–7
Double straight leg lowering test. **A,** Flexing the hips to 90°.
B, Start position with the knees straight. **C,** An example of leg
lowering. The examiner watches for anterior pelvic rotation, which
would indicate an inability to hold a neutral pelvis.

PURPOSE	To assess the strength of the abdominal muscles.
PATIENT POSITION	The patient lies supine and flexes the hips to 90° and then straightens the knees.
EXAMINER POSITION	The examiner is positioned so as to palpate the ASIS on one side and to observe for altered mechanics.
TEST PROCEDURE	The patient positions the pelvis in neutral (i.e., the PSISs are slightly superior to the ASISs) by doing a posterior pelvic tilt and holding the spinous processes tightly against the examining table. The straight legs then are eccentrically lowered.
INDICATIONS OF A POSITIVE TEST	As soon as the examiner feels the ASIS start to rotate forward during the leg lowering, the test is stopped and the examiner holds the patient's legs in that position while measuring the angle (plinth to thigh angle). The test must be done slowly, and the patient must not hold the breath. The test is graded as described in Table 8-4.

DOUBLE STRAIGHT LEG LOWERING TEST[6,11-13]—cont'd

Table 8-4

Double Straight Leg Lowering Test Grading

Grade	MMT Score	Patient Position
Normal	5	Able to reach 0° to 15° from the table before the pelvis tilts
Good	4	Able to reach 16° to 45° from the table before the pelvis tilts
Fair	3	Able to reach 46° to 75° from the table before the pelvis tilts
Poor	2	Able to reach 75° to 90° from the table before the pelvis tilts
Trace	1	Unable to hold the pelvis in neutral at all

MMT, Manual muscle test.

CLINICAL NOTES/CAUTIONS
- This test should be performed only if the patient receives a grade of "normal" in the dynamic abdominal endurance test or the abdominal isometric test.
- This is an abdominal eccentric test that can put a great deal of stress on the spine; therefore, the examiner must make sure the patient is able to hold a neutral pelvis before doing the exercise. If the patient cannot hold neutral spine or if the patient is symptomatic with the test, the test should not be completed. This test also causes greater abdominal activation than curl-ups.

RELIABILITY/SPECIFICITY/ SENSITIVITY   Unknown

DYNAMIC HORIZONTAL SIDE SUPPORT (SIDE BRIDGE OR SIDE PLANK) TEST[14,15]

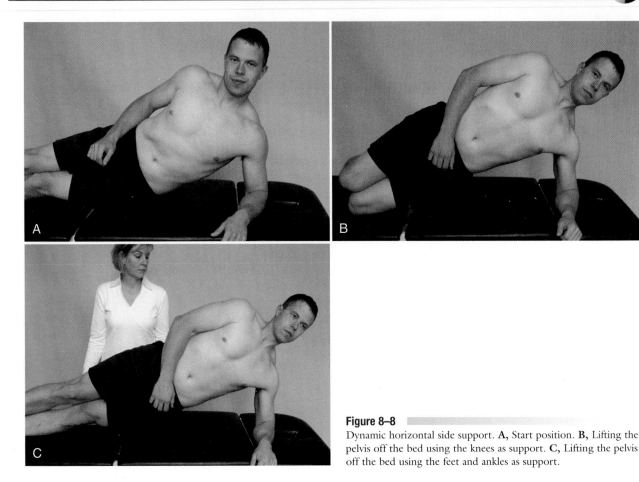

Figure 8–8

Dynamic horizontal side support. **A,** Start position. **B,** Lifting the pelvis off the bed using the knees as support. **C,** Lifting the pelvis off the bed using the feet and ankles as support.

PURPOSE	To test the quadratus lumborum muscle.
PATIENT POSITION	The patient is side lying, resting the upper body on the elbow.
EXAMINER POSITION	The examiner is positioned so as to observe for altered mechanics.
TEST PROCEDURE	To begin, the patient is side lying with the knees flexed to 90°. The examiner asks the patient to lift the pelvis off the examining table and straighten the spine. The weight of the body is supported by the forearm and elbow proximally and the lateral knee distally. If the patient can do the first test easily, the test can be made more difficult by having the patient keep the legs straight and then lift the knees and pelvis off the examining table with the feet as the base, so that the whole body is straight.
INDICATIONS OF A POSITIVE TEST	The patient should not roll forward or backward when doing the test. The examiner times how long the patient can hold the position without cheating. The test is graded as described in Table 8-5.

DYNAMIC HORIZONTAL SIDE SUPPORT (SIDE BRIDGE OR SIDE PLANK) TEST[14,15]—cont'd

Table 8-5
Dynamic Horizontal Side Support (Side Bridge) Test Grading

Grade	MMT Score	Patient Position
Normal	5	Able to lift the pelvis off the examining table and hold the spine straight (10- to 20-second hold)
Good	4	Able to lift the pelvis off the examining table but has difficulty holding the spine straight (5- to 10-second hold)
Fair	3	Able to lift the pelvis off the examining table but cannot hold the spine straight (<5-second hold)
Poor	2	Unable to lift the pelvis off examining table

MMT, Manual muscle test.

CLINICAL NOTES
- The test may also be done dynamically, to test endurance, by having the patient repeat the side bridging as many times as possible on each side.
- McGill et al.[15] reported that the side bridge should be able to be held 65% of the extensor time for men and 39% for women, and 99% of the flexor time for men and 79% for women.

RELIABILITY/SPECIFICITY/ SENSITIVITY
Unknown

PERIPHERAL JOINT SCANNING EXAMINATION

PERIPHERAL JOINT SCAN[16] DVD

PURPOSE   To rule out obvious pathological conditions in the lower extremities and to assess the peripheral joints of the lower extremity to determine whether more in-depth testing is required.

PATIENT POSITION   The patient is standing or supine, depending on the joint to be scanned.

EXAMINER POSITION   The examiner's position varies, depending on the joint to be scanned.

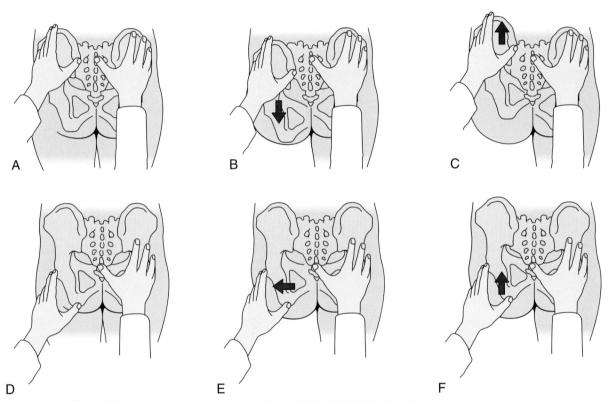

Figure 8–9

Tests to demonstrate left sacroiliac fixation. **A,** The examiner places the left thumb on the posterior superior iliac spine and the right thumb over one of the sacral spinous processes. **B,** With normal movement, the examiner's left thumb moves downward as the patient raises the left leg with full hip flexion. **C,** If the joint is fixed, the examiner's left thumb moves upward as the patient raises the left leg. **D,** The examiner places the left thumb over the ischial tuberosity and the right thumb over the apex of the sacrum. **E,** With normal movement, the examiner's left thumb moves laterally as the patient raises the left leg with full hip flexion. **F,** If the joint is fixed, the examiner's left thumb moves slightly upward as the patient raises the left leg. (Modified from Kirkaldy-Willis WH: *Managing low back pain,* p 94, New York, 1983, Churchill Livingstone.)

PERIPHERAL JOINT SCAN[16]—cont'd

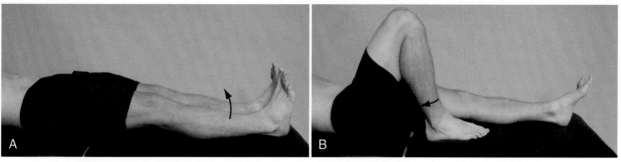

Figure 8–10
A, Knee extension. **B,** Knee flexion.

Sacroiliac Joints

TEST PROCEDURE

With the patient standing, the examiner palpates the PSIS on the test side with one thumb or finger and one of the sacral spines with the thumb or finger of the other hand. The patient then flexes the hip on the test side as far as possible. The examiner compares the findings with those of the other side. The examiner next places one thumb or finger on the patient's ischial tuberosity on the test side and one thumb or finger of the other hand on the sacral apex. The patient then is asked to flex the hip on the test side.

INDICATIONS OF A POSITIVE TEST

For the first part of the test, if the PSIS drops as it normally should, the test result is negative. Elevation of the PSIS indicates fixation of the sacroiliac joint on that side. If the second movement is normal, the thumb on the ischial tuberosity moves laterally. If the sacroiliac joint on that side is fixed, the thumb moves up. The other side then is tested for comparison. The unaffected side should be tested first.

CLINICAL NOTES

• This test has also been called *Gillet's test* or the *sacral fixation test*.
• If any positive signs occur, the examiner should do a detailed examination of the pelvic joints.

Hip Joints

TEST PROCEDURE

With the patient supine, the hip joints are actively moved through flexion, abduction, adduction, and medial and lateral rotation in as full ROM as possible. To test extension, the patient is positioned prone.

INDICATIONS OF A POSITIVE TEST

Any pattern of restriction or pain should be noted. ROM deficits and symptom reproduction both are indicators of a positive test result. The two sides should be compared, and any restriction of movement or abnormal signs and symptoms should be noted.

CLINICAL NOTES

• As the patient flexes the hip, the examiner may palpate the ilium, sacrum, and lumbar spine to determine when movement begins at the sacroiliac joint on that side and at the lumbar spine during the hip movement. The two sides should be compared.
• If any positive signs occur, the examiner should do a detailed examination of the hip joints.

Continued

PERIPHERAL JOINT SCAN[16]—*cont'd*

Knee Joints

TEST PROCEDURE The patient is supine, and the knee joint is actively moved through as full a range of flexion and extension as possible.

INDICATIONS OF A POSITIVE TEST Any restriction of movement or abnormal signs and symptoms should be noted. ROM deficits and symptom reproduction both are indicators of a positive test result. The two sides should be compared, and any restriction of movement or abnormal signs and symptoms should be noted.

CLINICAL NOTE • If any positive signs occur, the examiner should do a detailed examination of the knee joints.

Foot and Ankle Joints

TEST PROCEDURE With the patient supine, plantar flexion, dorsiflexion, supination, and pronation of the foot and ankle, as well as flexion and extension of the toes, are actively performed through a full ROM.

INDICATIONS OF A POSITIVE TEST Any alteration in signs and symptoms should be noted. ROM deficits and symptom reproduction both are indicators of a positive test result. The two sides should be compared, and any restriction of movement or abnormal signs and symptoms should be noted.

CLINICAL NOTES • It is important to note that the scanning process is meant to be a general clearing examination.
• If any positive signs occur, the examiner should do a detailed examination of the foot and ankle joints.

QUICK TEST OF THE LOWER PERIPHERAL JOINTS

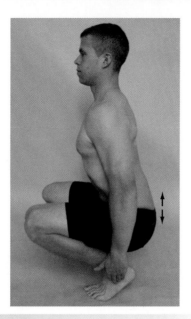

Figure 8–11
Quick test.

PURPOSE	The quick test is designed to enable the examiner to quickly assess the peripheral joints of the lower extremity and to determine whether more in-depth testing is required. This test can be substituted for the general lower limb peripheral joint scan, provided the patient believes that he or she can squat and return to standing and provided the examiner believes the patient is able to perform the test.
PATIENT POSITION	The patient is standing.
EXAMINER POSITION	The examiner is positioned to view the patient's motions and to observe any compensations that may occur during the squat and return to standing.
TEST PROCEDURE	The patient squats down as far as possible, bounces two or three times, and returns to the standing position. This action quickly tests the ankles, knees, and hips, as well as the sacrum, for any pathological condition.
INDICATIONS OF A POSITIVE TEST	If the patient can fully squat and bounce without any signs and symptoms, the peripheral joints probably are free of any pathological condition related to the complaint. If this test result is negative, the examiner need not test the general peripheral joints (general peripheral joint scan) with the patient in the lying position.
CLINICAL NOTE	• This test should be used only with caution and should not be done with patients suspected of having arthritis or a pathological condition in the lower limb joints, pregnant patients, or older patients who show weakness and hypomobility.
RELIABILITY/SPECIFICITY/ SENSITIVITY	Unknown

MYOTOME TESTING

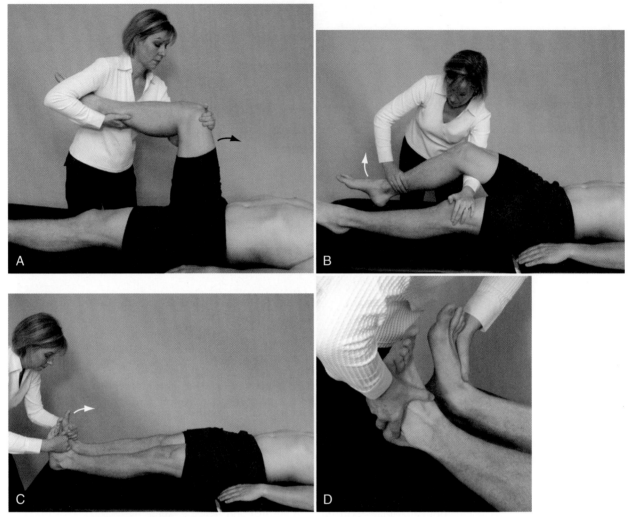

Figure 8–12
Positioning for testing myotomes. **A,** Hip flexion (L2). **B,** Knee extension (L3). **C,** Foot dorsiflexion (L4). **D,** Ankle eversion (S1).

PURPOSE	To assess the integrity of the lumbar spine nerve roots.
SUSPECTED INJURY	Spinal nerve root pathology
PATIENT POSITION	The patient is supine or prone, depending on the nerve root to be tested.
EXAMINER POSITION	The examiner is positioned directly adjacent to the patient's lower extremity.
TEST PROCEDURE	When testing myotomes, ideally the examiner should place the test joint or joints close to the neutral or resting position and then apply a resisted isometric pressure in a gradually increasing manner. The contraction should be held for at least 5 seconds to allow time for any myotomal weakness to become evident. The unaffected side is tested first.

MYOTOME TESTING—*cont'd*

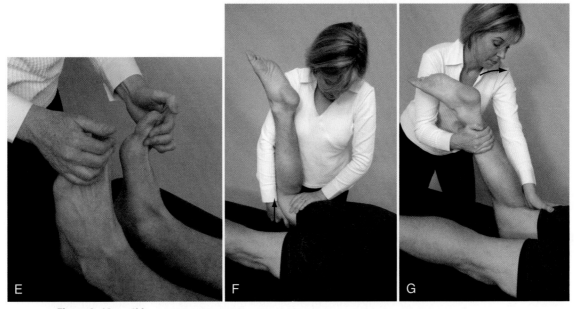

Figure 8–12 cont'd
E, Extension of the big toe (L5). **F,** Hip extension (S1). **G,** Knee flexion (S1-S2).

L2 myotome (hip flexion). The examiner flexes the patient's hip to 80° to 90° and then applies a resisted force into hip extension. The other side then is tested for comparison. To prevent excessive stress on the lumbar spine, the examiner must make sure the patient does not increase the lumbar lordosis while doing the test. The more the hip is flexed, the less is the stress on the lumbar spine. Only one leg is tested at a time.

L3 myotome (knee extension). The examiner flexes the patient's knee to 25° to 35° (over a pillow or the examiner's knee) and then applies a resisted flexion force at the midshaft of the tibia, making sure the heel is not resting on the examining table. The other side is tested for comparison.

L4 myotome (ankle dorsiflexion). The examiner asks the patient to place the feet at 90° relative to the leg (plantigrade position). The examiner applies a resisted force to the dorsum of each foot and compares the two sides. In this case, the two sides may be tested at the same time.

L5 myotome (toe extension). The patient is asked to hold both big toes in a neutral position. The examiner applies resistance to the nails of both toes and compares the two sides. It is imperative that the resistance be isometric; therefore, the amount of force in this case is less than that applied, for example, during knee extension. The two sides may be tested at the same time.

S1 myotome (ankle plantar flexion). The patient is asked to place the feet at 90° relative to the leg (plantigrade position). The examiner then applies resistance to the sole of the foot. Because of the strength of the plantar flexor muscles, this myotome is best tested with the patient standing. The patient slowly moves up and down on the toes of each foot (for at least 5 seconds) in turn (see modified Trendelenburg's test), and the examiner compares the differences between the two sides.

Continued

MYOTOME TESTING—*cont'd*

S1 myotome (ankle eversion). The patient is supine lying. The examiner applies a force to move the patient's foot into inversion while the patient isometrically resists.

S1 myotome (hip extension). The patient is prone lying, and the knee is flexed to 90°. The examiner then lifts the patient's thigh slightly off the examining table while stabilizing the leg. A downward force is applied to the posterior thigh with one hand while the other hand ensures that the patient's thigh is not resting on the table.

S1-S2 myotomes (knee flexion). The patient is prone with the knee flexed to 80° to 90°. The examiner applies an extension isometric force just above the ankle. Although the two knee flexors can be tested at the same time, this is not advisable because of the stress it places on the lumbar spine.

INDICATIONS OF A POSITIVE TEST Muscle weakness during testing indicates a positive test result.

CLINICAL NOTES/CAUTIONS
- For the S1 myotome, only one of the tests needs to be done.
- When appropriate, the examiner should test the two sides simultaneously for comparison. Simultaneous bilateral comparison is not possible for movements involving the hip and knee joints because of the weight of the limbs and the stress on the low back; therefore, in these cases the two sides must be done individually.
- The examiner should not apply pressure over the joints, because this may cause symptoms unrelated to the myotomes.
- The ankle movements should be tested with the knee flexed approximately 30°, especially if the patient complains of sciatic pain, because full dorsiflexion is considered a provocative maneuver for stretching neurological tissue. Likewise, the extended knee increases the stretch on the sciatic nerve and may result in false signs, such as weakness that results from pain rather than from pressure on the nerve root.
- Hamstring cramping may occur during testing of knee flexion. It does not indicate a positive test result, but the examiner should be aware that cramping may occur.
- If the patient is in extreme pain, all tests in the supine position should be completed before the patient is tested in the prone position. This reduces the amount of movement the patient must do, decreasing the patient's discomfort. Ideally, all tests in the standing position should be performed first, followed by tests in the sitting, supine, side-lying, and prone positions.

SPECIAL TESTS FOR NEUROLOGICAL DYSFUNCTION

Relevant Special Tests

Slump test
Straight leg raise test (Lasègue's test)
Prone knee bending test
Femoral nerve traction test
Bowstring test (Cram test or popliteal pressure sign)

Definition

Lumbar radiculopathy itself is not a cause of low back pain, but rather a result of some other lumbar pathological condition that affects one or more lumbar nerve roots. Impingement or inflammation of a lumbar nerve root can cause neurological symptoms into the lower extremity. The result of this process is a lumbar radiculopathy (pain from the spinal nerve root). Lumbar radiculopathy causes pain, numbness, tingling, and/or weakness in the lower extremity. These neurological symptoms occur in the areas supplied by the involved nerve root (dermatome and myotome).

Suspected Injury

Lumbar radiculopathy
Sciatic nerve entrapment
Femoral nerve entrapment

Epidemiology and Demographics

About 30% of patients with back pain have a radiculopathy associated with their low back pain. Between 1% and 10% of the general public will have a lumbar radiculopathy, and men and women are affected equally. Symptoms occur most often in men in their 40s and women in their 50s.[17-20]

Relevant History

The patient may report a history of low back pain or injury. Radicular symptoms generally are not noticed with the initial low back symptoms, but over time, the frequency of the low back pain increases, and the lower extremity radicular symptoms begin to appear. Some patients report that when the radicular leg pain begins, the back pain goes away.

Relevant Signs and Symptoms

- Radiculopathy can cause pain, numbness, tingling, and weakness in a nerve root distribution pattern. The pain may be described as sharp, shooting, or burning.
- The pain may begin in the low back or may start in the buttocks or posterior thigh.
- Most radiculopathies involve the lower lumbar nerve roots (L4-S1), sending symptoms below the level of the knee. Irritation of nerves from the upper lumbar nerve roots (L1-3) sends symptoms into the hip and anterior thigh above the level of the knee.
- The referral pattern varies, depending on the specific nerve root involved, but radicular pain results in numbness and tingling in the lower extremities in a dermatomal pattern. Sensory symptoms are more common with radiculopathy, but muscle weakness may be present, especially in more severe cases.
- Muscle weakness and reflex changes also occur in a specific myotomal pattern. A myotome is a motor function associated with a specific nerve root

Mechanism of Injury

Lumbar radiculopathy is the result of some other lumbar pathological condition. Impingement or irritation of a lumbar nerve root causes neurological signs and symptoms in the corresponding dermatome/myotome/sclerotome. Lumbar nerve root irritation or impingement may be caused by a herniated disc, degenerative disc disease (DDD), stenosis, spondylolisthesis, instability, or degenerative joint disease. Any of these pathological conditions can compromise the size of the intervertebral foramen and cause impingement on the lumbar nerve root.

Clinical Note

- These tests are potentially provocative assessment techniques; therefore, the examiner should increase tension on the system gradually and carefully. Continuous communication with the patient is required to ensure that symptoms are not exacerbated.

SLUMP TEST[21-26]

PURPOSE

The slump test has become the most common neurological test for the lower limb. It is performed to assess for movement restriction (impingement) of the dura and spinal cord and/or nerve roots.

PATIENT POSITION

The patient is seated on the edge of the examining table with the legs supported, the hips in neutral position (i.e., no rotation, abduction, or adduction), and the hands behind the back. In this position, the patient should have no symptoms.

EXAMINER POSITION

The examiner stands directly adjacent to the patient so as to control head and lower extremity motion.

TEST PROCEDURE

The examination is performed in sequential steps. First, the patient is asked to "slump" the back into thoracic and lumbar flexion. The examiner maintains the patient's chin in the neutral position to prevent neck and head flexion. If no symptoms are produced, the examiner places one hand on the patient's head and neck to control cervical and upper thoracic motion. The examiner then uses the same arm that has the hand resting on the head to apply overpressure across the shoulders to maintain flexion of the thoracic and lumbar spines. While this position is held, the patient is asked to actively flex the cervical spine and head as far as possible (i.e., chin to chest). The examiner then applies overpressure to maintain the cervical flexion of all three parts of the spine (cervical, thoracic, and lumbar), using the hand of the same arm to maintain overpressure in the cervical spine. Providing there are no symptoms, starting with the normal leg, the examiner's other hand is placed on the patient's foot or lower extremity to control lower extremity motion. The examiner then extends the patient's knee. If that does not produce symptoms, the examiner takes the patient's foot into maximum dorsiflexion. The test is repeated with the affected leg and then with both legs at the same time.

INDICATIONS OF A POSITIVE TEST

If the patient is unable to fully extend the knee because of pain, the examiner releases the overpressure to the cervical spine and the patient actively extends the neck. If the knee extends farther, the symptoms decrease with neck extension, or the positioning of the patient increases the symptoms, the test result is considered positive for increased tension in the neuromeningeal tract. During the slump test, the examiner looks for reproduction of the neuropathological symptoms, not just the production of symptoms. The test puts stress on certain tissues, so some discomfort or pain is not necessarily symptomatic for the problem. For example, nonpathological responses include pain or discomfort in the area of T8-T9 (in 50% of normal patients), pain or discomfort behind the extended knee and hamstrings, symmetrical restriction of knee extension, symmetrical restriction of ankle dorsiflexion, and symmetrical increased range of knee extension and ankle dorsiflexion on release of neck flexion.

CLINICAL NOTES

- The unaffected leg is always tested first.
- Butler[26] recommended doing bilateral knee extension in the slump position, on the grounds that any asymmetry in the amount of knee extension is easier to note this way.
- The effect of releasing neck flexion on the patient's symptoms should be noted. In hypermobile patients, more hip flexion (more than 90°), as well as hip adduction and medial rotation, may be required to elicit a positive response. If symptoms are produced in any phase of the sequence, it is important to stop the provocative maneuvers to prevent undue discomfort for the patient.
- Some people do knee extension last, because it often is easier to measure knee ROM to determine whether it has improved with treatment.
- Butler[26] has suggested modifications to the slump test to stress individual nerves (Table 8-6)

RELIABILITY/SPECIFICITY/ SENSITIVITY

Unknown

SLUMP TEST[21-26]—cont'd

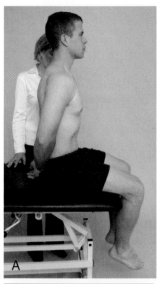

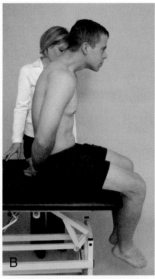

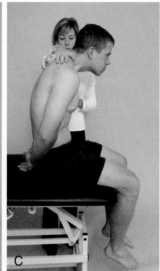

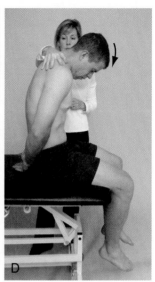

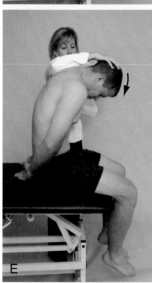

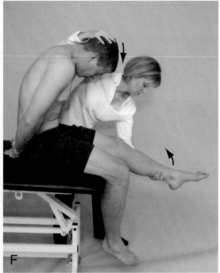

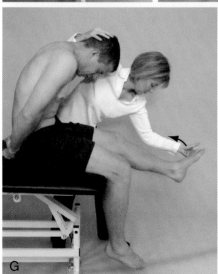

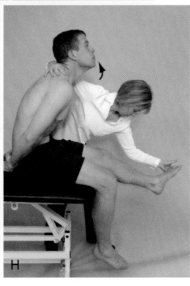

Figure 8–13

Sequence of subject postures in the slump test. **A,** The patient sits erect with the hands behind the back. **B,** The patient slumps the lumbar and thoracic spine while either the patient or the examiner keeps the head in neutral. **C,** The examiner pushes down on the shoulders while the patient holds the head in neutral. **D,** The patient flexes the head. **E,** The examiner carefully applies overpressure to the cervical spine. **F,** The examiner extends the patient's knee while holding the cervical spine flexed. **G,** While holding the knee extended and the cervical spine flexed, the examiner dorsiflexes the foot. **H,** The patient extends the head, which should relieve any symptoms. If symptoms are reproduced at any stage, further sequential movements are not attempted.

Continued

SLUMP TEST[21-26]—cont'd

Table 8-6

Slump Test and Modifications

	Slump Test (ST1)	Slump Test (ST2)	Side Lying Slump Test (ST3)	Long Sitting Slump Test (ST4)
Cervical spine	Flexion	Flexion	Flexion	Flexion, rotation
Thoracic and lumbar spine	Flexion (slump)	Flexion (slump)	Flexion (slump)	Flexion (slump)
Hip	Flexion (90°+)	Flexion (90°+), abduction	Flexion (20°)	Flexion (90°+)
Knee	Extension	Extension	Flexion	Extension
Ankle	Dorsiflexion	Dorsiflexion	Plantar flexion	Dorsiflexion
Foot	—	—	—	—
Toes	—	—	—	—
Nerve bias	Spinal cord, cervical and lumbar nerve roots, sciatic nerve	Obturator nerve	Femoral nerve	Spinal cord, cervical and lumbar nerve roots, sciatic nerve

Data from Butler DA: *Mobilisation of the nervous system,* Melbourne, 1991, Churchill Livingstone.

STRAIGHT LEG RAISE TEST (LASÈGUE'S TEST)[26-42]

DVD

PURPOSE To assess for impingement of the dura and spinal cord or nerve roots of the lower lumbar spine, especially the sciatic nerve.

PATIENT POSITION The patient lies supine. The hip is medially rotated and adducted, and the knee is extended. The head should be in a neutral position, and the hands should be at the sides.

EXAMINER POSITION The examiner stands adjacent to the pelvis of the test leg. The examiner places one hand on the patient's knee to stabilize it in extension. The other hand grasps the patient's ankle and is used to lift the leg upward.

TEST PROCEDURE The examiner flexes the patient's hip until the patient complains of pain or tightness in the back or back of the leg. The examiner then slowly and carefully lowers the leg back slightly (extends it) until the patient feels no pain or tightness. The examiner passively dorsiflexes the patient's foot or asks the patient to actively flex the neck so that the chin is on the chest; or, the two actions may be done simultaneously. Most commonly, foot dorsiflexion is done first.

INDICATIONS OF A POSITIVE TEST If the pain is primarily back pain, it is more likely a disc herniation from pressure on the anterior theca of the spinal cord, or the pathological condition causing the pressure is more centrally located. "Back pain only" patients who have a disc prolapse have smaller, more central prolapses. If the pain is primarily in the leg, the pathological condition causing the pressure on neurological tissues is more likely to be laterally located. A disc herniation or pathological condition causing pressure between the two extremes is more likely to cause pain in both areas.

STRAIGHT LEG RAISE TEST (LASÈGUE'S TEST)[26-42]—cont'd

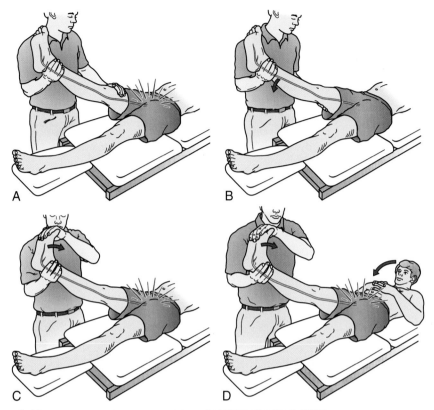

Figure 8–14

Straight leg raise test. **A,** Radicular symptoms are precipitated on the same side with straight leg raising. **B,** The leg is lowered slowly until pain is relieved. **C,** The foot then is dorsiflexed, causing a return of symptoms; this indicates a positive test result. **D,** To make the symptoms more provocative, the neck can be flexed by lifting the head at the same time the foot is dorsiflexed.

CLINICAL NOTES/CAUTIONS

- The uninvolved side should be tested first.
- Both the neck flexion and foot dorsiflexion are considered provocative or sensitizing tests for neurological tissue.
- Straight leg raise testing is one of the most common neurological tests of the lower limb.
- This test is a passive test, and each leg is tested individually; the normal leg is tested first.
- Modifications of the straight leg raise test can be used to stress different peripheral nerves to a greater degree; these are referred to as straight leg raise tests with a particular nerve bias (Table 8-7).
- The neck flexion movement has also been called *Hyndman's sign, Brudzinski's sign,* and *Lidner's sign.*
- A contralateral positive test result is called the *crossover sign* or *well leg test of Fajersztjan.* A positive crossover sign usually indicates a large disc protrusion and a poor prognosis for conservative treatment.

Continued

STRAIGHT LEG RAISE TEST (LASÈGUE'S TEST)[26-42]—cont'd

Table 8-7

Straight Leg Raise (SLR) Test and Modifications

	SLR (Basic)	SLR2	SLR3	SLR4	Cross (Well Leg) SLR5
Hip	Flexion and adduction	Flexion	Flexion	Flexion and medial rotation	Flexion
Knee	Extension	Extension	Extension	Extension	Extension
Ankle	Dorsiflexion	Dorsiflexion	Dorsiflexion	Plantar flexion	Dorsiflexion
Foot	—	Eversion	Inversion	Inversion	—
Toes	—	Extension	—	—	—
Nerve bias	Sciatic nerve and tibial nerve	Tibial nerve	Sural nerve	Common peroneal nerve	Nerve root (disc prolapse)

Data from Butler DA: *Mobilisation of the nervous system,* Melbourne, 1991, Churchill Livingstone.

RELIABILITY/SPECIFICITY/SENSITIVITY[40-42]
Reliability: 0.93
Validity: 98%
Specificity: 87%
Sensitivity: 33%

PRONE KNEE BENDING TEST[26,43,44]

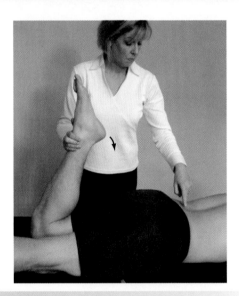

Figure 8–15
Prone knee bending test (PKB1), which stresses the femoral nerve and L2-L4 nerve root. The examiner points to the location in the lumbar spin where pain may be expected with a positive test result.

PRONE KNEE BENDING TEST[26,43,44]—cont'd

PURPOSE	To test for femoral nerve entrapment or L2-L3 nerve root involvement.
SUSPECTED INJURY	• Upper lumbar radiculopathy • Femoral nerve entrapment
PATIENT POSITION	The patient lies prone.
EXAMINER POSITION	The examiner stands adjacent to the pelvis on the side of the test limb.
TEST PROCEDURE	One of the examiner's hands is placed on the patient's pelvis to feel for compensations. The examiner's other hand grasps the ankle of the lower extremity being tested. The examiner passively flexes the knee as far as possible so that the patient's heel rests against the buttock. At the same time, the examiner makes sure the patient's hip is not rotated. The flexed knee position should be maintained for 45 to 60 seconds.
INDICATIONS OF A POSITIVE TEST	Unilateral neurological pain in the lumbar area, buttock, or anterior thigh may indicate an L2 or L3 nerve root lesion. This test also stretches the femoral nerve. Pain in the anterior thigh may indicate tight quadriceps muscles or stretching of the femoral nerve. A careful history and pain differentiation help delineate the problem.
CLINICAL NOTES/CAUTIONS	• If the examiner is unable to flex the patient's knee past 90° because of a pathological condition in the knee, the test may be performed by passive extension of the hip while the knee is flexed as much as possible. • If the rectus femoris is tight, the examiner should remember that taking the heel to the buttock may cause anterior torsion to the ilium, which could lead to sacroiliac or lumbar pain. • The test may be modified to stress different peripheral nerves (Table 8-8).
RELIABILITY/SPECIFICITY/SENSITIVITY	Unknown

Table 8-8

Prone Knee Bending (PBK) Test and Modifications

	Basic Prone Knee Bending (PKB1)	Prone Knee Bending (PKB2)	Prone Knee Extension (PKE)
Cervical spine	Rotation to test side	Rotation to test side	—
Thoracic and lumbar spine	Neutral	Neutral	Neutral
Hip	Neutral	Extension, adduction	Extension, abduction, lateral rotation
Knee	Flexion	Flexion	Extension
Ankle	—	—	Dorsiflexion
Foot	—	—	Eversion
Toes	—	—	—
Nerve bias	Femoral nerve, L2-L4 nerve root	Lateral femoral cutaneous nerve	Saphenous nerve

Data from Butler DA: *Mobilisation of the nervous system,* Melbourne, 1991, Churchill Livingstone.

FEMORAL NERVE TRACTION TEST[45,46]

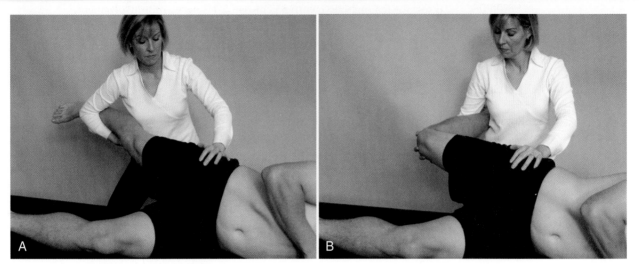

Figure 8–16
Femoral nerve traction test. **A,** Hip and knee are extended. **B,** Then knee is flexed.

PURPOSE	To test for femoral nerve entrapment or a pathological condition of the L2-L4 nerve root.
PATIENT POSITION	The patient lies on the side. Initially, for testing of the uninvolved leg, the patient lies on the involved side with the affected limb flexed slightly at the hip and knee to prevent pelvic rotation. The back should be straight, not hyperextended. The head should be slightly flexed and placed on a pillow to keep it in neutral alignment. For testing of the affected side, the patient lies on the unaffected side and the test is repeated.
EXAMINER POSITION	The examiner stands behind the patient's gluteal region.
TEST PROCEDURE	One of the examiner's hands is placed on the patient's pelvis to provide stability to the trunk and prevent hip and lumbar rotation. The examiner's other arm cradles the patient's test knee and leg. The examiner extends the knee while gently extending the hip approximately 15°. The patient's knee is then flexed on the affected side; this movement further stretches the femoral nerve.
INDICATIONS OF A POSITIVE TEST	Neurological pain radiates down the anterior thigh if the test result is positive.
CLINICAL NOTES/CAUTIONS	• This is also a traction test for the nerve roots at the midlumbar area (L2-L4). • As with the straight leg raise test, there is also a contralateral positive test. That is, when the test is performed, the symptoms occur in the opposite limb. This is called the crossed femoral stretching test. • Pain in the groin and hip that radiates along the anterior medial thigh indicates an L3 nerve root problem; pain extending to the midtibia indicates an L4 nerve root problem. • This test is similar to Ober's test for a tight iliotibial band, so the examiner must be able to differentiate between the two conditions. If the iliotibial band is tight, the test leg does not adduct but remains elevated away from the table, because the tight tendon riding over the greater trochanter keeps the leg abducted. • Femoral nerve injury presents with a different history, and the referred pain (anteriorly) tends to be stronger.
RELIABILITY/SPECIFICITY/ SENSITIVITY	Unknown

BOWSTRING TEST (CRAM TEST OR POPLITEAL PRESSURE SIGN)[47-51]

DVD

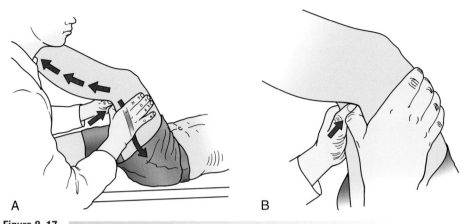

Figure 8–17

Bowstring test. **A,** The examiner does a straight leg raise test. If the test result is positive, the examiner relieves the pain by flexing the knee slightly. The examiner then pushes into the popliteal space (**B**) to increase the stress on the sciatic nerve and looks for a return of the symptoms seen with the straight leg raise test.

PURPOSE	To detect tension or pressure on the sciatic nerve (this test is a modification of the straight leg raise test).
PATIENT POSITION	The patient is supine with the hip slightly medially rotated and adducted and the knee extended. Care should be taken to make sure the head is in a neutral position and the arms are resting comfortably at the sides.
EXAMINER POSITION	The examiner stands directly adjacent to the test limb.
TEST PROCEDURE	The patient's ankle is placed on the examiner's shoulder. Both of the examiner's hands are placed around the patient's knee. The examiner's thumbs are placed in the popliteal area of the patient's knee. The examiner flexes the patient's hip until the patient complains of pain or tightness in the back or back of the leg. While maintaining the thigh in this position, the examiner flexes the knee slightly (20°), reducing the symptoms. Thumb or finger pressure then is applied to the popliteal area to re-establish the painful radicular symptoms.
INDICATIONS OF A POSITIVE TEST	Pain or symptoms such as tightness or tingling as a result of these maneuvers indicate a positive test result and pressure or tension on the sciatic nerve.
CLINICAL NOTE	• The test also may be done with the patient in the sitting position and the examiner passively extending the knee to produce pain. The examiner then slightly flexes the knee so that the pain and symptoms disappear. The examiner holds this slightly flexed position by clasping the patient's leg between the examiner's knees. The examiner then presses the fingers of both hands into the popliteal space. In this case, the test is called the *sciatic tension test* or *Deyerle's sign*.
RELIABILITY/SPECIFICITY/ SENSITIVITY	Unknown

SPECIAL TESTS FOR LUMBAR INSTABILITY[52-59]

Relevant Special Tests

H and I stability tests
Test of anterior lumbar spine stability
Test of posterior lumbar spine instability
Specific lumbar spine torsion test

Definition

The term *lumbar instability* refers to excess motion in the lumbar spine segments, in which the spinal segment or segments move more than normal under a typical external force or load. The excess motion results in pain or symptom reproduction. On x-ray, excessive motion is defined as an excessive rotational segmental angle or segmental translation greater than 3 mm.

Suspected Injury

Lumbar muscle spasm
Lumbar instability
Lumbar spondylolithesis
Lumbar spondylolysis
Lumbar ligament laxity

Epidemiology and Demographics

Typically, patients with lumbar instability fall into two categories: younger adults and older adults. Younger patients with the condition usually are between 20 and 30 years of age, and the problem is often related to lack of muscle control. Adults over age 60 often have instability caused by degenerative changes.

Relevant History

Younger patients may report a history of back injury or trauma. The trauma may have occurred in such a way that the passive ligamentous structures and joint capsule did not fully heal or there was resulting muscle weakness. The resultant scar tissue and collagen are weak, and the collagen is not as regularly aligned as normal collagen; therefore, the scar tissue and collagen are not strong enough to restrain outside forces. This, combined with muscle atrophy, especially in the deep muscles because of pain, results in laxity around the joint. Injury also may have resulted in a fracture or aggravation of the pars interarticularis. The patient often reports a lack of response to or only temporary symptom relief with intervention. Older adult patients often report a long history of episodic back pain that is increasing in frequency and intensity. The past history also may include trauma or injury to the lumbar region.

Relevant Signs and Symptoms

- Patients with lumbar instability usually report a history of recurrent/episodic locking, catching, or giving way of the low back during active motion. They may use terms such as "clicking," "clunking," or "slipping" or may report a feeling of instability.
- Patients may report a sharp pain with motion or a painful arc of motion.
- Patients usually feel decreased pain with activity (the muscles of the spine act to stabilize the instability) and increased pain with static positions (the muscles relax, and the spine shifts).
- Patients may report aching in the lumbar spine for several days after an episode of instability and usually report increased back pain after prolonged positioning and/or pain at end range of lumbar motion or on the return to neutral.
- The intensity of the pain may seem excessive relative to the provoking force or activity. Symptom onset occurs after what seems to be a simple activity with minimal provocation, and the symptoms often resolve rapidly.
- There is no consistent pattern of dysfunction or symptom onset.
- The pain is located in the lumbar region and may radiate into one or both buttocks or posterior thighs if the adjacent nerve root is irritated.
- Patients often report no relief or only temporary relief from previous interventions.

Mechanism of Injury

Lumbar instability may be caused by a severe sprain, fracture, spondylolisthesis, or previous lumbar surgery. Degenerative mechanisms include degenerative joint disease (DJD [osteoarthritis]) and degenerative disc disease (DDD [spondylosis]). Panjabi et al.[59] theorized that joint stability was achieved by the coordinated actions of three systems: the passive, active, and motor control neurological systems. Disruption or injury to any of these three systems could affect the other systems by forcing them to work harder to provide stability to the joint. In the case of trauma, ligaments that provide passive support to the spinal vertebrae could be sprained, resulting in joint laxity and instability. Motion and activity encourage activation of the active systems, thus joint stability is maintained; however, over time, the muscles also have a tendency to weakness or tightness, upsetting the normal neutral pelvis alignment. Static positions or positions of relative rest allow the lumbar musculature to turn off. When the muscles are not activated, lumbar dynamic stability can be lost. As the spinal segment loses stability, the instability aggravates pain-producing structures.

H AND I STABILITY TESTS[60,61]

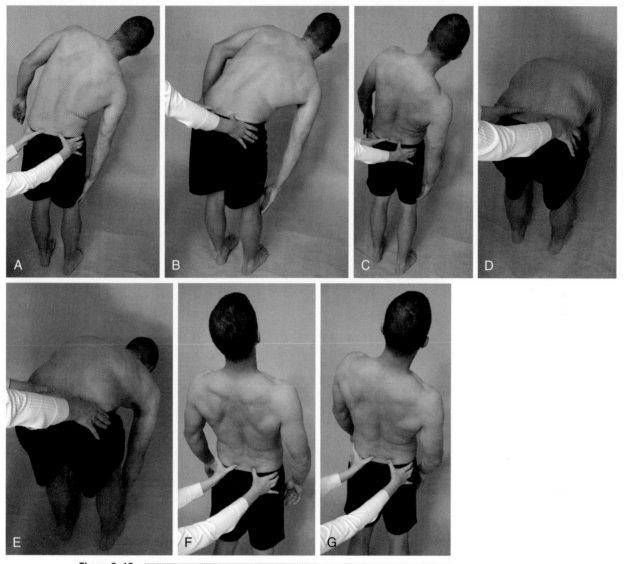

Figure 8–18
H and I stability tests. **A,** H test—side flexion. **B,** H test—side flexion followed by forward flexion.
C, H test—side flexion followed by extension. **D,** I test—forward flexion. **E,** I test—forward flexion
and side flexion. **F,** I test—extension. **G,** I test—extension and side flexion.

PURPOSE	To test for hypomobility and instability in the lumbar spine.
PATIENT POSITION	The patient stands in the normal resting position.
EXAMINER POSITION	The examiner kneels or stands directly behind the patient.
TEST PROCEDURE	The examiner's hands are placed on the patient's pelvis on the posterior superior iliac spines.

The first part of the test is the "H" movement. The patient stands in the normal resting position, which would be considered the center of the "H". The pain-free side is tested first. The patient is asked, with guidance from the examiner, to side-flex as far as possible (the side of the "H"). While in this position, the patient is asked to flex (the front of the "H") while the examiner notes how far the patient moves. The patient then

Continued

H AND I STABILITY TESTS[60,61]—*cont'd*

is moved into extension (the back of the "H"), and the examiner notes how far the patient moves. If flexion was more painful than extension, extension would be done before flexion. The patient then returns to neutral and repeats the movements to the other side. If necessary, the examiner may stabilize the pelvis with one hand and guide the movement with the other hand on the shoulder.

The second part of the test is the "I" movement. The patient stands in the normal resting position, which would be considered the center of the "I". Pain-free movement (flexion or extension) is tested first. With guidance from the examiner, the patient is asked to forward-flex the lumbar spine until the hips start to move (top part of the "I"). Once in flexion, the patient is guided into side bending (to the pain-free side first "I") while the examiner notes how far the patient moved. The patient then returns to the neutral starting position. The process is repeated to the symptomatic side. The patient is next tested into extension, and a similar process of extension and side flexion ensues. Note that the process can be completed by testing extension first followed by flexion. The decision should be driven by patient symptoms. If the patient is more symptomatic with flexion, then it should be tested last. If the patient is more symptomatic with extension, then extension will be tested last.

INDICATIONS OF A POSITIVE TEST   If a hypomobile segment is present, at least two of the movements (the movements into the same quadrant [e.g., the top right of the H and I]) are limited. If instability is present, one quadrant again is affected, but by only one of the movements (i.e., by the "H" movement or the "I" movement, but not both). For example, if the patient had spondylolisthesis instability in anterior shear (a component of forward flexion) and the "I" is attempted, the shear or slip occurs on forward flexion and little movement occurs during the attempted side bending. If the "H" is attempted, the side bending is normal, and the following forward flexion is full because the shear occurs in the second phase. So, in this case, the "I" movement is limited but not the "H" movement.

CLINICAL NOTE/CAUTION   • The "H" and "I" monikers relate to the movements that occur.
• This test is primarily for structural instability, but an instability jog may be evident during one of the movements if loss of control occurs. In this case, the end range is commonly normal, but loss of control occurs somewhere in the available ROM.

RELIABILITY/SPECIFICITY/ SENSITIVITY   Unknown

TEST OF ANTERIOR LUMBAR SPINE INSTABILITY[61]   DVD

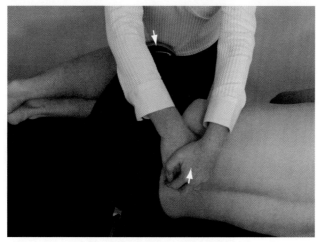

Figure 8–19
Test of anterior lumbar spine stability.

PURPOSE	To assess for anterior spinal instability of individual segments of the lumbar spine.
PATIENT POSITION	The patient is side lying with the hips flexed to 70° and the knees flexed about 90°.
EXAMINER POSITION	The examiner stands in front of the patient and adjacent to the pelvis.
TEST PROCEDURE	The examiner's hands are placed over the test segment. The patient's knees are placed into the crease of the examiner's hip. The examiner palpates and stabilizes the target spinous process (e.g., L4). By pushing the patient's knees posteriorly through the examiner's hip and along the line of the femur, the examiner can feel the relative movement of the L5 spinous process posteriorly relative to L4. Other levels of the spine may be tested in a similar fashion.
INDICATIONS OF A POSITIVE TEST	Normally, little or no movement occurs. With a positive test result, the examiner feels L4 slip forward or an increased muscle spasm occurs.
CLINICAL NOTE	• A problem with this test is that the examiner must make sure the posterior ligaments of the spine are relatively loose or relaxed before beginning. This can be controlled by altering the amount of hip flexion. With greater hip flexion, the posterior ligaments tighten more from the bottom (sacrum) up.
RELIABILITY/SPECIFICITY/ SENSITIVITY	Unknown

TEST OF POSTERIOR LUMBAR SPINE INSTABILITY[61]

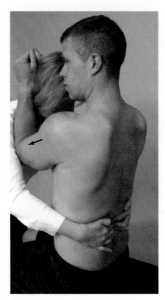

Figure 8–20
Test of posterior lumbar spine instability.

PURPOSE	To assess for posterior spinal instability of the lumbar spine.
PATIENT POSITION	The patient sits on the edge of the examining table.
EXAMINER POSITION	The examiner stands directly in front of the patient.
TEST PROCEDURE	The patient places the pronated arms, with the elbows bent, on the anterior aspect of the examiner's shoulders. The examiner puts both hands around the patient so that the fingers rest over the lumbar spine, and with the heels of the hands, gently pulling the lumbar spine into full lordosis. To stress L5 on S1, the examiner stabilizes the sacrum with the fingers of both hands and asks the patient to push through the forearms while maintaining the lordotic posture. Other levels of the spine may be tested in a similar fashion.
INDICATIONS OF A POSITIVE TEST	Excessive motion of the spinal segment or protective muscle spasm indicates a positive test result. Pain is not an indicator of a positive test result. In the case above, the examiner will feel L5 move posteriorly in a positive case.
CLINICAL NOTE	• This test is designed to produce a posterior shear of one vertebra on another (in this case, L5 on S1).
RELIABILITY/SPECIFICITY/ SENSITIVITY	Unknown

SPECIFIC LUMBAR SPINE TORSION TEST[60,61]

DVD

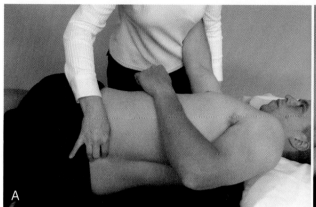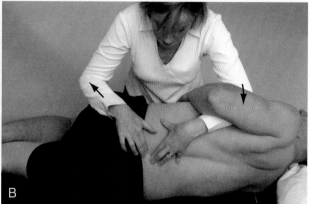

Figure 8–21
Specific lumbar spine torsion test (to L5-S1). **A,** Start position. **B,** Final position.

PURPOSE	To stress specific levels of the lumbar spine into spinal rotation.
PATIENT POSITION	The patient is placed in a right or left side-lying position with the lumbar spine in slight extension (slight lordosis). As the unaffected side should be tested first, it should be uppermost.
EXAMINER POSITION	The examiner is positioned in front of the patient and adjacent to the abdomen.
TEST PROCEDURE	One of the examiner's hands grasps the wrist of the patient's upper extremity in contact with the treatment table. The examiner's other hand is positioned on the lumbar spine. The examiner's fingers should be placed so as to palpate the desired spinous process. The examiner pulls the lower arm upward and forward at a 45° angle until movement is felt at the upper spinous process (L4) of the segment (e.g., L4-L5) being tested. This "locks" all the vertebrae above that spinous level. The examiner then stabilizes the spinous process by holding the left shoulder back with the examiner's elbow while rotating the pelvis and sacrum forward with the arm of the hand that is now palpating the lower (L5) spinous process until the lower spinous process starts to move. This means maximum stress is now being applied to that specific segment.
INDICATIONS OF A POSITIVE TEST	Minimal movement should occur, and a normal capsular tissue stretch should be felt when the segment is stressed by carefully pushing the shoulder back with the elbow while rotating the pelvis forward with the other arm/hand. Excessive movement or pain are signs of a positive test result.
CLINICAL NOTE/CAUTION	• This test position is a common position used to manipulate the spine; therefore, the examiner should take care not to overstress the rotation during assessment. In some cases, the examiner may hear a "click" or "pop" when doing this test; these are the same sounds that are heard with a manipulation.
RELIABILITY/SPECIFICITY/ SENSITIVITY	Unknown

SPECIAL TESTS FOR JOINT DYSFUNCTION[62-64]

Relevant Special Tests

Quadrant test
One-leg standing (stork standing) lumbar extension test

Definition

Lumbar spine joint dysfunction is not a pathological condition, but rather a movement or physiological disorder. Lumbar joint dysfunction can be the result of a broad range of orthopedic pathology. From a simplistic standpoint, the terms can be used to define any pathology or clinical presentation that is the result of malfunctioning joints in the lumbar spine.

Suspected Injury

Lumbar facet dysfunction (facet syndrome)
Degenerative disc disease (spondylosis)
Foraminal stenosis
Central stenosis
Degenerative joint disease (osteoarthritis)

Epidemiology and Demographics

Lumbar stenosis is the most common cause of neurological leg pain in older adults. The onset of symptoms occurs in the fifth or sixth decade, and stenosis is evenly distributed in men and women.

Relevant History

Younger adult patients commonly have a history of low back stiffness. A past history of trauma may predispose the patient to the current lumbar symptoms. Other contributing factors, such as leg length discrepancies, injuries to the lower extremity, or repetitive activities (e.g., gymnastics or bending backward), also may be associated with the joint dysfunction. Older adult patients may also have a history of low back pain that has progressively worsened. The patient also may have a prior history of trauma or lumbar instability.

Relevant Signs and Symptoms

- Younger adult patients may report a unilateral low back pain that radiates into the ipsilateral gluteal region.
- Patients may report that they began experiencing lumbar pain after bending forward. When they straightened up, they felt a sharp pain that has limited their motion since that time.
- Symptoms usually are increased with positions that require lumbar extension coupled with ipsilateral side bend and/or rotation.
- Symptoms often are alleviated by lumbar flexion.
- Symptoms generally are mechanical in nature. Specific activities worsen the symptoms, and specific activities alleviate the pain.
- Older adults with joint arthritis or stenosis usually report an insidious onset of low back pain and stiffness.
- Patients with either central or lateral stenosis have a low tolerance for trunk extension postures or activities. In patients with central stenosis, pain into the low back and gluteal region can occur bilaterally.
- Patients with lateral stenosis may report pain or sensory changes in one or both lower extremities. Pain may be located below the buttocks or below the knees. Functionally, walking usually is limited by low back pain or gluteal pain or both.

Mechanism of Injury

In younger adults, degeneration generally is not the cause of symptoms. Although the exact mechanism is unknown, it has been hypothesized that the source of pain is irritation or entrapment of pain-generating structures, such as the joint capsule or menscoid-like structures. These structures become impinged between the two opposing surfaces of the zygapophyseal (facet) joint or an ensuing inflammatory process, and pain may be generated.

In older adults, lumbar stenosis generally is a degenerative process, with hypertrophy of the lamina, degenerative hypertrophy of the facets, or buckling or hypertrophy of the ligamentum flavum. The intervertebral disc may undergo degenerative changes. This degeneration causes disc collapse and facet arthritis, narrowing the intervertebral foramen.

Central stenosis is a narrowing of the central vertebral canal and may be congenital or acquired. Lateral stenosis is a narrowing of the intervertebral foramen. Central stenosis may compromise the spinal cord or cauda equina (dural sac), whereas lateral stenosis may compromise the nerve root or dorsal root ganglia.

QUADRANT TEST[65-67]

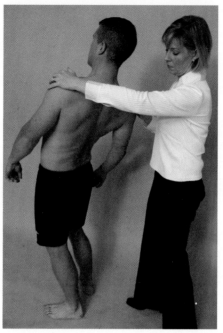

Figure 8–22
Quadrant test for the lumbar spine.

PURPOSE	To assess the response to maximum narrowing of the intervertebral foramen and to stress the facet joint.
PATIENT POSITION	The patient stands, unsupported.
EXAMINER POSITION	The examiner stands behind the patient and slightly to the side to be tested.
TEST PROCEDURE	The uninvolved side is tested first. The examiner's hands are placed on the patient's shoulders. The patient extends, side flexes, and rotates the spine while the examiner controls the movement by holding the shoulders. Overpressure may then be applied. The movement is continued until the limit of range is reached or until symptoms are produced. The amount of movement on the two sides is compared.
INDICATIONS OF A POSITIVE TEST	The test result is positive if the patient's symptoms are reproduced.
CLINICAL NOTES/CAUTIONS	• The position causes maximum narrowing of the intervertebral foramen and stress on the facet joint to the side on which rotation and side flexion occur. • Cipriano[67] described a similar test as Kemp's test. • A treatment table may be placed directly in front of the patient. For the initial start position, the patient places the front of the hips in direct contact with the table. The table stabilizes the hips and allows motion to occur more locally at the lumbar spine.
RELIABILITY/SPECIFICITY/ SENSITIVITY	Unknown

ONE-LEG STANDING (STORK STANDING) LUMBAR EXTENSION TEST[68-70]

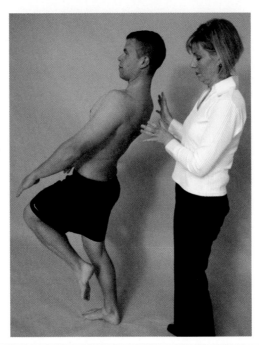

Figure 8–23
One-leg standing lumbar extension test.

PURPOSE	To assess for lumbar joint dysfunction (a positive test result may be associated with a pars interarticularis stress fracture or spondylolithesis).
PATIENT POSITION	The patient stands on one leg.
EXAMINER POSITION	The examiner is positioned directly behind the patient. This is an observational test; therefore, no manual contact is required. The examiner should be positioned close enough to the patient to provide stability if the patient requires assistance or loses balance.
TEST PROCEDURE	While standing on one leg, the patient extends the spine. The test is repeated with the patient standing on the opposite leg.
INDICATIONS OF A POSITIVE TEST	A positive test result is indicated by pain in the back.
CLINICAL NOTE/CAUTION	• If the stress fracture is unilateral, standing on the ipsilateral leg causes more pain. If rotation is combined with extension and pain results, this indicates a possible facet joint pathological condition on the side to which rotation occurs.
RELIABILITY/SPECIFICITY/ SENSITIVITY	Unknown

JOINT PLAY MOVEMENTS

SEGMENTAL FLEXION

DVD

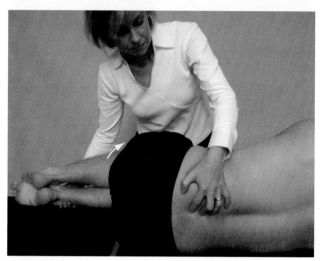

Figure 8–24
Segmental flexion.

PATIENT POSITION	The patient is side lying.
EXAMINER POSITION	The examiner stands facing the patient and is positioned adjacent to the abdomen.
TEST PROCEDURE	The examiner palpates between the spinous processes of the lumbar vertebrae with one hand (one finger on the spinous process, one finger above, and one finger below the process). The examiner then passively flexes both of the patient's knees and hips to 90°+. From this start position, the examiner passively flexes the knees toward the chest by flexing the hips. The examiner's body weight shift is used to cause the movement. The assessment begins at the S1 spinal segment and progresses upward to L1, with increased hip flexion as the examiner moves up the spine palpating the different segments for movement.
INDICATIONS OF A POSITIVE TEST	The examiner should feel the spinous processes move apart on flexion. If this gapping does not occur between two spinous processes or if gapping motion is less than the other spinal segments, the segment is considered hypomobile. If gapping occurs in excess or if the gapping motion in more than the other spinal segments, the segment is considered hypermobile.
CLINICAL NOTES	• The results of this test depend on the examiner's skill; interrater reliability studies have shown only average reliability. • An alternative means of palpation is to place just one finger in the interspinous space (between two spinous processes). • Motion is assessed by palpating when the supraspinous ligament becomes taut. • The patient's lower extremities can be heavy and difficult to hold and maneuver. Placing the patient's knees in the crease of the examiner's hip and using the examiner's legs to help lift and maneuver the legs make the technique easier to accomplish.

SEGMENTAL EXTENSION

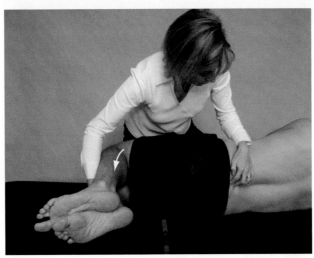

Figure 8–25
Segmental extension.

PATIENT POSITION	The patient is side lying.
EXAMINER POSITION	The examiner stands facing the patient and is positioned adjacent to the abdomen.
TEST PROCEDURE	The examiner palpates between the spinous processes of the lumbar vertebrae with one hand (one finger on the spinous process, one finger above, and one finger below the process). The examiner passively flexes both hips and knees to 90°+. From this position, the examiner uses the patient's knees to push posteriorly. The posterior force produces extension through the lumbar spine. The examiner gradually pushes through the patient's knees and extension is felt at the palpated spinal segment. The examiner assesses each spinal segment motion, starting at S1 and progresses upward to L1, with increased hip extension as the examiner palpates the different segments for movement.
INDICATIONS OF A POSITIVE TEST	The examiner should feel the spinous processes move together on extension. If this closing does not occur between the two spinous processes or if closing motion is less than the other spinal segments, the segment is considered hypomobile. If closing occurs in excess or if the closing motion is more than the other spinal segments, the segment is considered hypermobile.
CLINICAL NOTES/CAUTIONS	• The results of the test depend on the examiner's skill; interrater reliability studies have shown only average reliability. • An alternative means of palpation is to place one finger in the interspinous space (between two spinous processes) and feeling the spinous processes come together. • Motion is assessed by palpating when the supraspinous ligament becomes lax or the spinous processes reach their maximum approximation. • The patient's lower extremities can be heavy and difficult to hold and maneuver. Placing the patient's knees in the crease of the examiner's hip and using the examiner's legs to help lift and maneuver the legs make the technique easier to accomplish.

SEGMENTAL SIDE FLEXION

DVD

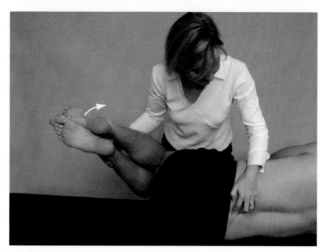

Figure 8–26
Segmental side flexion.

PATIENT POSITION	The patient is side lying.
EXAMINER POSITION	The examiner stands facing the patient and is positioned adjacent to the abdomen.
TEST PROCEDURE	The examiner palpates between the spinous processes of the lumbar vertebrae with one hand (one finger on the spinous process, one finger above, and one finger below the process). The examiner passively flexes both hips and knees to 90°. From this position, the examiner grasps the patient's ankles. The examiner passively rotates the limb upward. This motion produces side flexion at the lumbar spine. The examiner assesses each spinal segment motion, starting at S1 and progressing upwards to L1 while palpating the different segments for movement. The opposite side is then tested.
INDICATIONS OF A POSITIVE TEST	The examiner should feel the spinous processes side-flex and rotate. If this does not occur between two spinous processes or if it is excessive in relation to the other spinal segment movements, the segment is hypomobile or hypermobile, respectively.
CLINICAL NOTE	• Pathological conditions of the hip must be ruled out before this test is performed.

POSTERIOR-ANTERIOR CENTRAL VERTEBRAL PRESSURE (PACVP)

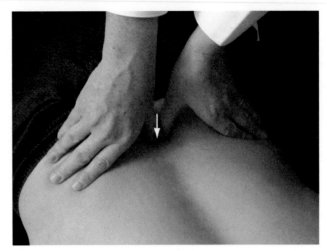

Figure 8–27
Posterior-anterior central vertebral pressure.

PATIENT POSITION	The patient is prone. Pillows or cushions may be used to put the lumbar spine in a neutral position.
EXAMINER POSITION	The examiner stands adjacent to the lumbar spine.
TEST PROCEDURE	The examiner places the tips of both thumbs on the spinous process of the vertebra to be tested. Starting at the L5 spinous process and working upward to the L1 spinous process, a posteroanterior pressure is applied through the examiner's thumbs, with the examiner pushing carefully from the shoulders, not from the thumbs. Each vertebra is pushed anteriorly. The examiner must take care to apply pressure slowly, with carefully controlled movements, to "feel" the movement, which actually is minimal. This "springing test" may be repeated several times to determine the quality of the movement and the end feel.
INDICATIONS OF A POSITIVE TEST	End range can be determined by feeling the adjacent spinous process (above or below). When the adjacent spinous process begins to move, the end range of the vertebral motion for the targeted spinal segment has been reached. As the joint play movements are performed, the examiner should note any decreased ROM, pain, or difference in end feel. Variations or symptom reproduction is considered a positive test result.
CLINICAL NOTES	• If the examiner plans to test end feel over several occasions, the same examining table should be used to improve reliability. Likewise, the patient should be positioned the same way each time. • The greatest movement occurs with the spine in neutral. The interrater reliability of these techniques is often low.

POSTERIOR-ANTERIOR UNILATERAL VERTEBRAL PRESSURE (PAUVP)

DVD

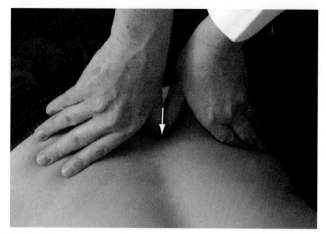

Figure 8–28
Posterior-anterior unilateral vertebral pressure.

PATIENT POSITION	The patient is prone. Pillows or cushions may be used to put the lumbar spine in a neutral position.
EXAMINER POSITION	The examiner stands adjacent to the lumbar spine.
TEST PROCEDURE	The examiner moves the thumbs laterally away from the tip of the spinous process so that the thumbs rest on the muscles overlying the lamina or the transverse process of the lumbar vertebra. The examiner places the tip of both thumbs on the lamina or transverse process, about 2.5 to 4 cm (1 to 1.5 inches) lateral to the spinous process of the lumbar vertebra. Starting at the L5 spinous process and working upward to the L1 spinous process, pressure is applied through the examiner's thumbs, with the examiner pushing carefully from the shoulders, and each vertebra is pushed anteriorly in a consecutive fashion. The examiner must take care to apply pressure slowly, with carefully controlled movements, to feel the movement, which actually is minimal. This springing test may be repeated several times to determine the quality of the movement and the end feel.
INDICATIONS OF A POSITIVE TEST	As the joint play movements are performed, the examiner should note any decreased ROM, pain, or difference in end feel. The same anterior springing pressure is applied as in the central pressure technique. This springing pressure causes a slight rotation of the vertebra in the opposite direction, which can be confirmed by palpating the spinous process while performing the technique. The two sides should be evaluated and compared. Variations or symptom reproduction is considered a positive test result.
CLINICAL NOTES	• The lumbar musculature often is guarded and tight (i.e., in spasm) in patients with a pathological low back condition; therefore, tenderness and stiffness from muscle tightness may influence the stiffness of joints and therefore affect the examiner's test results. • These techniques are specific to each vertebra and are applied to each vertebra in turn, or at least to the ones the examination has indicated may be affected by a pathological condition.

TRANSVERSE VERTEBRAL PRESSURE (TVP)

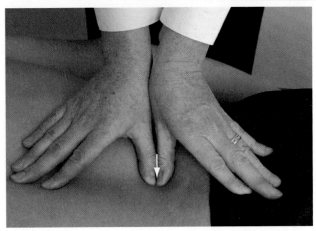

Figure 8–29
Transverse vertebral pressure.

PATIENT POSITION	The patient is prone. Pillows or cushions may be used to put the lumbar spine in a neutral position.
EXAMINER POSITION	The examiner stands adjacent to the lumbar spine.
TEST PROCEDURE	The examiner's thumbs are placed along the side of the spinous process of the lumbar spine. The examiner applies a transverse springing pressure to the side of the spinous process, which causes the vertebra to rotate in the direction of the pressure. The examiner feels for the quality of movement. Pressure should be applied to both sides of the spinous process to compare the quality of movement through the range available and the end feel. The examiner should begin the assessment at the L5 spinous process and work upward to the L1 spinous process. Each vertebra is tested consecutively.
INDICATIONS OF A POSITIVE TEST	TVP causes minimal rotation of the vertebral body; the end range can be determined by feeling for rotation of the adjacent spinous process. As the joint play movements are performed, the examiner should note any decreased ROM, pain, or difference in end feel. A difference in end feel, either hypermobility or hypomobility, is considered a positive test finding.
CLINICAL NOTE	• These techniques are specific to each vertebra and are applied to each vertebra in turn, or at least to the ones that the examination has indicated may be affected by a pathological condition.

References

1. McKenzie RA: *The lumbar spine: mechanical diagnosis and therapy*, Waikanae, New Zealand, 1981, Spinal Publications.
2. Bourdillon JF, Day EA: *Spinal manipulation*, London, 1987, William Heinemann Medical Books.
3. Moreau CE, Green BN, Johnson CD et al: Isometric back extension endurance tests: a review of the literature, *J Manip Physiol Ther* 24:110-122, 2001.
4. Kendall F: *Muscles, testing and function*, ed 3, Baltimore, 1983, Williams & Wilkins.
5. Moreland J, Finch E, Stratord P et al: Interrater reliability of six tests of trunk muscle function and endurance, *J Orthop Sports Phys Ther* 26:200-208, 1997.
6. Reese NB: *Muscle and sensory testing*, Philadelphia, 1999, Saunders.
7. Jorgensen K, Nicolaisen T: Trunk extensor endurance: determination and relation to low-back trouble, *Ergonomics* 30:259-267, 1987.
8. Ito T, Shirado O, Suzuki H et al: Lumbar trunk muscle endurance testing: an inexpensive alternative to a machine for evaluation, *Arch Phys Med Rehabil* 77:75-79, 1996.
9. Ng JK, Richardson CA, Jull GA: Electromyographic amplitude and frequency changes in the iliocostalis lumborum and multifidus muscles during a trunk holding exercise, *Phys Ther* 77:954-961, 1987.
10. Moffroid MT: Endurance of trunk muscles in persons with chronic low back pain: assessment, performance, training, *J Rehab Res Train* 34:440-447, 1997.
11. Clarkson HM: *Musculoskeletal assessment*, ed 2, Philadelphia, 2000, Lippincott Williams & Wilkins.
12. Youdas JW, Garrett TR, Egan KS et al: Lumbar lordosis and pelvic inclination in adults with chronic low back pain, *Phys Ther* 80:261-275, 2000.
13. Shields RK, DG Heiss: An electromyographic comparison of abdominal muscle synergies during curl and double straight leg lowering exercises with control of the pelvic position, *Spine* 22:1873-1879, 1999.
14. McGill SM: Low back exercises: evidence for improving exercise regimes, *Phys Ther* 78:754-765, 1998.
15. McGill SM, Childs A, Liebenson C: Endurance times for low back stabilization exercises: clinical targets for testing and training from a normal database, *Arch Phys Med Rehabil* 80:941-944, 1999.
16. Cyriax J: Textbook for orthopaedic medicine, vol I, Diagnosis of soft tissue lesions, London, 1975, Baillière Tindall.
17. Lipetz JS: Pathophysiology of inflammatory, degenerative, and compressive radiculopathies, Phys Med Rehabil Clin North Am 13:439-449, 2002.
18. Tsao B: The electrodiagnosis of cervical and lumbosacral radiculopathy, Neurol Clin 25:473-494, 2007.
19. van Rijn JC, Klemetso N, Reitsma JB et al: Symptomatic and asymptomatic abnormalities in patients with lumbosacral radicular syndrome: clinical examination compared with MRI, Clin Neurol Neurosurg 108:553-557, 2006.
20. Sueki D: Lumbar disc herniation. In Sueki D, Brechter J (eds): Orthopedic rehabilitation clinical advisor, St Louis, 2010, Mosby.
21. Maitland GD: The slump test: examination and treatment, *Aust J Physiother* 31:215-219, 1985.
22. Philip K, Lew P, Matyas TA: The inter-therapist reliability of the slump test, *Aust J Physiother* 35:89-94, 1989.
23. Maitland GD: Negative disc exploration: positive canal signs, *Aust J Physiother* 25:129-134, 1979.
24. Butler D, Gifford L: The concept of adverse mechanical tension in the nervous system, *Physiotherapy* 75:622-636, 1989.
25. Johnson EK, Chiarello CM: The slump test: the effects of head and lower extremity position on knee extension, *J Orthop Sports Phys Ther* 26:310-317, 1997.
26. Butler DA: *Mobilisation of the nervous system*, Melbourne, 1991, Churchill Livingstone.
27. Breig A, Troup JDG: Biomechanical considerations in straight-leg-raising test: cadaveric and clinical studies of the effects of medical hip rotation, *Spine* 4:242-250, 1979.
28. Charnley J: Orthopedic signs in the diagnosis of disc protrusion with special reference to the straight-leg-raising test, *Lancet* 1:186-192, 1951.
29. Edgar MA, Park WM: Induced pain patterns on passive straight-leg-raising in lower lumbar disc protrusion, *J Bone Joint Surg Br* 56:658-667, 1974.
30. Fahrni WH: Observations on straight-leg-raising with special reference to nerve root adhesions, *Can J Surg* 9:44-48, 1966.
31. Goddard BS, JD Reid: Movements induced by straight-leg-raising in the lumbosacral roots, nerves, and plexus and in the intrapelvic section of the sciatic nerve, *J Neurol Neurosurg Psychiatry* 28:12-18, 1965.
32. Scham SM, Taylor TKF: Tension signs in lumbar disc prolapse, *Clin Orthop* 75:195-204, 1971.
33. Urban LM: The straight-leg-raising test: a review, *J Orthop Sports Phys Ther* 2:117-133, 1981.
34. Wilkins RH, Brody IA: Lasègue's sign, *Arch Neurol* 21:219-220, 1969.
35. Summers B, Malhan K, Cassar-Pullicino V: Low back pain on passive straight leg raising: the anterior theca as a source of pain, *Spine* 30:342-345, 2005.
36. Spengler DM: *Low back pain: assessment and management*, Orlando, Fla, 1982, Grune & Stratton.
37. Woodhall R, Hayes GJ: The well-leg-raising test of Fajersztajn in the diagnosis of ruptured lumbar intervertebral disc, *J Bone Joint Surg Am* 32:786-792, 1950.
38. Khuffash B, Porter RW: Cross leg pain and trunk list, *Spine* 14:602-603, 1989.
39. Vucetic N, Svensson O: Physical signs in lumbar disc hernia, *Clin Orthop Relat Res* 333:192-201, 1996.
40. Gabbe BJ, Bennell KL, Majswelner H et al: Reliability of common lower extremity musculoskeletal screening tests. *Phys Ther Sports* 5:90-97, 2004.
41. Shiqing X, Quanzhi Z, Dehao F: Significance of the straight-leg-raising test in the diagnosis and clinical evaluation of lower lumbar intervertebral disc protrusion, *J Bone Joint Surg Am* 69:517-522, 1987.
42. Kosteljanetz M, Bang F. Schmidt-Olsen S: The clinical significance of straight leg raising (Lasègue's sign) in the diagnosis of prolapsed lumber disc: interobserver variation and correlation with surgical finding, *Spine* 13:393-395, 1988.

43. Herron LD, Pheasant HC: Prone knee-flexion provocative testing for lumbar disc protrusion, *Spine* 5:65-67, 1980.

44. Postacchini F, Cinotti G, Gumina S: The knee flexion test: a new test for lumbosacral root tension, *J Bone Joint Surg Br* 75:834-835, 1993.

45. Dyck P: The femoral nerve traction test with lumbar disc protrusion, *Surg Neurol* 6:163-166, 1976.

46. Kreitz BG, Coté P, Yong-Hing K: Crossed femoral stretching test: a case report, *Spine* I 21:1584-1586, 1996.

47. Macnab I: *Backache*, Baltimore, 1977, Williams & Wilkins.

48. Evans RC: *Illustrated essentials in orthopedic physical assessment*, St Louis, 1994, Mosby.

49. Brudzinski J: A new sign of the lower extremities in meningitis of children (neck sign), *Arch Neurol* 21:217, 1969.

50. Cram RH: A sign of sciatic nerve root pressure, *J Bone Joint Surg Br* 35:192-195, 1953.

51. Deyerle WM, May VR: Sciatic tension test, *South Med J* 49:999-1005, 1956.

52. Abbott JH, McCane B, Herbison P et al: Lumbar segmental instability: a criterion-related validity study of manual therapy assessment, *BMC Musculoskelet Disord* 7:56, 2005.

53. Cleland J: *Orthopaedic clinical examination: an evidence-based approach for physical therapists*, Carlstadt, NJ, 2005, Icon Learning Systems.

54. Fritz JM, Whitman JM, Childs JD: Lumbar spine segmental mobility assessment: an examination of validity for determining intervention strategies in patients with low back pain, *Arch Phys Med Rehabil* 86:1745-1752, 2005.

55. Fritz JM, Piva SR, Childs JD: Accuracy of the clinical examination to predict radiographic instability of the lumbar spine, *Eur Spine J* 14:743-750, 2005.

56. Hicks GE, Fritz JM, Delitto A, Mishock J: Interrater reliability of clinical examination measures for identification of lumbar segmental instability, *Arch Phys Med Rehabil* 84:1858-1864, 2003.

57. Kasai Y, Morishita K, Awakit E et al: A new evaluation method for lumbar spinal instability: passive lumbar extension test, *Phys Ther* 86:1661-1667, 2006.

58. Kikilus P: Lumbar instability. In Sueki D, Brechter J (eds): *Orthopedic rehabilitation clinical advisor*, St Louis, 2010, Mosby.

59. Panjabi MM, Aumi K, Duranceau J, Oxland T: Spinal stability and intersegmental muscle forces, *Spine* 14:194-200, 1989.

60. Meadows JT: *Orthopedic differential diagnosis in physical therapy: a case study approach*, New York, 1999, McGraw-Hill.

61. Dobbs AC: Evaluation of instabilities of the lumbar spine, *Orthop Phys Ther Clin North Am* 8:387-400, 1999.

62. Chad DA: Lumbar spinal stenosis, *Neurol Clin* 25(2):407-418, 2007.

63. Fritz JM, Delitto A, Welch WC, Erhard RD: Lumbar spinal stenosis: a review of current concepts in evaluation, management and outcome measurements, *Arch Phys Med Rehabil* 79:700-708, 1998.

64. Katz JN, Harris MB: Clinical practice lumbar spinal stenosis, *N Engl J Med* 358:815-825, 2008.

65. Lyle MA, Manes S, McGuinness M et al: Relationship of physical examination findings and self-reported symptoms severity and physical function in patients with degenerative lumbar conditions, *Phys Ther* 85:120-133, 2005.

66. Corrigan B, Maitland GD: *Practical orthopedic medicine*, London, 1985, Butterworths.

67. Cipriano JJ: *Photographic manual of regional orthopedic tests*, Baltimore, 1985 Williams & Wilkins.

68. Garrick JG, Webb DR: *Sports injuries: diagnosis and management*, Philadelphia, 1990, Saunders.

69. Jackson DW, Ciullo JV: Injuries of the spine in the skeletally immature athlete. In Nicholas JA, Hershmann EB (eds): *The lower extremity and spine in sports medicine*, vol 2, St Louis, 1986, Mosby.

70. Jackson DW, Wiltse LL, Dingeman RD et al: Stress reactions involving the pars interarticularis in young athletes, *Am J Sports Med* 9:304-312, 1981.

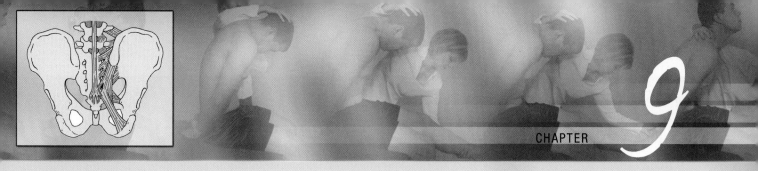

PELVIS

Précis of the Pelvis Assessment*

History (sitting)
Observation (standing)
Examination
   Active movements (standing)
      Flexion of the spine
      Extension of the spine
      Rotation of the spine (left and right)
      Side flexion of the spine (left and right)
      Flexion of the hip
      Abduction of the hip
      Adduction of the hip
      Extension of the hip
      Medial rotation of the hip
      Lateral rotation of the hip
   Special tests (standing)
      Gillet's (sacral fixation) test
      Ipsilateral anterior rotation test
      Flamingo test or maneuver
      Trendelenburg's sign
      Functional limb length test
   Special tests (sitting)
   Passive movements (supine)
      Sacral apex pressure test
      Thoracolumbar fascia length test
   Resisted isometric movements (supine)
      Forward flexion of the spine
      Flexion of the hip
      Abduction of the hip
      Adduction of the hip
      Extension of the hip
   Special tests (supine)
      Functional test of supine active straight leg raise test
      Leg length
      Sacroiliac rocking (knee-to-shoulder) test
      Gapping (transverse anterior stress) test

      Sign of the buttock
      Functional hamstring length
   Passive movements (side lying)
      Approximation test
      Passive extension and medial rotation of ilium on sacrum
      Passive flexion and lateral rotation of ilium on sacrum
   Reflexes and cutaneous distribution (supine, then prone)
   Passive movements (prone)
      Ipsilateral prone kinetic test
      Sacral apex pressure test
   Special tests (prone)
      Functional test for prone active straight leg raise test
      Prone knee bending test
   Joint play movements (prone)
      Cephalad movement of the sacrum with caudal movement of the ilium
      Cephalad movement of the ilium with caudal movement of the sacrum
   Palpation (prone, then supine)
   Diagnostic imaging

---

*The examination is shown in an order that limits the amount of moving or position changing the patient must do, yet ensures that all necessary structures are tested.

Assessment of the sacroiliac joints and symphysis pubis is done only after an assessment of the lumbar spine and hips unless specific trauma has occurred to the sacroiliac joints or symphysis pubis. The examination of the sacroiliac joints and symphysis pubis, therefore, may involve only passive movements, special tests, joint play movements, and palpation, because the other tests would have been completed during the assessment of the other joints.

After any examination, the patient should be warned of the possibility of exacerbation of symptoms as a result of the assessment.

SELECTED MOVEMENTS

NUTATION AND COUNTERNUTATION[1-4]

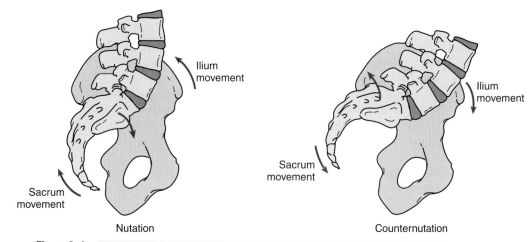

Ilium
movement

Sacrum
movement

Nutation

Ilium
movement

Sacrum
movement

Counternutation

Figure 9–1
Movements of nutation and counternutation occurring at the sacroiliac joint.

PURPOSE	Nutation and counternutation movements are used to assess the sacrum's ability to nutate (lock) and counternutate (unlock) on the innominates.

Nutation

PATIENT POSITION	The patient is sitting.
EXAMINER POSITION	The examiner sits or kneels directly behind the patient and palpates the inferior aspect of the posterior superior iliac spine (PSIS) on one side with one thumb while using the other thumb to palpate the sacral base (i.e., the thumbs are parallel).
TEST PROCEDURE	The patient is asked to bend forward. As the patient bends forward, the examiner notes how much flexion has occurred just as sacral nutation begins.
INDICATIONS OF A POSITIVE TEST	In the first 45° of forward flexion, the sacral base moves forward (nutates); however, near 60° (normally), the sacral base begins to counternutate, or move backward. During counternutation, the two PSISs should move upward equally in relation to the sacrum and toward each other, or approximate. At the same time, the anterior superior sacroiliac spine (ASIS) tends to flare out.

Counternutation

PATIENT POSITION	To test backward bending, the patient stands with the weight equally distributed on both legs.
EXAMINER POSITION	The examiner sits or kneels behind the patient and palpates both PSISs.
TEST PROCEDURE	The patient is asked to bend backward, and the examiner notes any asymmetry.

Continued

NUTATION AND COUNTERNUTATION[1-4]—*cont'd*

INDICATIONS OF A POSITIVE TEST	Normally, the PSISs move inferiorly on extension. The examiner palpates both sides of the sacrum at the level of S1. As the patient extends, the sacral base should move forward; this is called the *sacral flexion test*.
CLINICAL NOTES/CAUTIONS	• During extension, or backward bending, of the trunk, the innominate bones (i.e., the pelvic girdle) as a whole unit rotate posteriorly (nutation) on the femoral heads bilaterally. If one leg is actively flexed at the hip, the innominate on that side unilaterally rotates posteriorly. • During the posterior rotation of the innominate bones, the innominate slides anteriorly along the long arm of the sacral joint and superiorly up the short arm of the sacral joint. This movement is the same as sacral nutation. With backward bending, the two PSISs move inferiorly an equal amount.
RELIABILITY/SPECIFICITY/ SENSITIVITY	Unknown

COMMON STRESS TESTS (PASSIVE MOVEMENTS)

IPSILATERAL PRONE KINETIC TEST

DVD

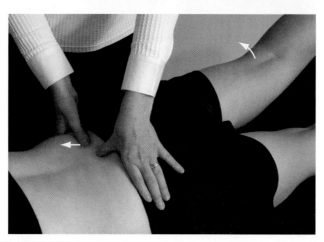

Figure 9–2

Ipsilateral prone kinetic test. On extension, the posterior superior iliac spine and sacral crest move superiorly and laterally.

PURPOSE	To assess the ability of the ilium to flex and to rotate laterally or posteriorly.
PATIENT POSITION	The patient lies prone.
EXAMINER POSITION	The examiner stands adjacent to the patient's pelvis.
TEST PROCEDURE	The examiner places one thumb on one PSIS and the other thumb parallel to it on the sacrum starting with the unaffected side. The patient then is asked to actively extend the leg on the side the examiner palpates. The test is then repeated on the affected side.
INDICATIONS OF A POSITIVE TEST	Normally, the PSIS moves superiorly and laterally when the patient extends the leg. If it does not, it indicates hypomobility with a posteriorly rotated ilium, or outflare.
CLINICAL NOTE	• This is a test of motion and movement; pain may be produced by the test, but it is not a sign of a positive test result.
RELIABILITY/SPECIFICITY/ SENSITIVITY	Unknown

PASSIVE EXTENSION AND MEDIAL ROTATION OF THE ILIUM ON THE SACRUM[1,5]

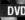

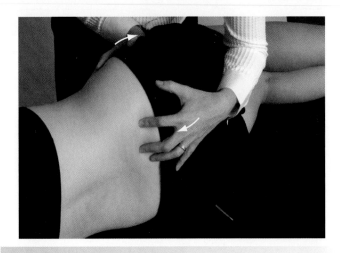

Figure 9–3
Passive extension and medial rotation of the ilium on the sacrum. The innominate bone is held in extension and medial rotation. The examiner palpates the sacrum and ilium with the fingers while rotating the ilium forward. With hypomobility, the relative movement is less than on the unaffected side, indicating an outflare.

PURPOSE	To assess for hypomobility and a posteriorly rotated ilium, or outflare of the pelvis.
PATIENT POSITION	The patient is side lying on the non-test side.
EXAMINER POSITION	The examiner stands adjacent to the patient's pelvis.
TEST PROCEDURE	On the unaffected side, the examiner places one hand over the ASIS area of the anterior ilium. The other hand is placed over the PSIS so that the fingers palpate the posterior ilium and sacrum. The examiner pulls the ilium down toward the knees with the hand over the ASIS and pushes the posterior ilium up with the other hand while feeling the relative movement of the ilium on the sacrum. The affected side then is tested for comparison.
INDICATIONS OF A POSITIVE TEST	If less movement occurs on the affected side, it indicates hypomobility and a posteriorly rotated ilium, or outflare.
CLINICAL NOTE	• If positive results are seen on both this test and the test of passive flexion and lateral rotation of the ilium on the sacrum, an upslip has occurred to the ilium relative to the sacrum.
RELIABILITY/SPECIFICITY/ SENSITIVITY	Unknown

PASSIVE FLEXION AND LATERAL ROTATION OF THE ILIUM ON THE SACRUM[1,5]   DVD

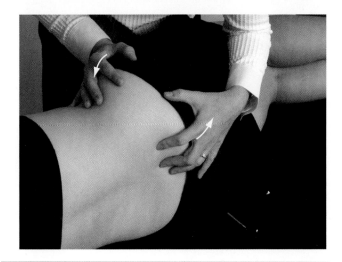

Figure 9–4
Passive flexion and lateral rotation of the ilium on the sacrum. The innominate bone is held in flexion
and lateral rotation. The examiner palpates the sacrum and ilium with the left fingers while rotating the
ilium backward. With hypomobility, the relative movement is less than on the unaffected side, indicating
an inflare.

PURPOSE	To assess for hypomobility and an anteriorly rotated ilium, or inflare of the pelvis.
PATIENT POSITION	The patient is side lying on the non-test side.
EXAMINER POSITION	The examiner stands adjacent to the patient's pelvis.
TEST PROCEDURE	On the unaffected side, the examiner places one hand over the ASIS area of the anterior ilium. The other hand is placed over the PSIS so that the fingers palpate the posterior ilium and sacrum. The examiner pushes the anterior ilium backward (up) with the anterior hand and pulls the ilium down with the posterior hand and arm while palpating the relative movement. The affected side then is tested for comparison.
INDICATIONS OF A POSITIVE TEST	If less movement occurs on the affected side, it is a sign of hypomobility and an anteriorly rotated ilium, or inflare.
CLINICAL NOTE/CAUTION	• If positive results are seen on both this test and the test of passive extension and medial rotation of the ilium on the sacrum, an upslip has occurred to the ilium relative to the sacrum.
RELIABILITY/SPECIFICITY/ SENSITIVITY	Unknown

GAPPING (TRANSVERSE ANTERIOR STRESS) TEST[1,6,7]

 DVD

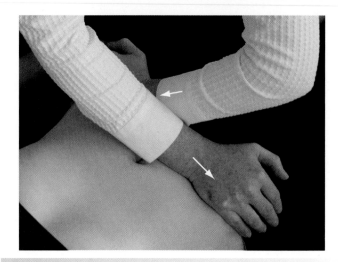

Figure 9–5
Gapping test.

PURPOSE	To assess the ability of the sacroiliac joints to gap anteriorly (this test also assesses the integrity of the anterior sacroiliac ligaments).
PATIENT POSITION	The patient lies supine.
EXAMINER POSITION	The examiner stands adjacent to the patient's pelvis.
TEST PROCEDURE	Crossing his or her arms, the examiner places a palm on each ASIS. The examiner then applies crossed-arm pressure to the ASISs, pushing down and outward with the arms.
INDICATIONS OF A POSITIVE TEST	The test result is positive only if unilateral gluteal or posterior leg pain is produced, indicating a sprain of the anterior sacroiliac ligaments.
CLINICAL NOTE/CAUTION	• Care must be taken in performing this test. Pushing against the ASISs can elicit pain, because the soft tissue is compressed between the examiner's hands and the patient's pelvis. If this is the case, the patient can be instructed to place his or her hands on each ASIS. The examiner then can push through the patient's hands.
RELIABILITY/SPECIFICITY/ SENSITIVITY	Unknown

SACROILIAC ROCKING (KNEE TO SHOULDER) TEST[1,8]   DVD

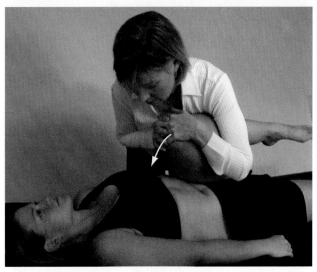

Figure 9–6
Sacroiliac rocking (knee to shoulder) test.

PURPOSE	To assess the integrity of the sacrotuberous ligament.
PATIENT POSITION	The patient lies supine.
EXAMINER POSITION	The examiner is positioned adjacent to the patient's pelvis.
TEST PROCEDURE	The examiner flexes the patient's knee and hip fully and then adducts the hip. The sacroiliac joint is "rocked" by flexion and adduction of the patient's hip. To do the test properly, the examiner moves the knee toward the patient's opposite shoulder. Some authors believe the hip should be medially rotated as it is flexed and adducted to increase the stress on the sacroiliac joint. Simultaneously, the sacrotuberous ligament may be palpated for tenderness.
INDICATIONS OF A POSITIVE TEST	Pain in the sacroiliac joints indicates a positive test result. While performing the test, the examiner may palpate the sacroiliac joint on the test side to feel for the slight amount of movement that normally is present.
CLINICAL NOTES/CAUTIONS	• This test is also called the *sacrotuberous ligament stress test*. • For proper performance of this test, both the hip and the knee must demonstrate no pathological conditions and must have full range of motion. • Care must be taken when performing this test, because it puts a great deal of stress on the hip and sacroiliac joints. If a longitudinal force is applied through the hip in a slow, steady manner (for 15 to 20 seconds) in an oblique and lateral direction, further stress is applied to the sacrotuberous ligament.
RELIABILITY/SPECIFICITY/SENSITIVITY	Unknown

SPECIAL TEST FOR NEUROLOGICAL INVOLVEMENT

PRONE KNEE BENDING (NACHLAS) TEST[9-11]

DVD

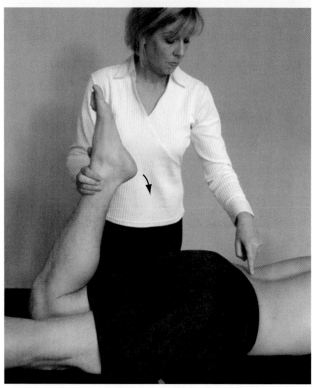

Figure 9–7
Prone knee bending test. The examiner is pointing where pain would be felt if the lumbar spine was involved.

PURPOSE	Normally, to test for a tight rectus femoris, an upper lumbar joint lesion, an upper spine nerve root lesion, or a hypomobile sacroiliac joint.
PATIENT POSITION	The patient lies prone.
EXAMINER POSITION	The examiner stands adjacent to the pelvis of the test limb.
TEST PROCEDURE	The examiner places one hand on the patient's pelvis to palpate the sacroiliac joint on the same side for compensations. The examiner's other hand grasps the ankle of the lower extremity that is being tested. The examiner passively flexes the knee as far as possible so that the patient's heel rests against the buttock (the examiner should make sure the patient's hip is not rotated). The flexed knee position should be maintained for 45 to 60 seconds.
INDICATIONS OF A POSITIVE TEST	• If pain is felt in the front of the thigh before full range is reached, the problem is in the rectus femoris muscle. • If pain is felt in the lumbar spine, the problem is in the lumbar spine, usually the L3 nerve root, especially if radicular symptoms are noted.

PRONE KNEE BENDING (NACHLAS) TEST[9-11]—*cont'd*

- If the problem is a hypomobile sacroiliac joint, the ipsilateral pelvic rim (ASIS) will rotate forward, usually before the knee reaches 90° of flexion.
- This test also stretches the femoral nerve. Pain in the anterior thigh may indicate tight quadriceps muscles or stretching of the femoral nerve. A careful history and pain differentiation help delineate the problem.

CLINICAL NOTES/CAUTIONS
- If the examiner is unable to flex the patient's knee past 90° because of a pathological condition in the knee, the test may be performed by passive extension of the hip while the knee is flexed as much as possible.
- If the rectus femoris is tight, the examiner should remember that taking the patient's heel to the buttock may cause anterior torsion to the ilium, which could lead to sacroiliac or lumbar pain.
- The test may be modified to stress different peripheral nerves (see Table 8-8).

RELIABILITY/SPECIFICITY/ SENSITIVITY
Unknown

SPECIAL TESTS FOR SACROILIAC JOINT DYSFUNCTION[6,7]

Relevant Special Tests

Gillet's test (sacral fixation test)
Functional test of supine active straight leg raise
Functional test of prone active straight leg raise
Prone knee bending (Nachlas) test
Ipsilateral anterior rotation test
Flamingo test or maneuver

Definition

Pathological conditions of the sacroiliac joints typically are considered a subclassification of the broader category of pelvic pain. Sacroiliac joint dysfunction refers to pathological motion or movement that occurs between the sacrum and the innominate.

Suspected Injury

Sacroiliac joint dysfunction

Epidemiology and Demographics

The incidence of pathological conditions of the sacroiliac joints is estimated to be 15%. Women seem to be more at risk than men. Men may be afflicted less frequently as they age, because bony fusion of the sacroiliac joints occurs more in men than women.[6,7]

Relevant History

The patient may report an event such as stepping into a hole or a traumatic fall onto one or both buttocks that preceded the onset of symptoms. Frequently, the initial onset in women occurs during or after pregnancy.

Relevant Signs and Symptoms

- The patient complains of pain in the region of the sacral sulcus, just medial to the posterior superior iliac spine. The pain may travel distally into the buttock and posterior thigh.
- Symptoms typically do not extend to or beyond the knee.
- Pain of sacroiliac joint origin does not generally refer proximally to the lumbar spine.

Mechanism of Injury

The most common correlation with the development of pelvic pain is pregnancy. Other mechanisms of injury typically include activities that require opposing innominate motion in which one innominate is posteriorly rotated and the other is relatively anteriorly rotated. Falling onto the buttocks or stepping unexpectedly into a pothole may result in the innominate being driven superiorly in relation to the sacrum.

GILLET'S TEST (SACRAL FIXATION TEST)[12-15]

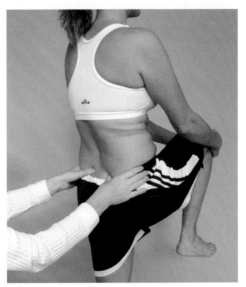

Figure 9–8
Gillet's (sacral fixation) test.

PURPOSE	To assess for sacral motion into nutation and counternutation.
PATIENT POSITION	The patient is standing.
EXAMINER POSITION	The examiner is either seated or kneeling directly behind the patient.
TEST PROCEDURE	The uninvolved side is tested first. The examiner palpates one of the PSISs with one thumb while holding the other thumb on the sacrum, parallel to the first thumb. The patient is asked to stand on one leg while pulling the opposite knee up toward the chest. This causes the innominate bone on the same side to rotate posteriorly. The test is repeated with the other leg, and the examiner palpates the other PSIS.
INDICATIONS OF A POSITIVE TEST	If the sacroiliac joint (PSIS) on the side on which the knee is flexed (i.e., the ipsilateral side) moves minimally or up, the joint is said to be hypomobile, or "blocked," indicating a positive test result. On the unaffected side, the test PSIS moves down or inferiorly. This test is similar to the test performed during hip flexion in active movement; the only difference is the points of palpation during the movement.
CLINICAL NOTES/CAUTIONS	• This test is also called the *ipsilateral posterior rotation test*. • Jackson[15] has suggested a modification of the test. After completing Gillet's test, the examiner palpates the same PSIS and sacrum and asks the patient to do a repeat Gillet's test using the other leg; this causes the opposite innominate bone to rotate posteriorly. As the patient flexes the hip and knee, the lumbar spine begins to flex, causing the sacrum to move inferiorly; as a result, the test innominate (the side opposite the leg being flexed) rotates anteriorly.
RELIABILITY/SPECIFICITY/ SENSITIVITY[13,14]	Intrarater reliability range: 0.08-0.18 Interrater reliability range: 0.00-0.02

FUNCTIONAL TEST OF SUPINE ACTIVE STRAIGHT LEG RAISE[1,16-18]

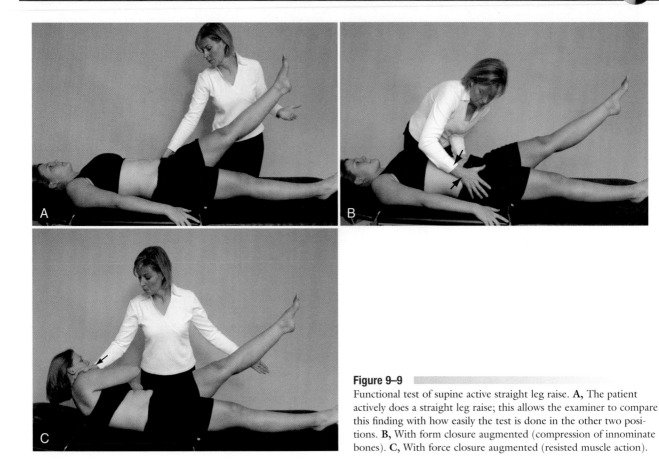

Figure 9-9

Functional test of supine active straight leg raise. **A,** The patient actively does a straight leg raise; this allows the examiner to compare this finding with how easily the test is done in the other two positions. **B,** With form closure augmented (compression of innominate bones). **C,** With force closure augmented (resisted muscle action).

PURPOSE	To assess whether stabilizing the sacroiliac joint actively or passively diminishes the patient's symptoms; also, to test force and form closure at the sacroiliac joints.
PATIENT POSITION	The patient is supine lying. The patient's head is in a neutral alignment, and no pillows should be use to support the head. The patient's hands should be placed at the sides.
EXAMINER POSITION	The examiner stands adjacent to the pelvis on the side of the test limb. The examiner should face the patient's head.
TEST PROCEDURE	The assessment involves two active leg lifts for each leg, first on the uninvolved side and then on the involved side. With the initial leg lift, the examiner places one hand on the ASIS to monitor the pelvis and to make sure no rotation occurs. This hand also may monitor the contraction of the transverse abdominis muscle. On the second leg lift, the examiner places both hands on the lateral aspect of both innominates and pushes in medially, compressing the innominates. With the first leg lift, the patient actively lifts one leg and then the other, and the examiner asks whether the patient notices any "effort differences" between the two sides. The examiner then stabilizes and compresses the pelvis while the patient actively does the straight leg raise (SLR), providing form closure of the sacroiliac joints by squeezing the innominate bones together anteriorly. The test is repeated on the other leg, and the patient is asked to compare the two legs regarding the effort required to raise the leg.

FUNCTIONAL TEST OF SUPINE ACTIVE STRAIGHT LEG RAISE[1,16-18]—*cont'd*

INDICATIONS OF A POSITIVE TEST

If the pain decreases or the SLR is easier with form closure (with no increased signs or symptoms), the test result is considered positive for possible sacroiliac joint problems. At the same time, the examiner can check the contraction of the pelvic floor/transverse abdominis/multifidus force couple by palpating medial to the ASIS bilaterally. If the force couple functions properly, tension is felt symmetrically and the abdomen moves inward. If superficial tension is felt, the internal obliques are contracting and a force couple imbalance exists. The multifidus may be palpated close to the spinous process posteriorly; it should contract when the pelvic floor contracts.

CLINICAL NOTES

- A modification tests force closure at the sacroiliac joints. The patient is asked to flex and rotate the trunk toward the side on which the straight leg raise (SLR) was actively being performed, and the examiner resists the trunk motion. The two sides are compared for any difference.
- Force closure tests the muscles' ability to stabilize the sacroiliac joints during movement.

RELIABILITY/SPECIFICITY/ SENSITIVITY

Unknown

FUNCTIONAL TEST OF PRONE ACTIVE STRAIGHT LEG RAISE[1]

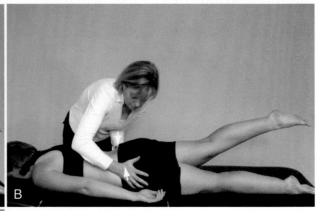

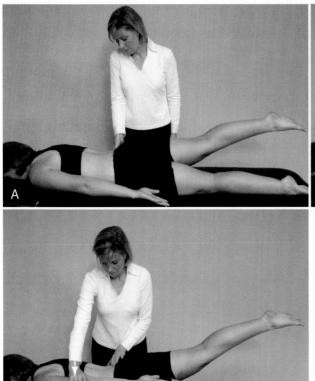

Figure 9–10

Functional test of prone active straight leg raise. **A,** The patient actively extends the straight leg; this allows the examiner to compare this finding with how easily the test is done in the other two position. **B,** With form closure augmented (compression of innominate bones). **C,** With force closure augmented (resisted muscle action).

PURPOSE	To assess whether stabilizing the sacroiliac joint actively or passively diminishes the patient's symptoms.
PATIENT POSITION	The patient is prone lying with the head in a neutral alignment. The patient's hands should be positioned at the sides.
EXAMINER POSITION	The examiner stands adjacent to the patient's pelvis and should be turned to face the patient's feet.
TEST PROCEDURE	The uninvolved side is tested first. The patient is assessed under three conditions. First, there is no examiner contact. Second, the examiner's hands are placed on the lateral aspects of the pelvis to provide a medially directed force to the pelvis. Third, the examiner grasps and supports the contralateral upper arm. To do the test, the patient actively extends the hip under each of these three conditions. The first condition is hip extension. The second condition involves the same movement as the first, with the examiner applying manual compression to the innominate bones (form closure). In the third condition, the examiner resists extension of the contralateral, medially rotated arm (force closure) as the patient extends the straight leg.
INDICATIONS OF A POSITIVE TEST	A positive test result is indicated if pain is produced with the first condition and if either of the other two conditions results in a decrease in symptoms. A decrease in pain with compression of the innominate indicates a form closure problem, probably ligamentous in nature. A decrease in pain in the third phase of the test indicates a force closure problem, and contractile stability is the issue.

FUNCTIONAL TEST OF PRONE ACTIVE STRAIGHT LEG RAISE[1]—*cont'd*

CLINICAL NOTE   • If function improves when force closure stabilization is used, exercise probably will benefit the patient.

RELIABILITY/SPECIFICITY/ SENSITVITY   Unknown

IPSILATERAL ANTERIOR ROTATION TEST[1]

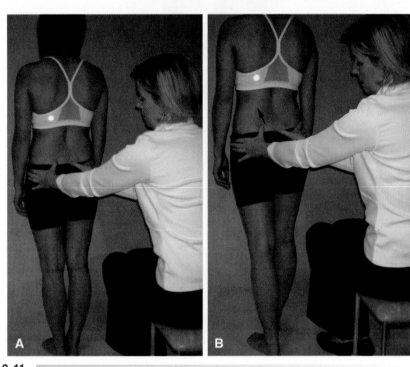

Figure 9–11
Ipsilateral anterior rotation test. **A,** Start position. **B,** Leg extended.

PURPOSE   To assess whether the innominate on the test side is able to rotate anteriorly (nutates) while the sacrum rotates to the opposite side.

PATIENT POSITION   The patient is standing with the weight equally distributed on both feet.

EXAMINER POSITION   The examiner sits behind the patient.

TEST PROCEDURE   The examiner palpates one PSIS with one thumb and the sacrum, on a parallel line, with the other thumb. The patient is asked to extend the ipsilateral leg. The other side is tested for comparison.

INDICATIONS OF A POSITIVE TEST   A positive test result is indicated by the absence of anterior rotation of the innominate relative to the sacrum.

CLINICAL NOTE   • Normally, the PSIS moves superiorly and laterally.

RELIABILITY/SPECIFICITY/ SENSITVITY   Unknown

FLAMINGO TEST OR MANEUVER[3]

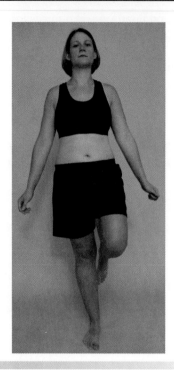

Figure 9–12
Flamingo test.

PURPOSE	To assess for injury to the sacroiliac joints and symphysis pubis.
PATIENT POSITION	The patient stands on one leg.
EXAMINER POSITION	The examiner stands behind the patient to observe the sacroiliac joints.
TEST PROCEDURE	When the patient stands on one leg, the weight of the trunk causes the sacrum to shift and rotate forward and distally (caudally). The ilium moves in the opposite direction. On the non-weight-bearing side, the opposite occurs, but the stress is greatest on the stance side.
INDICATIONS OF A POSITIVE TEST	Pain in the symphysis pubis or sacroiliac joint indicates a positive test result for lesions in whichever structure is painful.
CLINICAL NOTES	• The stress on the joints may be increased by having the patient hop on one leg. • This position is also used to take a stress radiograph of the symphysis pubis.
RELIABILITY/SPECIFICITY/ SENSITVITY	Unknown

SPECIAL TESTS FOR LEG LENGTH

Relevant Special Tests

Leg length test
Functional limb length test

Definition

The term "leg length discrepancies" refers to a difference in the longitudinal length of one leg compared to the other leg. Leg length discrepancies can fall into two classifications. One category is the actual, or true, leg length discrepancy. In these cases, the length of one leg truly is different from the length of the other leg. The other category is apparent, or functional, leg length discrepancy. In this case, one leg appears different from the other leg, but when the legs are measured, the lengths are identical. The cause of the apparent length discrepancy may be biomechanical factors, such as pelvic rotation or foot pronation.

Suspected Injury

Leg length discrepancy can occur because of trauma, such as fractures or surgery (e.g., arthroplasty), or simply as the result of varied rates of development of the two legs.

Epidemiology and Demographics

Freiberg[19] studied patients with low back pain and discovered that patients with a leg length discrepancy greater than 15 mm were five times more likely to experience low back pain. Hip and sciatic pain occurred in the longer leg 78% of the time. In patients with leg length discrepancies greater than 3 cm, an asymmetrical lateral side bend of the spine occurs on the side of the longer leg; this results in abnormal loading mechanics of the spine. Leg length discrepancies of this magnitude are present in 40% of the general population.[20]

ten Brinke et al.[20] reported that in 64 (62%) of 104 patients with a leg length discrepancy of 1 mm or greater, the back pain radiated into the shorter leg.

Relevant History

The patient may have a history of trauma to or a fracture of the lower extremity. Falls onto the buttock may result in apparent leg length discrepancies.

Relevant Signs and Symptoms

- Leg length differences themselves are not usually painful.
- Difference is clinically relevant as a contributing cause of symptoms and pathological conditions in other regions, such as the lumbar spine, pelvis, sacroiliac joint, or lower extremity.
- Objective examination of any of these regions should include an examination of leg length.

Mechanism of Injury

Actual leg length changes can be caused by falls, surgery, or by trauma. This is especially relevant if the fracture occurred in a child and the fracture was through the growth plate. A patient also may have a history of total joint replacement, which may have resulted in changes in actual leg length. Arthritic changes in the joints of the lower extremity can be a source of total leg length differences. Patients with apparent leg length discrepancies may have a history of trauma to the lumbar spine, pelvis, hip, knee, or ankle.

LEG LENGTH TEST[21,22]

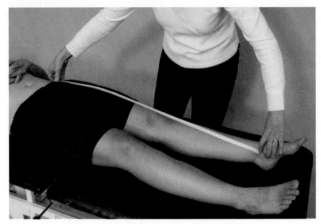

Figure 9–13
Measuring leg length (anterior superior iliac spine to medial malleolus).

PURPOSE	To assess for leg length discrepancies.
PATIENT POSITION	The patient is supine lying with the ASISs level; the patient's lower limbs are perpendicular to the line joining the ASISs.
EXAMINER POSITION	The examiner stands adjacent to the limb to be tested.
TEST PROCEDURE	Using a flexible tape measure, the examiner measures the distance from the ASIS to the medial or lateral malleolus on the same side. The measurement is repeated on the other side, and the results are compared.
INDICATIONS OF A POSITIVE TEST	A difference of 1 to 1.5 cm (0.4 to 0.6 inch) is considered normal. The examiner should keep in mind, however, that leg length differences within this range also may be pathological if symptoms result.
CLINICAL NOTES/CAUTIONS	• Nutation (backward rotation) of the ilium on the sacrum results in a decrease in leg length, as does counternutation (anterior rotation) on the opposite side. • If the iliac bone on one side is lower, the leg on that side usually is longer.
RELIABILITY/SPECIFICITY/ SENSITIVITY	Unknown

FUNCTIONAL LIMB LENGTH TEST[23]

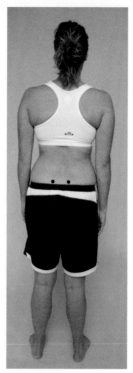

Figure 9–14
Functional leg length in the standing position. The dots on the back indicate the PSISs.

PURPOSE	To assess for leg length discrepancies while the patient is in a weight-bearing position.
PATIENT POSITION	The patient is standing.
EXAMINER POSITION	The examiner is seated or kneeling directly in front of the patient.
TEST PROCEDURE	The patient stands relaxed while the examiner palpates the level of the ASISs and PSISs, noting any asymmetry. The patient then is placed in the "correct" stance (i.e., subtalar joints neutral, knees fully extended, and toes facing straight ahead), and the ASISs and PSISs are palpated again; the examiner notes any changes that have occurred.
INDICATIONS OF A POSITIVE TEST	If the asymmetry has been corrected by "correcting" the position of the limb, the leg is structurally normal (i.e., the bones have proper length) but abnormal joint mechanics (i.e., a functional deficit) are producing a functional leg length difference (Table 9-1). Therefore, if the asymmetry is corrected by proper positioning, the test result is positive for a functional leg length difference.
CLINICAL NOTE	• Functional limb length testing helps the clinician determine whether leg length discrepancies play a role in the patient's pain and dysfunction in weight-bearing positions.
RELIABILITY/SPECIFICITY/ SENSITIVITY	Unknown

Continued

Table 9-1

Functional Limb Length Difference

Joint	Functional Lengthening	Functional Shortening
Foot	Supination	Pronation
Knee	Extension	Flexion
Hip	Lowering	Lifting
	Extension	Flexion
	Lateral rotation	Medial rotation
Sacroiliac	Anterior rotation	Posterior rotation

Modified from Wallace LA: Lower quarter pain: mechanical evaluation and treatment. In Grieve GP (ed): *Modern manual therapy of the vertebral column,* p 467, Edinburgh, 1986, Churchill Livingstone.

OTHER SPECIAL TESTS

SIGN OF THE BUTTOCK TEST

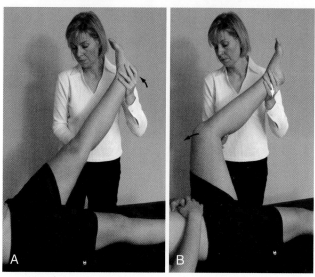

Figure 9–15

Sign of the buttock test. **A,** The hip is flexed with the knee straight until resistance or pain is felt. **B,** The knee then is flexed to see whether further hip flexion can be achieved; if so, the test result is negative.

PURPOSE	To assess whether the patient's symptoms are related to lumbar and hamstring pathological conditions or to a pathological condition in the buttock region.
PATIENT POSITION	The patient is supine.
EXAMINER POSITION	The examiner stands adjacent to the pelvis on the side of the test limb.
TEST PROCEDURE	The examiner grasps the patient's heel with one hand and places the other hand at the patient's knee to support and stabilize the leg. A passive unilateral straight leg raise test is done. If restriction or pain is found on one side, the examiner flexes the patient's knee while holding the thigh in the same position. Once the knee is flexed, the examiner tries to flex the hip further.
INDICATIONS OF A POSITIVE TEST	If the problem is in the lumbar spine or hamstrings, hip flexion increases. This finding indicates a negative result on the sign of the buttock test. If hip flexion does not increase when the knee is flexed, this is a positive result on the sign of the buttock test, and it indicates a pathological condition in the buttock, such as bursitis, tumor, or abscess.
CLINICAL NOTE/CAUTION	• A patient with this pathological condition also exhibits a noncapsular pattern of the hip.
RELIABILITY/SPECIFICITY/ SENSITIVITY	Unknown

TRENDELENBURG'S SIGN

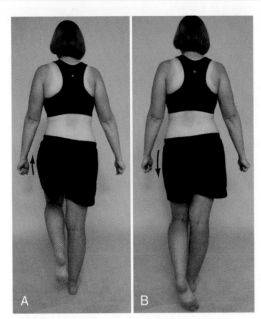

Figure 9–16
Trendelenburg's sign. **A,** Negative test result. **B,** Positive test result.

PURPOSE	To assess the stability of the hip and the ability of the hip abductors to stabilize the pelvis on the femur.
PATIENT POSITION	The patient stands, unsupported.
EXAMINER POSITION	The examiner is seated or kneeling directly in front of or directly behind the patient and is positioned to observe the position of the pelvis. This is an observational test; no manual contact is required.
TEST PROCEDURE	Starting with the unaffected side, the patient is asked to stand or balance first on one leg and then on the other leg. While the patient is balancing on one leg, the examiner watches the movement of the pelvis.
INDICATIONS OF A POSITIVE TEST	If the pelvis rises on the nonstance side, the test result is considered negative, because the gluteus medius muscle on the opposite (stance) side is lifting up the pelvis on the nonstance side, as it normally does in a one-legged stance. If the pelvis on the nonstance side falls, the test result is considered positive; this is an indication of weakness or instability of the hip abductor muscles, primarily the gluteus medius on the stance side.
CLINICAL NOTES/CAUTIONS	• This test should always be performed on the unaffected side first so that the patient understands what to do. • Although the examiner watches what happens on the nonstance side, it is the stance side that is being tested. • The patient also may try to compensate by lateral flexing toward the stance leg. This position is taken so that the patient's center of mass is placed over the stance limb. As a result, the demands on the gluteal muscle are less. This compensation should be corrected and the test repeated.
RELIABILITY/SPECIFICITY/ SENSITIVITY	Unknown

FUNCTIONAL HAMSTRING LENGTH TEST[1]

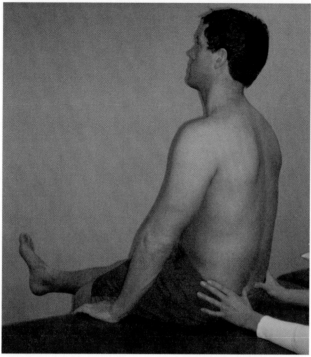

Figure 9–17
Test of the functional length of the hamstrings and the sacrotuberous ligament.

PURPOSE	To assess the length of the patient's hamstring muscle.
PATIENT POSITION	The patient sits on the examining table with the knees flexed to 90°, no weight on the feet, and the spine in neutral.
EXAMINER POSITION	The examiner sits behind the patient.
TEST PROCEDURE	The examiner palpates the PSIS with one thumb while the other thumb rests parallel on the sacrum. The patient is asked to slowly and actively extend the knee.
INDICATIONS OF A POSITIVE TEST	Normally, full knee extension is possible without posterior rotation of the pelvis or flexion of the lumbar spine.
CLINICAL NOTE/CAUTION	• Tight hamstrings cause the pelvis to rotate posteriorly and/or the spine to flex. Although not an actual pathology, limited hamstring length can contribute to dysfunction and a pathological condition at the lumbar spine and pelvis.
RELIABILITY/SPECIFICITY/ SENSITIVITY	Unknown

References

1. Lee D: *The pelvic girdle,* ed, Edinburgh, 1999, Churchill Livingstone.
2. Maigne R: *Orthopaedic medicine: a new approach to vertebral manipulation,* Springfield, IL, 1972, Charles C Thomas.
3. Ombregt L, Bisschop B, ter Veer HJ, Van de Velde T: *A system of orthopedic medicine,* London, 1995, Saunders.
4. Maigne R: *Diagnosis and treatment of pain of vertebral origin,* Baltimore, 1996, Williams & Wilkins.
5. Lee DG: Clinical manifestations of pelvic girdle dysfunction. In Boyling JD, Palastanga N (eds): *Grieve's modern manual therapy: the vertebral column,* ed 2, Edinburgh, 1994, Churchill Livingstone.
6. Bernard TN Jr, Kirkaldy-Willis WH: Recognizing specific characteristics of nonspecific low back pain, *Clin Orthop Relat Res* 217:266-280, 1987.
7. Schwarzer AC, Aprill CN, Bogduk N: The sacroiliac joint in chronic low back pain, *Spine* 20:31-37, 1995.
8. Porterfield JA, DeRosa C: *Mechanical low back pain: perspectives in functional anatomy,* Philadelphia, 1991, Saunders.
9. Butler DA: *Mobilisation of the nervous system,* Melbourne, 1991, Churchill Livingstone.
10. Herron LD, Pheasant HC: Prone knee-flexion provocative testing for lumbar disc protrusion, *Spine* 5:65-67, 1980.
11. Postacchini F, Cinotti G, Gumina S: The knee flexion test: a new test for lumbosacral root tension, *J Bone Joint Surg Br* 75:834-835, 1993.
12. Woerman AL: Evaluation and treatment of dysfunction in the lumbar-pelvic-hip complex. In Donatelli R, Wooden MJ (eds): *Orthopedic physical therapy,* Edinburgh, 1989, Churchill Livingstone.
13. Meijne W, van Neerbos K, Aufdemkampe G, van der Wurff P: Intraexaminer and interexaminer reliability of the Gillet test, *J Manip Physiol Ther* 22:4-9, 1999.
14. Carmichael JP: Inter and intra examiner reliability of palpation for sacroiliac joint dysfunction, *J Manip Physiol Ther* 10:164-171, 1987.
15. Jackson R: Diagnosis and treatment of pelvic girdle dysfunction, *Orthop Phys Ther Clin North Am* 7:413-445, 1998.
16. Mens JM, Vleeming A, Snijders CJ et al: The active straight leg raising test and mobility of the pelvic joints, *Eur Spine* 8:468-473, 1999.
17. Mens JM, Vleeming A, Snijders CJ et al: Reliability and validity of the active straight leg raise test in posterior pelvic pain since pregnancy, *Spine* 26:1167-1171, 2001.
18. Mens JM, Vleeming A, Snijders CJ et al: Validity of the active straight leg raise test for measuring disease severity in patients with posterior pelvic pain after pregnancy, *Spine* 27:196-200, 2002.
19. Friberg O: Clinical symptoms and biomechanics of lumbar spine and hip joint in leg length inequality, *Spine* 8: 643-651, 1983.
20. ten Brinke A, van der Aa HE, van der Palen J, Oosterveld F: Is leg length discrepancy associated with side of radiating pain in patients with a lumbar herniated disc? *Spine* 24:684-686, 1999.
21. DonTigny RL: Dysfunction of the sacroiliac joint and its treatment, *J Orthop Sports Phys Ther* 1:23-35, 1979.
22. Fischer P: Clinical measurement and significance of leg length and iliac crest height discrepancies, *J Man Manip Ther* 5:57-60, 1997.
23. Wallace LA: Limb length difference and back pain. In Grieve GP (ed): *Modern manual therapy of the vertebral column,* Edinburgh, 1986, Churchill Livingstone.

Hip

Précis of the Hip Assessment*

History
Observation
Examination
  Active movements (supine)
    Hip flexion
    Hip abduction
    Hip lateral rotation
    Hip medial rotation
  Passive movements (supine) as in active movements
  (if necessary)
  Resisted isometric movements (supine)
    Hip flexion
    Hip extension
    Hip adduction
    Hip abduction
    Hip medial rotation
    Hip lateral rotation
    Knee flexion
    Knee extension
  Special tests (supine)
    Patrick's test
    Flexion-adduction test
    Trendelenburg's sign
    Anterior labral tear test
    Posterior labral tear test
    Craig's test
    Thomas test
    Leg length tests
    Weber-Barstow maneuver
    Sign of the buttock
    Ely's test
    Rectus femoris contracture test
    90-90 straight leg raise test
    Abduction-adduction contracture tests
    Noble compression test

Reflexes and cutaneous distribution (supine)
  Reflexes
  Sensory scan
  Peripheral nerves
Joint play movements (supine)
  Caudal glide
  Compression
  Lateral distraction
  Quadrant test
Palpation (supine)
Active movement (prone)
  Hip extension
  Hip rotation
Passive movement (prone)
  Hip extension
Resisted isometric movements (prone)
  Hip medial rotation (if not previously done)
  Hip lateral rotation (if not previously done)
  Knee flexion (if not previously done)
  Knee extension (if not previously done)
Special tests (prone and side lying)
  Ober's test
  Prone lying test
Reflexes and cutaneous distribution (prone)
Palpation (prone)
Diagnostic imaging

---

*The examination is shown in an order that limits the amount of movement the patient must do but ensures that all necessary structures are tested. After the rest of the examination has been completed, the examiner may ask the patient to perform the appropriate functional test. Also, after any assessment, the patient should be warned that symptoms may be exacerbated by the assessment.

SELECTED MOVEMENTS

ACTIVE MOVEMENTS

DVD

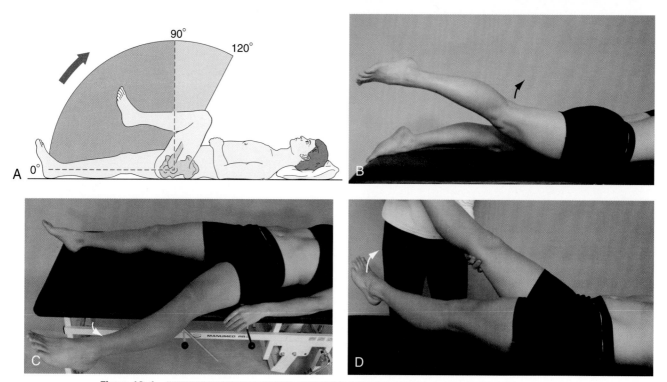

Figure 10–1

Active movements of the hip. **A,** Flexion. **B,** Extension. **C,** Abduction. **D,** Adduction.

Continued

GENERAL INFORMATION   The active movements of the hip are performed with the most painful ones being done last. Some movements are done with the patient supine and some with the patient prone. If the history indicates that repetitive movements, sustained postures, or combined movements have caused symptoms, the examiner should make sure these movements are tested as well. For example, sustained extension of the hip may provoke gluteal pain in the presence of claudication in the common or internal iliac artery.[1]

During the active movements, the examiner should always watch for the possibility of muscle or force couple imbalances that lead to abnormal muscle recruitment patterns. For example, during extension, the normal pattern is contraction of the gluteus maximus followed by the erector spinae on the opposite side and the hamstrings (depending on the load being extended). If the erector spinae contract first, the pelvis will rotate anteriorly, and hyperextension of the lumbar spine will occur.

During the active movements, the examiner should watch the pelvis and the anterior superior iliac spines (supine) and posterior superior iliac spines (prone). During hip movement, if the pelvic force couples are normal, the pelvis and anterior superior iliac spines (ASISs) and posterior superior iliac spines (PSISs) will not move. If they do, it may be an indication of muscle imbalance.

PATIENT POSITION   The patient is supine or prone, depending on the movement to be tested.

EXAMINER POSITION   The examiner is positioned at the patient's side to observe the movements and to palpate the ASISs (in supine) or the PSISs (in prone).

Continued

ACTIVE MOVEMENTS—*cont'd*

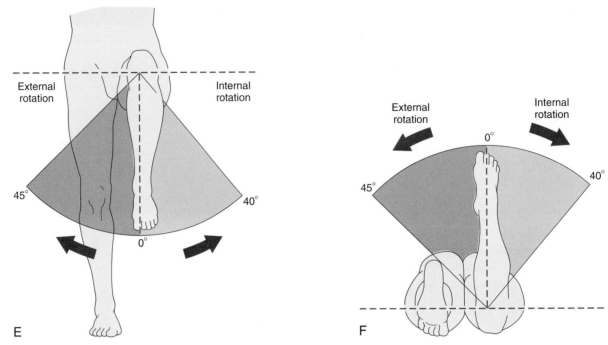

E

F

Figure 10–1 cont'd
E, Rotation in the supine position. **F,** Rotation in the prone position. (**A, E,** and **F** redrawn from
Beetham WP, Polley HF, Slocumb CH, Weaver WF: *Physical examination of the joints,* pp 134, 137,
138, Philadelphia, 1965, Saunders.)

Flexion (in Supine)

TEST PROCEDURE   The patient is asked to flex the hip up toward the chest as far as possible.

INDICATIONS OF A POSITIVE TEST   Hip flexion normally ranges from 110° to 120° with the knee flexed. If the ASIS on
the test side begins to move, the movement is stopped, because pelvic rotation is oc-
curring rather than hip flexion. The patient's knee is flexed during the test to prevent
limitation of movement caused by hamstring tightness. If the range of movement is less
than the above normal ROM or is less than the unaffected leg, the test result is positive.

CLINICAL NOTES/CAUTIONS   • During the movement, if the abdominals are weak, the pelvis will rotate anteriorly. If
the hip flexors are weak, the pelvis will rotate posteriorly.
• If sharp groin pain is elicited on flexion and medial rotation (combined movement),
the pain may be the result of anterior impingement of the femoral neck against the
acetabular rim.[2-6]

Abduction (in Supine)

TEST PROCEDURE   Before asking the patient to do the abduction or adduction movement, the examiner
should make sure the pelvis is "balanced" or level, with the ASISs level and the legs
perpendicular to a line joining the two ASISs. This ensures the angles measured for
adduction and abduction are measured from the same starting point for each leg. The
patient then is asked to abduct one leg at a time.

ACTIVE MOVEMENTS—*cont'd*

INDICATIONS OF A POSITIVE TEST
Hip abduction normally ranges from 30° to 50°. Abduction is stopped when the pelvis begins to move. If the range of movement is less than normal or is less than the unaffected leg, the test result is considered positive. Pelvic motion is detected by palpation of the ASIS and by telling the patient to stop the movement as soon as the ASIS on either side starts to move. Normally, the ASIS on the movement side elevates; the opposite ASIS may drop or elevate. When the patient abducts the leg, the opposite ASIS tends to move first; with an adduction contracture, this occurs earlier in the range of movement. If lateral rotation and slight flexion occur early in the abduction movement, the tensor fascia lata may be stronger and the gluteus medius and gluteus minimus weak. If lateral rotation occurs later in the ROM, the iliopsoas or piriformis may be overactive. If the pelvis tilts up at the beginning of movement, the quadratus lumborum is overactive. All these movements demonstrate imbalance patterns.

Adduction (in Supine)

TEST PROCEDURE
Hip adduction is measured from the same starting position as abduction. The patient is asked to adduct one leg over the other while the examiner makes sure the pelvis does not move. Adduction also may be measured by asking the patient to abduct one leg and leave it abducted, as the examiner makes sure the test leg is 90° to a line formed by the ASISs. The other leg then is tested for the amount of adduction present. The advantage of this method is that the test leg does not have to be flexed to clear the other leg before the adduction movement is done.

INDICATIONS OF A POSITIVE TEST
Hip adduction normally is 30°. When the patient adducts the leg, the ASIS on the same side moves first. The movement occurs earlier in the ROM if an abduction contracture is present.

Rotation (in Supine)

TEST PROCEDURE
In the supine position, the patient simply rotates the straight leg on a balanced pelvis. Turning the foot or leg outward tests lateral rotation; turning the foot or leg inward tests medial rotation. The examiner can then measure hip rotation by having the patient hold the foot in plantigrade and measuring the angle of the foot to a vertical line from the middle of the heel. In another supine test, the patient is asked to flex both the hip and knee to 90°, as the patient would do when tested in sitting.[7] When this method is used, it must be recognized that having the patient rotate the leg outward tests medial rotation, whereas having the patient rotate the leg inward tests lateral rotation.

INDICATIONS OF A POSITIVE TEST
Medial rotation normally ranges from 30° to 40° and lateral rotation from 40° to 60°. If the ASIS begins to move, the movement is stopped, because pelvic rotation is occurring rather than hip rotation. If the range of movement is less than normal or less than in the unaffected leg, the test result is considered positive.

Extension (in Prone)

TEST PROCEDURE
The patient is asked to extend the hip.

INDICATIONS OF A POSTIVE TEST
Extension of the hip normally ranges from 0° to 15°. If the range of movement is less than this or less than in the unaffected leg, the test result is positive. The examiner must be careful to differentiate between hip extension and spinal extension. Patients often have a tendency to extend the lumbar spine at the same time they extend the hip, giving the appearance of increased hip extension. Elevation of the pelvis or movement of the PSIS superiorly indicates that the patient has passed the end of hip extension.

Continued

ACTIVE MOVEMENTS—*cont'd*

Rotation (in Prone)

TEST PROCEDURE   With the patient prone, the pelvis is balanced by aligning the legs at right angles to a line joining the PSISs. The patient then flexes the knee to 90°. Medial rotation is tested when the leg is rotated outward, and lateral rotation is tested when the leg is rotated inward. Usually, this method (prone) is used to measure hip rotation, because it is easier to measure the angle during the test.

INDICATIONS OF A POSITIVE TEST   Medial rotation normally ranges from 30° to 40°, and lateral rotation from 40° to 60°. If the range of movement is less than these amounts or less than the unaffected leg, the test result is considered positive.

SPECIAL TESTS FOR HIP PATHOLOGY[8-13]

Relevant Special Tests

Patrick's test (flexion, abduction, and external rotation [FABER] or figure-four test)

Flexion-adduction test

Trendelenburg's sign

Anterior labral tear test (flexion, adduction, and internal rotation [FADDIR] test)

Posterior labral tear test

Craig's test

Definition

Historically, the diagnosis of hip injury and pathological conditions has been limited to diagnoses such as bursitis, arthritis, or genetic dysplasias. Recently, new imaging and surgical techniques have widened the range of pathological conditions routinely diagnosed in the hip region. Injuries to the labrum and the cartilage around the hip have become potential sources of symptoms and dysfunction. The larger scope of pathological conditions in and around the hip joint has made the diagnosis of such conditions much more challenging for the clinician.

Suspected Injury

Adductor tendinopathy

Anterior hip instability

Anterior-superior impingement syndrome

Posterior-inferior impingement

Avascular necrosis

Hip flexor/adductor strain

Iliopsoas tendinitis or spasm

Labral tears (hip)

Legg-Calvé-Perthes syndrome

Osteoarthritis

Slipped capital femoral epiphysis

Snapping hip syndrome

Epidemiology and Demographics

The epidemiology and demographics of patients with a pathological condition of the hip vary greatly, depending on the tissues injured or the pathology involved.

• Osteoarthritis affects 10% to 25% of the population over age 55.

• Osteonecrosis can occur in people of any age, but it is most common in people in their 30s, 40s, and 50s.

• In children, the most common cause of hip pain is acute transient synovitis. The incidence of slipped capital femoral epiphysis is about 6.1 per 10,000 in boys and 3 per 10,000 in girls. The incidence of Legg-Calvé-Perthes disease is about 1.5 to 5 per 10,000.

• In newborns, the prevalence of developmental dysplasia of the hip (DDH) has been reported in screened populations at rates of 2.5 to 20 per 1000 births; however, it reaches 40 to 90 per 1000 births in some communities.

Relevant History

Previous musculoskeletal injuries can contribute to biomechanical changes and stresses placed on the hip region. Ankle, knee, abdominal, groin, thoracic, and lumbar spine injuries all can lead to movement compensations, which change the normal mechanics of the hip. Over time, these changes result in abnormal wear on hip joint structures, leading to deterioration and degeneration.

Relevant Signs and Symptoms

In the elderly, arthritis is a common source of hip pain. Patients with hip osteoarthritis experience two distinct types of pain: a dull, aching pain, which becomes more constant over time, and short episodes of a more intense, often unpredictable, emotionally draining pain. Both of these pains can occur at the same time. Hip pain tends to be on the medial and anterior aspect of the hip. Posterior and lateral pain often is referred from the lumbar spine or sacroiliac joints. In children, pathological conditions of the hip can be pain free or can manifest as pain in the knee, especially on the medial side. A child with a pathological condition of the hip commonly presents with a limp and Trendelenburg weakness.

Mechanism of Injury

The mechanism of injury plays a large role in the differential diagnosis of patients with acute hip and thigh pathological conditions and a lesser role for chronic pain. Acute traumatic injuries often can be traced back to the movement or motion that occurred at the time of injury. Muscle strains around the hip and thigh region often occur during eccentric deceleration movements. Trauma to the hip may produce a fracture, subluxation, dislocation, compartment syndrome, muscle strain, contusion, or labral tear.

A gradual onset of symptoms often indicates tendinopathy, bursitis, hernia, osteitis pubis, femoral acetabular impingement, or a stress fracture. An insidious onset often indicates degenerative joint disease or referred pain. Acute symptoms generally are the result of trauma to the tissue; chronic or insidious hip pain may be associated with a previous injury to the hip or lower extremity. Compensation begins to occur, and eventually the body breaks down around the hip region.

PATRICK'S TEST (FLEXION, ABDUCTION, AND EXTERNAL ROTATION [FABER] OR FIGURE-FOUR TEST)[14-16]

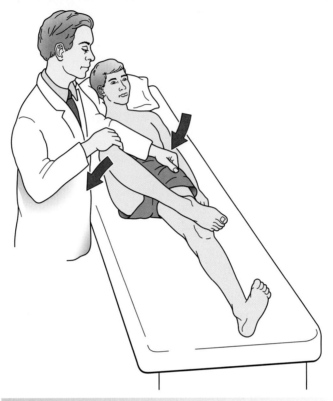

Figure 10–2

Patrick's test (FABER or figure-four test) for detecting limitation of motion in the hip. (Redrawn from Beetham WP, Polley HF, Slocumb CH, Weaver WF: *Physical examination of the joints,* p 139, Philadelphia, 1965, Saunders.)

PURPOSE   To assess for pathological conditions of the hip joint, iliopsoas spasm, or sacroiliac joint dysfunction.

SUSPECTED INJURY   • Hip joint pathological conditions
• Iliopsoas spasm
• Sacroiliac joint dysfunction

PATIENT POSITION   The patient is supine. The test leg is flexed, and the contralateral leg is straight.

EXAMINER POSITION   The examiner stands adjacent to the patient's test hip.

TEST PROCEDURE   One of the examiner's hands is placed on the knee of the test limb. The examiner's other hand is placed on the contralateral ASIS and will be used to stabilize the contralateral pelvis. The examiner places the patient's test leg so that the foot of the test leg is on top of the knee of the opposite leg. The examiner then slowly lowers the knee of the test leg toward the examining table.

PATRICK'S TEST (FLEXION, ABDUCTION, AND EXTERNAL ROTATION [FABER] OR FIGURE-FOUR TEST)[14-16]—cont'd

INDICATIONS OF A POSITIVE TEST   A negative test result is indicated if the knee of the test leg falls to the table or at least is parallel to the opposite leg. A positive test result is indicated if the knee of the test leg remains above the opposite straight leg. If the result is positive, the test indicates that the hip joint may be affected, that iliopsoas spasm may be present, or that the sacroiliac joint may be affected (if the patient has posterior pain).

CLINICAL NOTE/CAUTION

- FABER is the position of the hip when the patient begins the test. This test sometimes is referred to as *Jansen's test*.

RELIABILITY/SPECIFICITY/ SENSITIVITY[15,16]   Reliability: Test-retest ICC: 0.93
Intrarater: 0.87

FLEXION-ADDUCTION TEST[17,18]

DVD

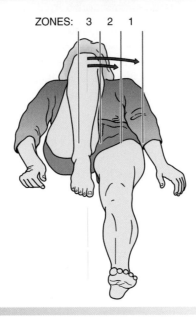

ZONES: 3   2   1

Figure 10–3

The normal hip permits the ipsilateral knee to move convincingly across the midline of the body without rolling the pelvis. The knee should enter zone 1 by overlapping the opposite hip and, in a youthful or supple patient, reaches a position lateral to the thigh. Progressive pathological changes in the hip limit adduction to zones 2 and 3, with the production of pain by this maneuver. (Redrawn from Woods D, Macnicol M: The flexion-adduction test: an early sign of hip disease, *J Pediatr Orthop* 10:181, 2001.)

PURPOSE	To assess for pathological conditions of the hip in older children and young adults.
SUSPECTED INJURY	• Slipped capital femoral epiphysis • Anterior hip impingement of the adductor longus, pectineus, iliopsoas, sartorius, or tensor fascia lata • Anterior labral pathological conditions
PATIENT POSITION	The patient is supine, and the contralateral lower extremity should be straight.
EXAMINER POSITION	The examiner stands adjacent to the pelvis on the side of the test hip.
TEST PROCEDURE	One of the examiner's hands grasps the patient's knee. The examiner flexes the patient's hip to at least 90° with the knee flexed. The examiner then adducts the flexed leg.
INDICATIONS OF A POSITIVE TEST	Normally, the knee passes over the opposite hip without pelvic movement. In hips with a pathological condition, adduction is limited and accompanied by pain or discomfort, and the pelvis rotates laterally toward the straight leg.
CLINICAL NOTE/CAUTION	• Maitland[18] called this test the quadrant, or scouring, test if the hip was fully flexed. He believed that the test stressed or compressed the femoral neck against the acetabulum, or pinched the adductor longus, pectineus, iliopsoas, sartorius, or tensor fascia lata.
RELIABILITY/SPECIFICITY/ SENSITIVITY	Unknown

TRENDELENBURG'S SIGN[19]

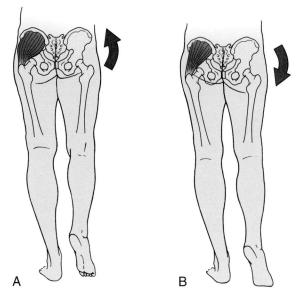

Figure 10–4

Trendelenburg's sign. **A,** Negative test. **B,** Positive test.

PURPOSE	To assess the stability of the hip and the ability of the hip abductors to stabilize the pelvis on the femur.
SUSPECTED INJURY	• Weakness of the hip abductors
PATIENT POSITION	The patient stands, unsupported.
EXAMINER POSITION	The examiner is seated or kneeling directly in front of or directly behind the patient. The examiner should be positioned so as to observe the position of the pelvis. No manual contact is required; this is an observational test.
TEST PROCEDURE	The patient is asked to stand on one lower limb, starting with the uninvolved side.
INDICATIONS OF A POSITIVE TEST	Normally, when a person stands on one leg with no additional support, the pelvis rises on the opposite side; this indicates a negative test result. A positive test result is indicated if the pelvis on the opposite side (nonstance side) drops when the patient stands on the affected leg. Dropping of the pelvis on the opposite side indicates a weak gluteus medius or an unstable hip (e.g., as a result of hip dislocation) on the affected or stance side.
CLINICAL NOTE/CAUTION	• The test should always be performed on the unaffected side first so that the patient understands what to do.
RELIABILITY/SPECIFICITY/ SENSITIVITY	Unknown

ANTERIOR LABRAL TEAR TEST (FLEXION, ADDUCTION, AND INTERNAL ROTATION [FADDIR] TEST)[20,21]

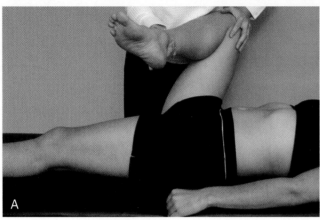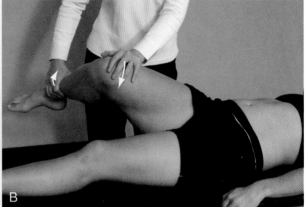

Figure 10–5
Anterior labral tear test. **A,** Starting position. **B,** End position.

PURPOSE	To test for anterior-superior impingement syndrome or an anterior labral tear in the hip, as well as iliopsoas tendinitis.
SUSPECTED INJURY	• Anterior-superior impingement syndrome • Anterior labral tear • Iliopsoas tendinitis
PATIENT POSITION	The patient is supine. The contralateral leg should be positioned in full hip and knee extension.
EXAMINER POSITION	The examiner is positioned adjacent to the pelvis on the test hip side.
TEST PROCEDURE	One of the examiner's hands grasps the patient's knee, and the other hand grasps the ankle. The examiner takes the hip into full flexion, lateral rotation, and full abduction as a starting position. The examiner then takes the hip into extension combined with medial rotation and adduction.
INDICATIONS OF A POSITIVE TEST	A positive test result is indicated if pain is produced or if the patient's symptoms are reproduced, with or without a click.
CLINICAL NOTE/CAUTION	• The examiner should hold and stabilize the lower extremity being tested securely to minimize guarding by the patient.
RELIABILITY/SPECIFICITY/ SENSITIVITY	Unknown

POSTERIOR LABRAL TEAR TEST[20]

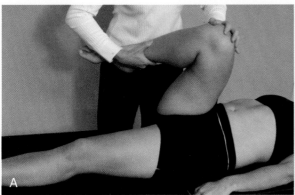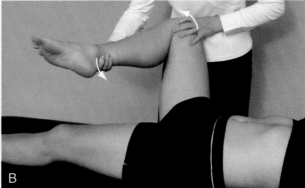

Figure 10–6
Posterior labral tear test. **A,** Starting position. **B,** End position.

PURPOSE	To assess for a labral tear, anterior hip instability, or posterior-inferior impingement.
SUSPECTED INJURY	• Labral tear • Anterior hip instability • Posterior-inferior impingement
PATIENT POSITION	The patient lies supine, and the contralateral leg should be straight.
EXAMINER POSITION	The examiner is positioned adjacent to the pelvis on the test hip side.
TEST PROCEDURE	One of the examiner's hands grasps the patient's knee, and the other hand grasps the ankle. The examiner takes the hip into full flexion, adduction, and medial rotation as a starting position. The examiner then takes the hip into extension combined with abduction and lateral rotation.
INDICATIONS OF A POSITIVE TEST	A positive test result is indicated if groin pain or patient apprehension is produced, or if the patient's symptoms are reproduced, with or without a click.
CLINICAL NOTE/CAUTION	• The test is sometimes called the *apprehension test* if apprehension occurs toward the end of ROM.
RELIABILITY/SPECIFICITY/ SENSITIVITY	Unknown

CRAIG'S TEST[22-29]

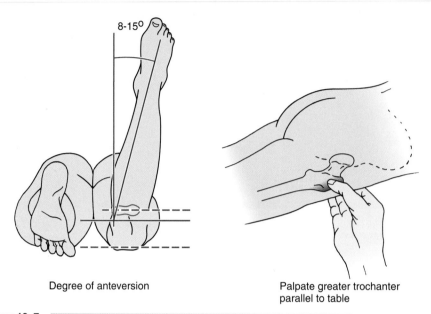

Degree of anteversion

Palpate greater trochanter parallel to table

Figure 10–7
Craig's test to measure femoral anteversion.

PURPOSE	To measure femoral anteversion or forward torsion of the femoral neck.
SUSPECTED DEFORMITY	• Femoral anteversion • Femoral neck torsion
PATIENT POSITION	The patient lies prone with the knee flexed to 90°. The hips and thigh are aligned with the trunk and parallel to each other, with the legs at 90° to a line joining the posterior-superior iliac spines.
EXAMINER POSITION	The examiner stands adjacent to the test hip.
TEST PROCEDURE	The examiner palpates the posterior aspect of the greater trochanter of the patient's femur with one hand and grasps the ankle with the other hand. The hip then is slowly and passively rotated medially and laterally until the greater trochanter is parallel with the examining table or reaches its most lateral position (the trochanter is parallel when it can be felt most lateral in reference to midline of the body). The degree of anteversion can then be estimated, based on the angle of the lower leg with the vertical.

Continued

CRAIG'S TEST[22-29]—*cont'd*

INDICATIONS OF A POSITIVE TEST   At birth, the mean angle is approximately 30°; in the adult, the mean angle is 8° to 15°.

CLINICAL NOTES/CAUTIONS

- Craig's test has been found to correlate well with radiographic findings (within 4°) in children.
- The test is also called the *Ryder method* for measuring anteversion or retroversion.
- Anteversion of the hip is measured by the angle made by the femoral neck with the femoral condyles. It is the degree of forward projection of the femoral neck from the coronal plane of the shaft, and it decreases during the growing period.
- Increased anteversion leads to squinting patellae and toeing-in. Excessive anteversion is twice as common in girls as in boys. A common clinical finding of excessive anteversion is excessive medial hip rotation (more than 60°) and decreased lateral rotation in extension. Gelberman et al.[29] pointed out, however, that rotation should be viewed both in neutral (as in the Craig's test) and with 90° of hip flexion, because rotation shows greater variability in flexion. These researchers felt that greater medial rotation than lateral rotation in both positions was a better indicator of increased femoral anteversion.
- With retroversion, the plane of the femoral neck rotates backward in relation to the coronal condylar plane, or the acetabulum itself may be retroverted.

RELIABILITY/SPECIFICITY/ SENSITIVITY[28]

Reliability: Intrarater: 0.94
Interrater: 0.85

SPECIAL TESTS FOR LEG LENGTH

Relevant Special Tests

True leg length
Weber-Barstow maneuver (visual method)
Functional leg length

Definition

A *leg length discrepancy* is the difference in the longitudinal length of one leg compared with the other. Leg length discrepancies can be classified in two ways: as actual (true) leg length discrepancies or as apparent (functional) leg length discrepancies. In true leg length discrepancies, the length of one leg is truly different from the length of the other leg. In functional leg length discrepancies, one leg appears different from the other, but when the two legs are measured, the lengths are identical. The apparent length discrepancy can be caused by biomechanical factors (e.g., pelvic rotation) or foot pronation (see Table 9-1).

Suspected Injury

Leg length discrepancy can be the result of trauma, such as fractures or surgery (e.g., arthroplasty), or simply varied rates of development of the two legs.

Epidemiology and Demographics

Freiberg[30] studied patients with low back pain and discovered that those with a leg length discrepancy greater than 15 mm were five times more likely to have low back pain. Hip and sciatic pain occurred in the longer leg 78% of the time. In patients with leg length discrepancies greater than 3 cm, an asymmetrical lateral side bend of the spine occurs on the side of the longer leg. This results in abnormal loading mechanics of the spine. Leg length discrepancies of this magnitude are present in 40% of the general population.[31]

ten Brinke et al.[31] reported that in 64 (62%) of 104 patients with a leg length discrepancy of 1 mm or more, the back pain radiated into the shorter leg.

Relevant History

The patients may have a history of trauma or a fracture of the lower extremity. Falls onto the buttock also may result in apparent leg length discrepancies.

Relevant Signs and Symptoms

- Leg length differences themselves are not usually painful.
- Difference is clinically relevant as a contributing cause of symptoms and pathological conditions in other regions, such as the lumbar spine, pelvis, sacroiliac joint, or lower extremity.
- An objective examination of any of these regions should include an examination of leg length.

Mechanism of Injury

Actual leg length changes can be caused by falls, surgery, or trauma. This is especially relevant if the fracture occurred in a child, and the fracture was through the growth plate. A patient also may have a history of total joint replacement, which may cause alterations in actual leg length. Arthritic changes in the joints of the lower extremity can give rise to total leg length differences.

Patients with apparent leg length discrepancies may have a history of trauma to the lumbar spine, pelvis, hip, knee, or ankle.

TRUE LEG LENGTH[32-37]

DVD

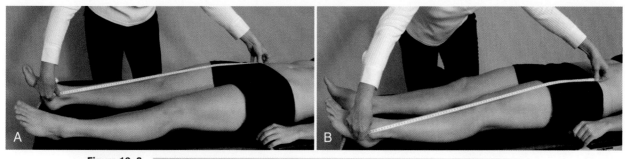

Figure 10–8

Measuring true leg length. **A,** Measuring to the medial malleolus. **B,** Measuring to the lateral malleolus.

PURPOSE	To assess for differences in leg length and leg asymmetries.
PATIENT POSITION	Patient is supine. The legs should be 15 to 20 cm (4 to 8 inches) apart and parallel to each other. If the legs are not placed in proper relation to the pelvis, apparent shortening of a limb may occur. The lower limbs must be placed in comparable positions relative to the pelvis, because abduction of the hip brings the medial malleolus closer to the ASIS on the same side, and adduction of the hip takes the medial malleolus farther from the ASIS on the same side. If one hip is fixed in abduction or adduction as a result of contracture or some other cause, the normal hip should be adducted or abducted an equal amount to ensure accurate leg length measurement.
EXAMINER POSITION	Before any measuring is done, the examiner must set the patient's pelvis square, level, or in balance with the lower limbs (see Patient Position). The examiner stands adjacent to the lower extremity of the leg being measured.
TEST PROCEDURE	To obtain the leg length, the examiner measures from the ASIS to the lateral or medial malleolus. The flat metal end of the tape measure is placed immediately distal to the ASIS and pushed up against it. The thumb then presses the tape end firmly against the bone, rigidly fixing the tape measure against the bone. The index finger of the other hand is placed immediately distal to the lateral or medial malleolus and pushed against it. The thumbnail is brought down against the tip of the index finger so that the tape measure is pinched between them.
INDICATIONS OF A POSITIVE TEST	A slight difference (1 to 1.5 cm/0.4 to 0.6 inch) in leg length is considered normal; however, this difference still can cause symptoms.
CLINICAL NOTE/CAUTION	• In North America, the leg length measurement usually is taken from the ASIS to the medial malleolus. However, these values may be altered by muscle wasting or obesity. Measuring to the lateral malleolus is less likely to be affected by the muscle bulk.
RELIABILITY/SPECIFICITY/ SENSITIVITY[37]	Reliability: Interrater ICC: 0.94 Intrarater range: 0-1

WEBER-BARSTOW MANEUVER (VISUAL METHOD)[38]

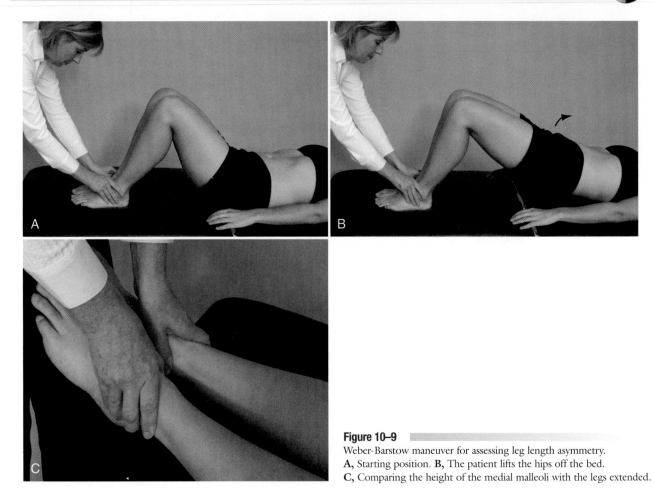

Figure 10–9

Weber-Barstow maneuver for assessing leg length asymmetry.
A, Starting position. **B,** The patient lifts the hips off the bed.
C, Comparing the height of the medial malleoli with the legs extended.

PURPOSE	To assess for differences in leg length and leg asymmetries.
PATIENT POSITION	The patient lies supine with the hips and knees flexed and the feet flat on the table (crook lying).
EXAMINER POSITION	The examiner stands at the patient's feet.
TEST PROCEDURE	The examiner palpates the distal aspect of the medial malleoli of both feet with the thumbs. The patient then actively lifts the pelvis from the examining table and returns to the starting position. Next, the examiner passively extends the patient's legs and compares the positions of the malleoli using the borders of the thumbs. Different levels indicate asymmetry.
INDICATIONS OF A POSITIVE TEST	If one leg is shorter than the other, the examiner can determine where the difference is by measuring the following:

- From the iliac crest to the greater trochanter of the femur (for coxa vara or coxa valga). The neck-shaft angle of the femur normally is 150° to 160° at birth and decreases to 120° to 135° in the adult. In an adult, if this angle is less than 120°, the condition is known as *coxa vara;* if it is more than 135°, it is known as *coxa valga.*
- From the greater trochanter of the femur to the knee joint line on the lateral aspect (for femoral shaft shortening).
- From the knee joint line on the medial side to the medial malleolus (for tibial shaft shortening).

WEBER-BARSTOW MANEUVER (VISUAL METHOD)[38]—cont'd

- The femoral lengths can be compared by having the patient lie supine with the hips and knees flexed to 90° (crook lying). If one femur is longer than the other, its height will be higher.
- The relative length of the tibia may also be examined with the patient lying prone. The examiner places the thumbs transversely across the soles of the feet just in front of the heels. The knees are flexed 90°, and the relative heights of the thumbs are noted. Care must be taken to ensure that the legs are perpendicular to the examining table.

CLINICAL NOTES/CAUTIONS
- Apparent or functional shortening of the leg is evident if the patient has a lateral pelvic tilt when the measurement is taken.
- Apparent or functional shortening of the limb is the result of adaptations the patient has made in response to a pathological condition or contracture somewhere in the spine, pelvis, or lower limbs. In reality, there is no structural or anatomical difference in bone lengths.

RELIABILITY/SPECIFICITY/ SENSITIVITY   Unknown

FUNCTIONAL LEG LENGTH[39]

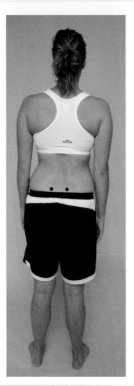

Figure 10–10

Functional leg length in standing position. The dots on the back indicate the posterior superior iliac spines.

PURPOSE

To assess for leg length discrepancies while the patient is in a weight-bearing position.

PATIENT POSITION

The patient is standing.

EXAMINER POSITION

The examiner is seated or kneeling directly in front of or behind the patient.

TEST PROCEDURE

The patient stands relaxed while the examiner palpates the level of the ASISs and PSISs, noting any asymmetry. The patient then is placed in the "correct" stance (i.e., subtalar joints neutral, knees fully extended, and toes facing straight ahead). The ASISs and PSISs are palpated again, and the examiner notes any changes.

INDICATIONS OF A POSITIVE TEST

If the asymmetry has been corrected by "correcting" the position of the limb, the leg is structurally normal (i.e., the bones are the proper length); however, abnormal joint mechanics (i.e., a functional deficit) are producing a functional leg length difference (see Table 9-1). Therefore, if the asymmetry is corrected by proper positioning, the test result is positive for a functional leg length difference.

CLINICAL NOTES

- Functional limb length testing helps the clinician determine whether leg length discrepancies play a role in the patient's pain and dysfunction when in weight-bearing positions.
- The amount of limb length discrepancy can be gauged by sequentially placing magazines or thin books under the patient's foot until the pelvis is level.

RELIABILITY/SPECIFICITY/ SENSITIVITY

Unknown

SPECIAL TESTS FOR MUSCLE TIGHTNESS

Relevant Special Tests

Sign of the buttock
Thomas test
Rectus femoris contracture test (Kendall test)
Ely's test (tight rectus femoris)
Ober's test
Prone lying test for iliotibial band contraction
Noble compression test
Adduction contracture test
Abduction contracture test
90-90 Straight leg raise test (hamstrings contracture)

Definition

Muscle tightness is not a pathological condition, but it can indicate such a condition or can lead to changes that themselves contribute to a pathological condition. Muscle as a tissue has a contractile ability. Given this quality, muscles are uniquely suited to facilitate movement and motion. They protect and guard the body. Therefore, muscles have two primary functions: the first is to move, and the second is to protect. Muscle tightness often is indicative of the protective function. It can indicate a pathological condition that the body is protecting and guarding. It also can indicate adaptive shortening as a result of postural changes or repetitive motion.

Suspected Injury

Any pathological condition of the hip; the lumbar, pelvic, or abdominal area; or the lower extremity can be the source of muscle tightness.

Epidemiology and Demographics

Because muscle tightness is not a pathological condition, no known studies exist that address the prevalence of muscle tightness epidemiologically or demographically. From a clinical perspective, muscle tightness plays a large role in the assessment of the patient. Clinicians consider it when hypothesizing about a pathological condition that the muscle guarding (protective spasm) may be protecting, and a pathological condition that the tightness may be creating or inducing in adjacent regions of the body.

Relevant History

The patients may complain of pain or injury in the hip joint or in regions adjacent to the hip joint. Not uncommonly, patients have a long history of low back and pelvic, abdominal, or lower extremity pain. The patient also may have a history of a childhood injury or a pathological condition at the hip joint.

Relevant Signs and Symptoms

Muscle tightness in and of itself is not generally painful. If it indicates a pathological condition of the hip or in other regions (most commonly the lumbar spine and pelvis), the signs and symptoms take on the characteristics of the particular pathological condition.

Mechanism of Injury

The means by which the muscle tightness appears may be due to injury or a pathological condition. Mechanisms may vary, but they take on the characteristics of the pathological condition producing the muscle tightness. Trauma, such as a fall, or a motor vehicle accident, can cause muscle tightness in the hip. Similarly, irritable bowel syndrome, ovarian cysts, and inguinal hernias are all pathological conditions that can lead to hip muscle tightness as the body attempts to protect the injured structures. Hip flexor tightness and the consequential anterior pelvic tilt is commonly seen in patients with pathological low back and pelvic conditions. Occupations that require prolonged sitting also can result in adaptive shortening of some of the hip musculature.

SIGN OF THE BUTTOCK TEST

DVD

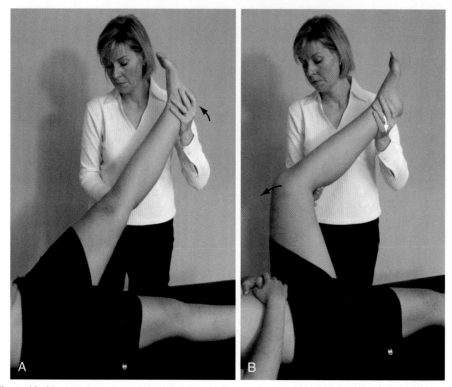

Figure 10–11
Sign of the buttock test. **A,** The hip is flexed with the knee straight until resistance or pain is felt. **B,** The knee then is flexed to see whether further hip flexion can be achieved; if so, the test result is negative.

PURPOSE	To assess whether the patient's symptoms are related to lumbar and hamstring pathological conditions or to a pathological condition in the buttock region.
PATIENT POSITION	The patient is supine.
EXAMINER POSITION	The examiner stands adjacent to the pelvis on the side of the test limb.
TEST PROCEDURE	One of the examiner's hands grasps the patient's heel, and the other hand is placed at the knee to support and stabilize the leg. The examiner performs a passive unilateral straight leg raise test. If restriction or pain is found on one side, the examiner flexes the patient's knee while holding the patient's thigh in the same position. Once the knee has been flexed, the examiner tries to flex the hip further.
INDICATIONS OF A POSITIVE TEST	If the problem is in the lumbar spine, hamstrings, or involves nerve mobility, hip flexion increases. This finding indicates a negative sign of the buttock test. If hip flexion does not increase when the knee is flexed, this is a positive sign of the buttock test and indicates a pathological condition in the buttock, such as bursitis, a tumor, or an abscess.
CLINICAL NOTE/CAUTION	• A patient with this pathological condition would also show a noncapsular pattern of the hip.
RELIABILITY/SPECIFICITY/ SENSITIVITY	Unknown

THOMAS TEST[40]

DVD

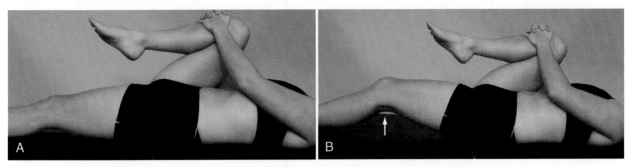

Figure 10–12
Thomas test. **A,** Negative test result. **B,** Positive test result.

PURPOSE	To assess for a hip flexor contracture, which is the most common type of contracture of the hip.
PATIENT POSITION	The patient lies supine.
EXAMINER POSITION	The examiner first checks the patient for excessive lordosis, which commonly is present with tight hip flexors. The examiner then positions himself or herself to view the patient's pelvis and the angle of the lower extremity. The test can be done actively by the patient or passively by the examiner (more common) while the examiner or patient stabilizes the contralateral leg into flexion.
TEST PROCEDURE	The examiner passively flexes one of the patient's hips, bringing the knee to the chest to flatten the lumbar spine and stabilize the pelvis. The patient holds the flexed hip against the chest while leaving the test leg relaxed in the start position.
INDICATIONS OF A POSITIVE TEST	If the patient does not have a flexion contracture, the test hip (the straight leg) remains on the examining table. If a contracture is present, the straight leg raises off the table as the other leg is flexed to the chest, and the patient feels a muscle stretch end feel. The angle of contracture can be measured. If the examiner pushes the lower limb down onto the table, the patient may show an increased lordosis, which also indicates a positive test result.
CLINICAL NOTES/CAUTIONS	• If measurements are taken during the test, the examiner must be sure the restriction is in the hip and not the pelvis or lumbar spine. If the leg does not lift off the table but abducts as the other leg is flexed to the chest, this is called the J sign or stroke and indicates a tight iliotibial band on the extended leg side. • The examiner also may passively hold the flexed limb in position instead of having the patient hold the knee to the chest. When a patient actively holds the knee to the chest, some contraction of the hip flexors may be present and the patient may not be able to fully relax the test limb.
RELIABILITY/SPECIFICITY/ SENSITIVITY	Unknown

RECTUS FEMORIS CONTRACTURE TEST (KENDALL TEST)

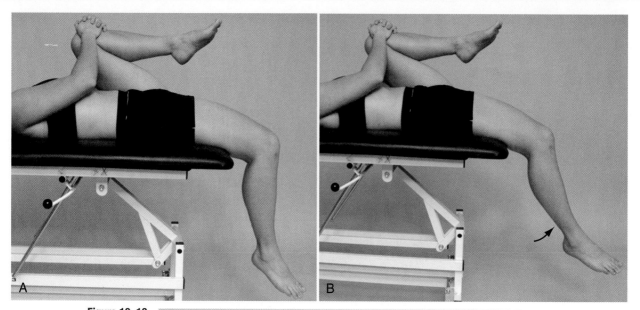

Figure 10–13
Rectus femoris contracture. **A,** The movement leg is brought to the chest. The test leg remains bent over the end of the examining table, indicating a negative test result. **B,** The test knee extends, indicating a positive test result.

PURPOSE	To assess for contractures or tightness of the rectus femoris muscle.
PATIENT POSITION	The patient lies supine with the knees bent over the end or edge of the examining table.
EXAMINER POSITION	The examiner is positioned to view the patient's pelvis and the angle of the lower extremity. No manual contact is required.
TEST PROCEDURE	The two sides are tested and compared. Starting with the unaffected side, the patient flexes one knee onto the chest and holds it while the examiner watches what happens to the leg left bent over the end of the examining table (the test leg).
INDICATIONS OF A POSITIVE TEST	The angle of the test knee, which is bent over the end of the examining table, should remain at approximately 90° when the opposite knee is flexed to the chest. If it does not (i.e., the test knee extends slightly), a contracture probably is present.
CLINICAL NOTES/CAUTIONS	• The examiner may attempt to passively flex the knee to see whether it remains at 90° of its own volition and to test the end feel. • The examiner should always palpate for muscle tightness when doing any contracture test. If no palpable tightness is noted, the probable cause of restriction is tight joint structures (e.g., the capsule), and the end feel will be different (muscle stretch versus capsular end feel).
RELIABILITY/SPECIFICITY/ SENSITIVITY	Unknown

ELY'S TEST (TIGHT RECTUS FEMORIS)[41]   DVD

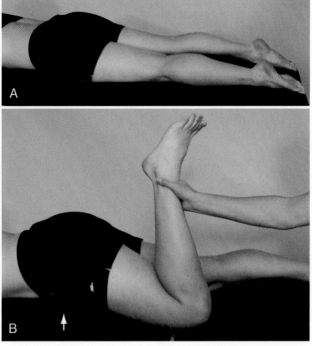

Figure 10–14
Ely's test for a tight rectus femoris. **A,** Position for the test. **B,** Posture test shown by hip flexion when the knee is flexed.

PURPOSE	To assess for contractures or tightness of the rectus femoris muscle.
PATIENT POSITION	The patient lies prone.
EXAMINER POSITION	The examiner is positioned at the patient's feet.
TEST PROCEDURE	One of the examiner's hands grasps the ankle of the test limb. The examiner passively flexes the patient's knee. The other hand can be placed on the posterior aspect of the patient's pelvis to assess for sacral movement.
INDICATIONS OF A POSITIVE TEST	On flexion of the knee, a positive test result is indicated if the hip on the same side spontaneously flexes; this means that the rectus femoris muscle is tight on that side.
CLINICAL NOTE/CAUTION	• The two sides should be tested and compared, starting with the unaffected side.
RELIABILITY/SPECIFICITY/ SENSITIVITY	Unknown

OBER'S TEST[42]

DVD

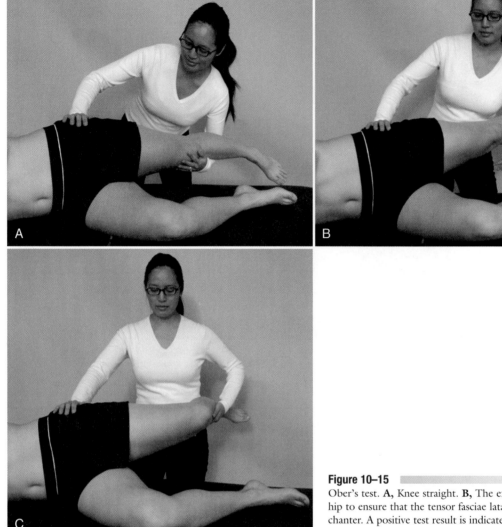

Figure 10–15

Ober's test. **A,** Knee straight. **B,** The examiner passively extends the hip to ensure that the tensor fasciae latae runs over the greater trochanter. A positive test result is indicated if the leg remains abducted while the muscles are relaxed. **C,** Test done with the knee flexed.

PURPOSE	To assess the tensor fascia latae (iliotibial band) for tightness.
PATIENT POSITION	The patient is in the side-lying position with the lower leg flexed at the hip and knee for stability. The upper leg is the test leg.
EXAMINER POSITION	The examiner stands behind the thigh.
TEST PROCEDURE	One of the examiner's hands is placed beneath the patient's knee to lift and support it, and the other hand is placed on the pelvis to stabilize it and to assess for motion. The examiner then passively abducts and extends the patient's upper leg with the knee straight or flexed to 90°. The examiner slowly lowers the upper limb. For this test, it is important to extend the hip slightly so that the iliotibial band passes over the greater trochanter of the femur. To do this, the examiner stabilizes the pelvis when doing the test to prevent the pelvis from "falling backward." The examiner also watches the pelvis to make sure that it does not side-tilt as the upper leg is lowered toward the treatment table.

OBER'S TEST[42]—cont'd

INDICATIONS OF A POSITIVE TEST

If a contracture is present, the leg remains abducted and does not fall to the table. With a normal iliotibial band length, the foot should be able to touch the table without the pelvis tilting.

CLINICAL NOTES/CAUTIONS

- Ober originally described the test with the knee flexed.[42] However, a greater stretch is put on the iliotibial band when doing the test with the knee extended. Also, when the knee is flexed during the test, greater stress is placed on the femoral nerve. If neurological signs (i.e., neurological pain, paresthesia) occur during the test, the examiner should consider a pathological condition affecting the femoral nerve.
- Tenderness over the greater trochanter should lead the examiner to consider trochanteric bursitis.

RELIABILITY/SPECIFICITY/ SENSITIVITY

Unknown

PRONE LYING TEST FOR ILIOTIBIAL BAND CONTRACTURE[43]

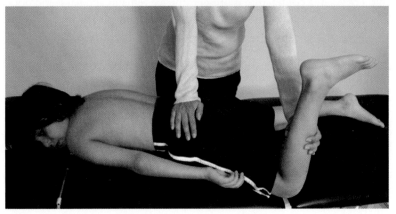

Figure 10–16
Prone lying test for iliotibial band contracture.

PURPOSE	To assess the tensor fascia latae (iliotibial band) for tightness.
PATIENT POSITION	The patient lies prone.
EXAMINER POSITION	The examiner stands on the opposite side to the leg being tested.
TEST PROCEDURE	With one hand, the examiner holds the ankle of the test leg and maximally abducts the leg at the hip; the other hand is used to apply pressure to the buttock on the same side as the test leg to flatten the pelvis and correct any hip flexion deformity. While maintaining the hip in neutral rotation and the knee flexed to 90°, the examiner adducts the hip until there is a firm end feel. The angle is measured relative to the body's vertical axis, and the results are compared with those for the other side.
INDICATIONS OF A POSITIVE TEST	A positive test result is indicated by a difference in the measurements on the test side and the contralateral, uninvolved side.
CLINICAL NOTE	• This test is more commonly done in children.
RELIABILITY/SPECIFICITY/ SENSITIVITY	Unknown

NOBLE COMPRESSION TEST[44]

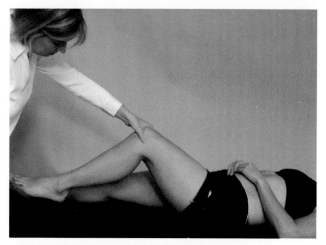

Figure 10–17

Noble compression test for iliotibial band friction syndrome. The patient extends the knee. The examiner indicates where pain is felt, at about 30° of flexion.

PURPOSE	To assess whether iliotibial band friction syndrome (tendinitis) exists near the knee.
PATIENT POSITION	The patient lies supine. The knee is flexed to 90° and accompanied by hip flexion (crook lying).
EXAMINER POSITION	The examiner stands adjacent to the test limb.
TEST PROCEDURE	The unaffected leg is tested first. The examiner places a thumb of one hand on the lateral femoral epicondyle so the thumb is also over the distal end of the iliotibial band. The examiner's other hand helps stabilize the thigh. The examiner flexes the patient's knee to 90°, accompanied by hip flexion. The examiner then applies pressure to the lateral femoral epicondyle or 1 to 2 cm (0.4 to 0.8 inch) proximal to it with the thumb. While the pressure is maintained, the patient's knee is passively extended or the patient may extend the knee actively. The two legs are compared.
INDICATIONS OF A POSITIVE TEST	With a positive test result, the patient complains of severe pain over the lateral femoral condyle at approximately 30° of flexion (0° being a straight leg). The patient usually says it is the same pain that accompanies the patient's activity (e.g., running).
CLINICAL NOTE/CAUTION	• Iliotibial band friction syndrome is a chronic inflammation of the iliotibial band near its insertion, adjacent to the femoral condyle.
RELIABILITY/SPECIFICITY/ SENSITIVITY	Unknown

ADDUCTION CONTRACTURE TEST[45]

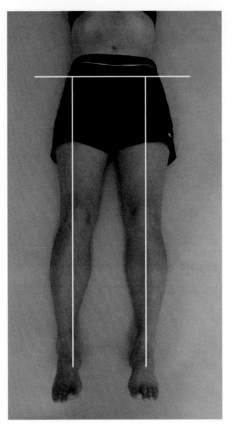

Figure 10–18
Balancing the pelvis on the legs (femora).

PURPOSE   To assess the length of the adductor muscles (adductor longus, brevis, and magnus; and pectineus) of the hip.

PATIENT POSITION   The patient lies supine with the ASISs level. Both legs should be placed in 0° of hip and knee extension.

EXAMINER POSITION   The examiner is positioned to view the patient's pelvis and the angle of the lower extremity. No manual contact is required.

TEST PROCEDURE   Normally, the examiner can easily "balance" the pelvis on the legs. This balancing implies a line joining the ASISs that is perpendicular to the two lines formed by the straight legs. If an adduction contracture is present, the affected leg forms an angle of less than 90° with the line joining the two ASISs. If the examiner then attempts to balance the lower limb with the pelvis, the pelvis (i.e., ASISs) shifts up on the affected side or down on the unaffected side, and balancing is not possible.

ADDUCTION CONTRACTURE TEST[45]—*cont'd*

INDICATIONS OF A POSITIVE TEST Normally, hip abduction should be 30° to 50° before the ASIS moves. If the ASIS moves before this, the adductors are tight if a muscle stretch end feel is felt. This type of contracture can lead to functional shortening of the limb rather than true shortening.

CLINICAL NOTE • Patients, especially children, with adductor spasticity may also be tested by abduction. The patient is supine. The examiner quickly abducts the leg. If a "grab" or "kicking in" of the stretch reflex occurs at less than 30°, the test result is considered positive for adductor spasticity. The test should be repeated with the knee flexed to rule out medial hamstring contracture.

RELIABILITY/SPECIFICITY/ SENSITIVITY Unknown

ABDUCTION CONTRACTURE TEST   DVD

PURPOSE To assess the length of the abductor muscles (gluteus medius and minimus) of the hip.

PATIENT POSITION The patient lies supine with the ASISs level. Both legs should be placed in 0° of hip and knee extension (see Figure 10-18).

EXAMINER POSITION The examiner is positioned to view the patient's pelvis and the angle of the lower extremity. No manual contact is required.

TEST PROCEDURE The examiner attempts to balance the lower limb with the pelvis. The pelvis (i.e., the ASIS) shifts down on the affected side or up on the unaffected side, and balancing is not possible.

INDICATIONS OF A POSITIVE TEST If an abduction contracture is present, the affected leg forms an angle of more than 90° with a line joining the two ASISs. Normally, hip adduction should be about 30° before the ASIS moves. If the ASIS moves before this, the abductors are tight if a muscle stretch end feel is felt.

CLINICAL NOTE • This type of contracture can lead to functional lengthening of the limb rather than true lengthening.

RELIABILITY/SPECIFICITY/ SENSITIVITY Unknown

90-90 STRAIGHT LEG RAISE TEST (HAMSTRINGS CONTRACTURE)[46-48]

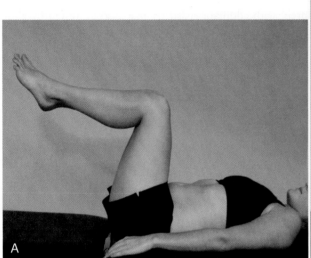
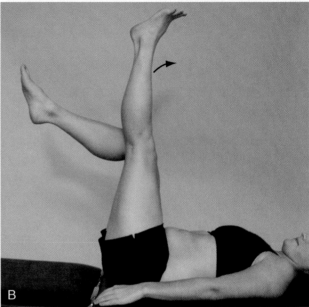

Figure 10–19
The 90-90 straight leg raise test.

PURPOSE	To assess for contracture, muscle guarding, or limitation of the hamstring muscle.
PATIENT POSITION	The patient lies supine. Both hips are flexed to 90°, and the knees are in relaxed flexion.
EXAMINER POSITION	The examiner is positioned to observe the motion of the knee and pelvis. No manual contact is required.
TEST PROCEDURE	The patient may grasp behind the knees with both hands to stabilize and ensure the hips remain at 90° of flexion or the patient's arms may remain resting at the side. Starting with the uninvolved side, the patient actively extends each knee in turn as far as possible.
INDICATIONS OF A POSITIVE TEST	For normal flexibility in the hamstrings, knee extension should be within 20° of full extension. Kuo et al.[48] called this angle the *popliteal angle* (the angle between two lines; one line along the shaft of the femur and one line along the line of the tibia). They reported this angle to be 180° from birth to age 2; the angle then decreased to about 155° by age 6 and remained fairly constant after that. If the angle was less than 125°, the hamstrings were considered tight.
CLINICAL NOTES	• Nerve root symptoms may also result, because this positioning is similar to the slump test or straight leg raise test. • The patient should be advised to straighten the leg slowly. If the ROM is limited by nerve root involvement, this test can easily exacerbate a patient's symptoms.
RELIABILITY/SPECIFICITY/ SENSITIVITY	Unknown

References

1. Ombregt L, Bissehop P, ter Veer HJ, Van de Velde T: *A system of orthopedic medicine,* London, 1995, Saunders.
2. Ito K, Minka M-A, Leung M et al: Femoroacetabular impingement and the cam-effect: an MRI-based quantitative anatomical study of the femoral head-neck offset, *J Bone Joint Surg Br* 83:171-176, 2001.
3. Leunig M, Werlen S, Ungersbock A et al: Evaluation of the acetabular labrum by MR arthrography, *J Bone Joint Surg Br* 79:230-234, 1997.
4. Klaue K, Durnin CW, Ganz R: The acetabular rim syndrome: a clinical presentation of dysplasia of the hip, *J Bone Joint Surg Br* 73:423-429, 1991.
5. Crawford JR, Villar RN: Current concepts in the management of femoroacetabular impingement, *J Bone Joint Surg Br* 87:1459-1462, 2005.
6. Ferguson TA, Matta J: Anterior femoroacetabular impingement: a clinical presentation, *Sports Med Arthro Rev* 10:134-140, 2002.
7. Simoneau GG, Hoenig KJ, Lepley JE, Papanek PE: Influence of hip position and gender on active hip internal and external rotation, *J Orthop Sports Phys Ther* 28:158-164, 1998.
8. Tepper S, Hochberg M: Factors associated with hip osteoarthritis: data from the First National Health and Nutrition Examination Survey (NHANES-I), *Am J Epidemiol* 137:1081-1088, 1993.
9. Felson D: Epidemiology of hip and knee osteoarthritis, *Epidemiol Rev* 10:1-28, 1988.
10. Hungerford D, Jones L: Asymptomatic osteonecrosis: should it be treated? *Clin Orthop Relat Res* 429:124-130, 2004.
11. Hägglund G, Hansson L, Ordeberg G: Epidemiology of slipped capital femoral epiphysis in southern Sweden, *Clin Orthop Relat Res* 191:82-94, 1984.
12. Margetts B, Perry C, Taylor J, Dangerfield P: The incidence and distribution of Legg-Calvé-Perthes disease in Liverpool, 1982-95, *Arch Dis Child* 84:351-35, 2001.
13. Peled E, Eidelman M, Katzman A, Bialik V: Neonatal incidence of hip dysplasia: ten years of experience, *Clin Orthop Relat Res* 466:771-775, 2008.
14. Evans RC: *Illustrated essentials in orthopedic physical assessment,* St Louis, 1994, Mosby.
15. Cliborne AV, Waineer RS, Rhon DI et al: Clinical hip tests and a functional squat test in patients with knee osteoarthritis: reliability, prevalence of positive test findings, and short-term response to hip mobilization, *J Orthop Sports Phys Ther* 34:676-685, 2004.
16. Ross MD, Nordeen MH, Barido M: Test-retest reliability of Patrick's hip range of motion test in healthy college-aged men, *J Strength Cond Res* 17:156-161, 2003.
17. Woods D, Macnicol M: The flexion-adduction test: an early sign of hip disease, *J Pediatr Orthop* 10:180-185, 2001.
18. Maitland GD: *The peripheral joints: examination and recording guide,* Adelaide, 1973, Virgo Press..
19. Trendelenburg F: Trendelenburg's test (1895), *Clin Orthop Relat Res* 355:3-7, 1998.
20. Fitzgerald RH: Acetabular labrum tears: diagnosis and treatment, *Clin Orthop Relat Res* 311:60-68, 1995.
21. Braly BA, Beall DP, Martin HD: Clinical examination of the athletic hip, *Clin Sports Med* 25:199-210, 2006.
22. Tonnis D, Heinecke A: Acetabular and femoral anteversion: relationship with osteoarthritis of the hip, *J Bone Joint Surg Am* 81:1747-1770, 1999.
23. Reynolds D, Lucas J, Klaue K: Retroversion of the acetabulum, *J Bone Joint Surg Br* 81:281-288, 1999.
24. Adams MC: *Outline of orthopaedics,* London, 1968, E & S Livingstone.
25. Adams MC: *Outline of orthopaedics,* London, 1968, E & S Livingstone.
26. Tachdjian MO: *Pediatric orthopedics,* Philadelphia, 1972, Saunders.
27. Staheli LT: Medial femoral torsion, *Orthop Clin North Am* 11:39-50, 1980.
28. Jonson SR, Gross MT: Intraexaminer reliability, interexaminer reliability, and mean values for nine lower extremity skeletal measures in healthy naval midshipmen, *J Orthop Sports Phys Ther* 25:253-263, 1997.
29. Gelberman RH, Cohen MS, Desai SS et al: Femoral anteversion: a clinical assessment of idiopathic in-toeing gait in children, *J Bone Joint Surg Br* 69:75-79, 1987.
30. Friberg O: Clinical symptoms and biomechanics of lumbar spine and hip joint in leg length inequality, *Spine* 8:643-651, 1983.
31. ten Brinke A, van der Aa HE, van der Palen J, Oosterveld F: Is leg length discrepancy associated with side of radiating pain in patients with a lumbar herniated disc? *Spine* 24:684-686, 1999.
32. Bolz S, Davies GJ: Leg length differences and correlation with total leg strength, *J Orthop Sports Phys Ther* 6:123-129, 1984.
33. Reider B: *The orthopedic physical examination,* Philadelphia, 1999, Saunders.
34. Clarke GR: Unequal leg length: An accurate method of detection and some clinical results, *Rheumatol Phys Med* 11:385-390, 1972.
35. Fisk JW, Balgent ML: Clinical and radiological assessment of leg length, *N Z Med J* 81:477-480, 1975.
36. Woerman AL, Binder-Macleod SA: Leg-length discrepancy assessment: accuracy and precision in five clinical methods of evaluation, *J Orthop Sports Phys Ther* 5:230-239, 1984.
37. Hinson R, Brown SH: Supine leg length differential estimation: an inter- and intra-examiner reliability study, *Chiropr Res J* 5:17-22, 1998.
38. Woerman AL: Evaluation and treatment of dysfunction in the lumbar-pelvic-hip complex. In Donatelli R, Wooden MJ (eds): *Orthopedic physical therapy,* Edinburgh, 1989, Churchill Livingstone.
39. Wallace LA: Limb length difference and back pain. In Grieve GP (ed): *Modern manual therapy of the vertebral column,* Edinburgh, 1986, Churchill Livingstone.
40. Thurston A: Assessment of fixed flexion deformity of the hip, *Clin Orthop* 169:186-189, 1982.
41. Gruebel-Lee DM: *Disorders of the hip,* Philadelphia, 1983, Lippincott.

42. Ober FB: The role of the iliotibial and fascia lata as a factor in the causation of low-back disabilities and sciatica, *J Bone Joint Surg* 18:105-110, 1936.

43. Gautam VK, Anand S: A new test for estimating iliotibial band contracture, *J Bone Joint Surg Br* 80:474-475, 1998.

44. Noble HB, Hajek MR, Porter M: Diagnosis and treatment of iliotibial band tightness in runners, *Phys Sportsmed* 10:67-68: 71-72, 74, 1982.

45. Crawford AH: Neurologic disorders. In Steinberg ME (ed): *The hip and its disorders,* Philadelphia, 1991, Saunders.

46. Saudek CE: The hip. In Gould JA (ed): *Orthopedic and sports physical therapy,* St Louis, 1990, Mosby.

47. Palmar ML, Epler M: *Clinical assessment procedures in physical therapy,* Philadelphia, 1990, Lippincott.

48. Kuo L, Chung W, Bates E, Stephen J: The hamstring index, *J Pediatr Orthop* 17:78-88, 1997.

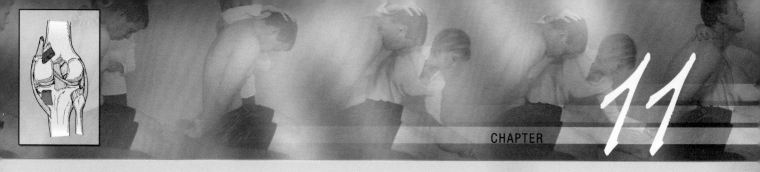

KNEE

Précis of the Knee Assessment*

History
Observation
Examination
Active movements
Knee flexion
Knee extension
Medial rotation of the tibia on the femur
Lateral rotation of the tibia on the femur
Patellar tracking
Passive movements (as in active movements)
Resisted isometric movements
Knee flexion
Knee extension
Ankle plantar flexion
Ankle dorsiflexion
Tests for ligament stability
Test for one-plane medial instability
Abduction (valgus stress) test
Hughston's valgus stress test
Test for one-plane lateral instability
Adduction (varus stress) test
Hughston's varus stress test
Tests for one-plane anterior and posterior instabilities
Posterior sag sign (gravity drawer test)
Godfrey (gravity) test
Lachman test
Drawer sign
Active drawer test
Tests for anteromedial and anterolateral rotary instabilities
Slocum test
Lateral pivot shift maneuver (test of MacIntosh)
Jerk test of Hughston
Slocum ALRI test
Crossover test of Arnold
Tests for posteromedial and posterolateral rotary instabilities
Hughston's posteromedial drawer sign
Hughston's posterolateral drawer sign
Posteromedial pivot shift
Jakob test (reverse pivot shift maneuver)
External rotation recurvatum test
Loomer's posterolateral rotary instability test

Special tests
Tests for meniscus injury
McMurray test
Apley's test
Bounce home test
Plica tests
Mediopatellar plica test
Hughston's plica test
Tests for patellofemoral dysfunction
Clarke's sign
McConnell test for chondromalacia patella
Tests for swelling
Brush, stroke, or bulge test
Indentation test
Fluctuation test
Patellar tap test (ballotable patella)
Other tests
Q-angle or patellofemoral angle
Fairbank's apprehension test
Noble compression test
Functional leg length
Reflexes and cutaneous distribution
Joint play movements
Backward and forward movements of the tibia on the femur
Medial and lateral translations of the tibia on the femur
Medial and lateral displacements of the patella
Depression (distal movement) of the patella
Anterior movement of the fibula on the tibia
Palpation
Diagnostic imaging

---

*Although an examination of the knee may be performed with the patient in the supine position, some of the tests may require the patient to move to other positions (e.g., standing, lying, prone, sitting). When these tests are used, the examination should be planned so that movements (and therefore the patient's discomfort) are kept to a minimum. The sequence should proceed from standing, to sitting, to supine lying, to side lying, and finally to prone lying. After any examination, the patient should be warned that the assessment may result in an exacerbation of symptoms.

SELECTED MOVEMENTS

ACTIVE MOVEMENTS[1,2]

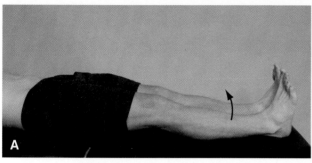
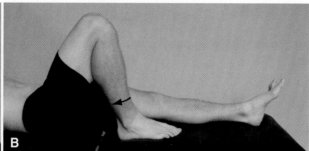

Figure 11–1
Active movements of the knee. **A,** Extension. **B,** Flexion.

GENERAL INFORMATION	During the active movements of the knee, the examiner should observe (1) the excursion of the patella, to make sure it tracks freely and smoothly; (2) the range of motion (ROM) available in the tibiofemoral and patellofemoral joints; (3) whether pain occurs during the movement, and if so, where and when; and (4) what appears to be limiting the movement. The active movements may be performed in the sitting or supine position; as always, the most painful movements should be done last, and the unaffected side is tested first.
PATIENT POSITION	The patient is supine or sitting
EXAMINER POSITION	The examiner stands to the side of the patient to instruct the person and observe the ROM.

Continued

ACTIVE MOVEMENTS[1,2]—cont'd

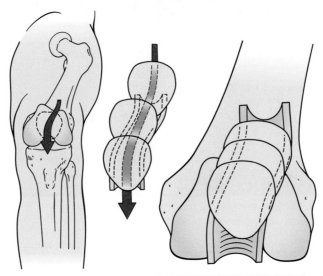

Figure 11–2
Multiplanar patellar path during knee flexion. (Redrawn from Stanitski CL, DeLee JC, Drez D [eds]: *Pediatric and adolescent sports medicine*, p 307, Philadelphia, 1994, Saunders.)

Flexion

TEST PROCEDURE   The patient is asked to flex the knee as far as possible.

INDICATIONS OF A POSITIVE TEST   Full knee flexion is 135° (0° being a straight knee). If the range of movement is less than this or is less than in the unaffected leg, the test result is positive. As the patient moves the knee through flexion and extension, the examiner should watch the movement of the patella as it "tracks" along the femoral trochlea. The examiner should note whether the movement is smooth from beginning to end or whether the patella shows a lag or abrupt jump as it attempts to center in the groove. The patella does not follow a straight path as the knee moves from extension to flexion. Normally, it follows a curved pattern, moving medially in early flexion and then laterally.

Extension

TEST PROCEDURE   The patient is asked to extend the knee.

INDICATIONS OF A POSITIVE TEST   Active knee extension is approximately 0° but may be −15°, especially in women, who are more likely to have hyperextended knees (genu recurvatum). If the range of movement is less than this or is less than in the unaffected leg, the test result is positive. The knee extensor muscles develop the greatest force near 60°, and the knee flexor muscles develop their greatest force between 45° and 10°. To complete the last 15° of knee extension, a 60% increase in the force of the quadriceps muscles is required. Therefore, the examiner should watch for evidence of quadriceps lag, which means the quadriceps muscles are not strong enough to fully extend the knee. The lag results from loss of mechanical advantage, muscle atrophy, decreasing power of the muscle as it shortens, adhesion formation, effusion, or reflex inhibition that results in instability of the knee.

PATELLAR MOBILITY[3,4]

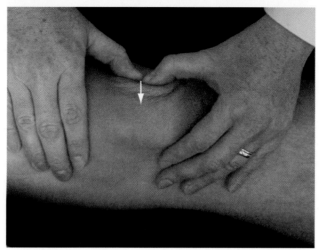

Figure 11–3
Patella medial glide.

PURPOSE	To assess the mobility of the patella.
SUSPECTED INJURY	Patellofemoral dysfunction
PATIENT POSITION	The patient is sitting or supine.
EXAMINER POSITION	The examiner is positioned directly adjacent to the knee to be tested.
TEST PROCEDURE	The examiner's hands are placed near the knee to stabilize the tibia and femur. The thumbs of the hands are placed on the side (either medial or lateral) of the patella. The examiner passively glides the patella medially and laterally. The amount, quality, and symptomology of the motion are noted. The side-to-side passive motion of the patella also should be tested in 45° of flexion; this is a more functional position and gives a better indication of the functional stability of the patella.
INDICATIONS OF A POSITIVE TEST	Normally, the patella should move up to half its width medially and laterally in extension. The end feel of these movements is tissue stretch. Lateral displacement must be performed with care, especially in patients who have experienced a dislocated patella.
CLINICAL NOTE/CAUTION	• When the patella is pushed medially or laterally, the examiner should note whether it stays parallel to the femoral condyles or tilts or rotates. For example, if the patella is pushed medially when the medial structures are tight, the lateral border of the patella tilts up. Likewise, with tight lateral structures, the medial border tilts up. If the lateral structures are tight superiorly, the inferior pole of the patella medially rotates. These are examples of dynamic tilt and rotation problems of the patella.
RELIABILITY/SPECIFICITY/ SENSITIVITY	Unknown

SPECIAL TESTS FOR ONE-PLANE MEDIAL INSTABILITY

Relevant Special Tests

Abduction (valgus stress) test
Hughston's valgus stress test

Definition

Sudden or violent shearing of the tibiofemoral joint can result in stretching or tearing of the tibial (medial) collateral ligament (MCL/TCL) and other, associated ligaments. The shear or excessive force causes the tibia to move away from the femur (i.e., gap) on the medial side.

Suspected Injury

Structures that may have been injured include:
Tibial collateral ligament (superficial and deep fibers)
Posterior oblique ligament
Posteromedial capsule
Anterior cruciate ligament
Posterior cruciate ligament
Medial quadriceps expansion
Semimembranosus muscle
NOTE: The structures damaged and the degree of injury depend on the forces applied. The more structures damaged, the more unstable the knee

Epidemiology and Demographics

The exact prevalence of MCL/TCL injuries in the general population is unknown. It is the most common ligament injury. The MCL/TCL often is injured in conjunction with other structures, such as the anterior cruciate ligament or medial meniscus.[5]

Relevant History

The patient may report a previous history of a knee injury that has affected the mechanics of the knee. Previous injuries to the ankle or hip also may predispose a person to increased stresses at the knee.

Relevant Signs and Symptoms

- Mild to moderate knee pain is present.
- The patient reports feeling a tearing in the knee, not a "pop."
- Bruising in the medial knee often is present, because the MCL/TCL is an extra-articular structure.
- Swelling builds up slowly over several days.
- The patient walks with a limp and has pain on knee extension, because extension stretches the ligament.
- Instability and "giving way" may be noted.
- Loss of knee motion and moderate stiffness may be present.
- Medial joint line pain or pain where the ligament attaches to the femur or tibia may be reported.

Mechanism of Injury

The MCL/TCL functions to restrain valgus stress and lateral rotation of the tibia. A blow to the outside of the knee most commonly injures the ligament. Contact injuries involving direct valgus loading to the knee are the usual mechanism in a complete tear. Noncontact, or indirect, injuries occur with deceleration, cutting, and pivoting motions. Anatomically, the MCL/TCL is composed of two layers, the superficial layer and the deep layer; the deep layers attach to the medial meniscus.

Avulsion of ligaments generally occurs between the unmineralized and mineralized fibrocartilage layers. MCL/TCL injury occurs most often at the femoral attachment (65% of cases).[6-11]

ABDUCTION (VALGUS STRESS) TEST[12,13]

DVD

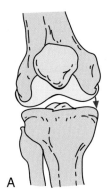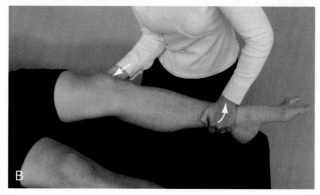

Figure 11–4
Abduction (valgus stress) test. **A,** "Gapping" on the medial aspect of the knee. **B,** Position for testing the medial collateral ligament (extended knee).

PURPOSE	To assess for one-plane (straight) medial instability, which means that the tibia moves away from the femur (i.e., gaps) on the medial side.
SUSPECTED INJURY	Structures that may have been injured include: Medial collateral ligament (superficial and deep fibers) Posterior oblique ligament Posteromedial capsule Anterior cruciate ligament Posterior cruciate ligament Medial quadriceps expansion Semimembranosus muscle
PATIENT POSITION	The patient is supine with the test knee in extension.
EXAMINER POSITION	The examiner stands adjacent to the lateral aspect of the knee.
TEST PROCEDURE	The unaffected knee is tested first. One of the examiner's hands grasps the patient's ankle, and the other hand supports the lateral aspect of the knee joint. The examiner applies a valgus stress at the knee (pushes the knee medially) while the ankle is stabilized in slight lateral rotation either with the hand or with the leg held between the examiner's arm and trunk. The knee is tested first in full extension and then in slight flexion (20° to 30°) so that it is "unlocked." The two legs are compared.
INDICATIONS OF A POSITIVE TEST	A positive test result is indicated if the tibia moves away from the femur excessively when a valgus stress is applied with the knee in extension. The normal abrupt end feel is lost with a positive test result. Increased gapping with the knee in extension indicates injury to the medial collateral ligament and the anterior cruciate ligament. Increased gapping with the knee slightly flexed indicates injury primarily to the medial collateral ligament. If the test result is positive when the knee is flexed to 20° to 30°, structures that may have been injured include: • Medial collateral ligament • Posterior oblique ligament • Posterior cruciate ligament • Posteromedial capsule

Continued

ABDUCTION (VALGUS STRESS) TEST[12,13]—*cont'd*

CLINICAL NOTES

- A positive test result on full extension is classified as a major disruption of the knee. The examiner usually finds that one or more of the rotary tests also produce a positive result.
- If the examiner applies lateral rotation to the foot when performing the test in extension and finds excessive lateral rotation on the affected side, this is a sign of possible anteromedial rotary instability.
- The flexed part of the valgus stress test is considered the true test for one-plane medial instability, because the cruciates are eliminated.

RELIABILITY/SPECIFICITY/
SENSITIVITY[13]

Reliability (interrater range): $k = 0.01$-0.38

HUGHSTON'S VALGUS STRESS TEST[12]

DVD

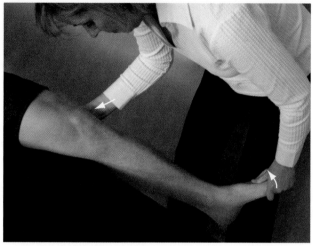

Figure 11–5
Hughston's valgus stress test.

PURPOSE	To assess for one-plane (straight) medial instability.
SUSPECTED INJURY	Structures that may have been injured include: Medial collateral ligament (superficial and deep fibers) Posterior oblique ligament Posteromedial capsule Anterior cruciate ligament Posterior cruciate ligament Medial quadriceps expansion Semimembranosus muscle
PATIENT POSITION	The patient is supine with the test knee in extension.
EXAMINER POSITION	The examiner stands adjacent to the lateral aspect of the knee.
TEST PROCEDURE	The normal knee is tested first. One of the examiner's hands grasps the patient's big toe, and the other hand supports the lateral aspect of the knee joint. Facing the patient's foot, the examiner abducts the hip so that the thigh lies on the plinth but the lower leg is free. The examiner grasps the patient's big toe and applies a valgus stress, allowing any natural rotation of the tibia. The two legs are compared.
INDICATIONS OF A POSITIVE TEST	A positive test result is indicated if the tibia moves away from the femur excessively when a valgus stress is applied with the knee in extension, and the end feel is changed. The structures tested are the same as in the abduction (valgus) stress test.
CLINICAL NOTE	• Doing the test with the thigh resting on the plinth often allows the patient to relax more and is less likely to lead to muscle spasm, which may limit movement.
RELIABILITY/SPECIFICITY/ SENSITIVITY	Unknown

SPECIAL TESTS FOR ONE-PLANE LATERAL INSTABILITY

Relevant Special Tests

Adduction (varus stress) test
Hughston's varus stress test (see Hughston's valgus stress test)

Definition

Sudden or violent shearing of the tibiofemoral joint can result in stretching or tearing of the lateral (fibular) collateral ligament (LCL/FCL) and other, associated ligaments. The shear or excessive force causes the tibia to move away from the femur (i.e., gap) on the lateral side.

Suspected Injury

Structures that may have been injured include:
Fibular or lateral collateral ligament
Posterolateral capsule
Arcuate-popliteus complex
Biceps femoris tendon
Posterior cruciate ligament
Anterior cruciate ligament
Lateral gastrocnemius muscle
Iliotibial band
Peroneal nerve

Epidemiology and Demographics

Injury to the LCL/FCL is the least common knee ligament injury. Injuries to the LCL/FCL are rare, accounting for only 2% of all knee injuries. The LCL/FCL is the least likely knee ligament to be sprained, because most LCL/FCL injuries are caused by a blow to the inside of the knee, and that area usually is shielded by the opposite leg.[6,7,9-11]

Relevant History

The patient may report a previous history of a knee injury that has affected the mechanics of the knee. Previous injuries to the ankle or hip may also predispose the patient to increased stresses at the knee.

Relevant Signs and Symptoms

- Mild to moderate knee pain is present.
- The patient may report feeling a pop in the knee.
- Loss of knee motion and moderate stiffness are present.
- Lateral joint line pain may be reported.
- Bruising in the lateral knee often is present, because the LCL/FCL is an extra-articular structure.
- Swelling builds up slowly over several days.
- Instability and giving way may be noted.

Mechanism of Injury

The LCL/FCL functions to control varus loading and lateral rotation of the tibia running from the femoral condyle to the head of the fibula. Contact injuries involve a direct varus load to the knee; this is the usual mechanism in a complete tear. The most common method of injury is a direct varus force with the foot plantar flexed and the knee in extension. Related injuries include injuries to the peroneal nerve, posterolateral capsule damage, or posterior cruciate ligament damage. The mechanism of knee adduction, flexion, and lateral rotation of the femur on the tibia is a much less common mechanism.

With excessive force, the LCL/FCL usually is disrupted initially, followed by the capsular ligaments, the arcuate ligament complex, the popliteus, the iliotibial band, the biceps femoris, and the common peroneal nerve; one or both cruciate ligaments may be disrupted.

Avulsion of ligaments generally occurs between the unmineralized and mineralized fibrocartilage layers. LCL/FCL injury occurs most commonly at the fibular attachment (75% of cases).[6,7,9-11]

ADDUCTION (VARUS STRESS) TEST

DVD

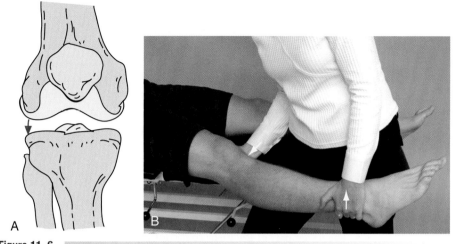

Figure 11–6

Adduction (varus stress) test. **A,** One-plane lateral instability "gapping" on the lateral aspect. **B,** Position for testing the lateral collateral ligament in extension.

PURPOSE To assess for one-plane lateral instability (i.e., the tibia moves away from the femur an excessive amount on the lateral aspect of the leg).

SUSPECTED INJURY Structures that may have been injured include:
Fibular or lateral collateral ligament
Posterolateral capsule
Arcuate-popliteus complex
Biceps femoris tendon
Posterior cruciate ligament
Anterior cruciate ligament
Lateral gastrocnemius muscle
Iliotibial band
Peroneal nerve

PATIENT POSITION The patient is supine with the test knee in extension.

EXAMINER POSITION The examiner stands adjacent to the medial aspect of the knee.

TEST PROCEDURE The unaffected side is tested first. One of the examiner's hands grasps the patient's ankle, and the other hand supports the medial aspect of the knee joint. The examiner applies a varus stress at the knee (pushes the knee laterally) while the ankle is stabilized. The test is done first with the knee in full extension and then with the knee in 20° to 30° of flexion. If the tibia is laterally rotated in full extension before the test, the cruciate ligaments will be uncoiled and maximum stress will be placed on the collateral ligaments. The two legs are compared.

MODIFICATION OF TEST Hughston's varus stress test may be used. In this case, the examiner grasps the fifth and fourth toes and applies a varus stress to the knee in extension and slightly flexed (20° to 30°). The two legs are compared.

Continued

ADDUCTION (VARUS STRESS) TEST—*cont'd*

INDICATIONS OF A POSITIVE TEST

The test result is positive if the tibia moves away from the femur more than on the normal side when a varus stress is applied and the end feel is modified (more mushy). If excessive gapping occurs when the knee is tested in full extension, primarily the lateral collateral ligament and anterior cruciate ligament have been injured. If excessive gapping occurs when the knee is flexed, primarily the lateral collateral ligament has been injured. If the test result is positive when the knee is flexed 20° to 30° with lateral rotation of the tibia, the structures that may have been injured are:
- Lateral collateral ligament
- Posterolateral capsule
- Arcuate-popliteus complex
- Iliotibial band
- Biceps femoris tendon

CLINICAL NOTES

- The examiner may also find that one or more of the rotary instability tests produce a positive result, especially if the test is positive in extension.
- The flexed part of the varus stress test is classified as the true test for one-plane lateral instability.
- If Hughston's valgus stress test is performed, the examiner can rest the patient's thigh on the plinth, which often allows the patient to relax more and is likely to lead to less muscle spasm.

RELIABILITY/SPECIFICITY/ SENSITIVITY

Unknown

SPECIAL TESTS FOR ONE-PLANE POSTERIOR INSTABILITY

Relevant Special Tests

Posterior sag sign (gravity drawer test)
Reverse Lachman test
Godfrey (gravity) test
Drawer sign (see Special Tests for One-Plane Anterior Instability)
Active drawer test (see Special Tests for One-Plane Anterior Instability)

Definition

A sudden or violent shearing of the tibiofemoral joint can result in stretching or tearing of the posterior cruciate ligament and other, associated ligaments. The excessive shearing causes the tibia to translate posteriorly on a fixed femur or the femur to translate anteriorly on a fixed tibia.

Suspected Injury

Structures that may have been injured include:
Posterior cruciate ligament (PCL)
Arcuate-popliteus complex
Posterior oblique ligament (POL)
Anterior cruciate ligament (ACL)
NOTE: The ligaments damaged and the degree of injury depend on the forces applied. The more structures damaged, the more unstable the knee.

Epidemiology and Demographics

The posterior cruciate ligament is the strongest of all the knee ligaments and the least frequently injured (3% to 20% of knee injuries).[5-7,10,11,14-17]

Relevant History

The patient may report a previous history of a knee injury that has affected the mechanics of the knee. Previous injuries to the ankle or hip also may predispose the patient to increased stresses at the knee.

Relevant Signs and Symptoms

- Mild knee pain is present.
- Feeling or hearing a pop is rare (unlike with ACL injuries).
- Moderate swelling or hemarthrosis is present.
- The patient may report a feeling of instability and giving way.
- Loss of knee motion and moderate stiffness are present.
- Medial joint line pain may be reported.
- Retropatellar pain symptoms are present.

Mechanism of Injury

A patient with an ACL tear usually reports an active mechanism of injury; most PCL injuries, however, occur when passive external forces are applied to the knee. A posteriorly directed force on a flexed knee (i.e., the anterior aspect of the flexed knee strikes the dashboard, or a person falls on another person's leg) may cause PCL injury. Also, a fall onto a flexed knee with the foot in plantar flexion and the tibial tubercle striking the ground first, directing a posterior force to the proximal tibia, may result in injury to the PCL.

Hyperextension alone may lead to an avulsion injury of the PCL from the origin; this kind of injury may be amenable to repair. An anterior force to the anterior tibia in a hyperextended knee with the foot planted results in combined injury to the knee ligaments, along with knee dislocation.[5-7,10,11,14-17]

POSTERIOR SAG SIGN (GRAVITY DRAWER TEST)[18-22]

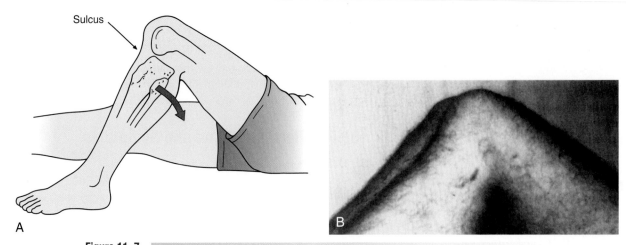

Sulcus

A

B

Figure 11–7
Sag sign. **A,** Illustration of the posterior sag sign. **B,** Note the profile of the two knees: the left (nearer) sags backward compared with the normal right knee, indicating a posterior cruciate ligament tear. (From O'Donoghue DH: *Treatment of injuries to athletes,* ed 4, p 450, Philadelphia, 1984, Saunders.)

PURPOSE	To assess for one-plane posterior instability.
SUSPECTED INJURY	Structures that may have been injured include: Posterior cruciate ligament Arcuate-popliteus complex Posterior oblique ligament Anterior cruciate ligament
PATIENT POSITION	The patient lies supine with the hip flexed to 45° and the knee flexed to 90°.
EXAMINER POSITION	The examiner is positioned so as to observe the patient's knee. This is an observational test; no manual contact is required.
TEST PROCEDURE	Once the test position has been established, the examiner asks the patient to relax and observes the position of the tibia in relation to the femur. The two legs are compared.
INDICATIONS OF A POSITIVE TEST	In the test position, if the PCL is torn, gravity causes the tibia to "drop back," or sag back on the femur. Posterior tibial displacement is more noticeable when the knee is flexed 90° to 110° than when the knee is only slightly flexed. Normally, the medial tibial plateau extends 1 cm anteriorly beyond the femoral condyle when the knee is flexed 90°. If this "step" is lost (which is what occurs with a positive posterior sag sign caused by a torn PCL), the step-off test, or thumb sign, is considered positive.
CLINICAL NOTES	• This test should always be done first when testing the cruciates to prevent a false positive test when doing the test for the anterior cruciate. • If the patient tests positive for the posterior sag sign, the individual should carefully extend the knee while the examiner holds the hip in 90° to 100° of flexion. This action is sometimes called the *voluntary anterior drawer sign,* and the results are similar to those of the active anterior drawer test. As the patient slowly extends the knee, the tibial plateau moves or shifts forward to its normal position, indicating that the tibia previously was posteriorly subluxated (posterior cruciate tear) on the femur.
RELIABILITY/SPECIFICITY/ SENSITIVITY	Unknown

REVERSE LACHMAN TEST[23]

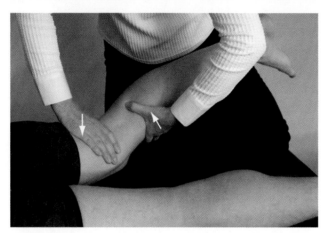

Figure 11–8
Reverse Lachman test.

PURPOSE	To assess for one-plane posterior instability.
SUSPECTED INJURY	Structures that may have been injured include: Posterior cruciate ligament Arcuate-popliteus complex Posterior oblique ligament Anterior cruciate ligament
PATIENT POSITION	The patient lies prone (the knee is flexed to 30° by the examiner).
EXAMINER POSITION	The examiner is positioned adjacent to the patient's shin.
TEST PROCEDURE	The unaffected leg is tested first. The examiner grasps the tibia with one hand while fixing the femur with the other hand. The examiner makes sure the hamstring muscles are relaxed by feeling the weight of the leg below the knee in the examiner's hand. The examiner then pulls the tibia up (posteriorly), noting the amount of movement and the quality of the end feel.
INDICATIONS OF A POSITIVE TEST	A positive test result is indicated by excessive motion compared to the contralateral, or unaffected, side.
CLINICAL NOTES/CAUTIONS	• The examiner should be cautious of a false-positive test result if the anterior cruciate ligament has been torn, because gravity may cause an anterior shift. • This test is not as accurate for the posterior cruciate ligament as is the posterior drawer or sag test; when the posterior cruciate ligament is torn, the greatest posterior displacement is at 90°. • In the case of acute trauma, swelling prevents the examiner from getting a true indication of the joint's mobility. The best time to assess joint laxity is immediately after an injury, before swelling occurs, or in the chronic state. The examiner may need to allow time for the swelling to reduce before true joint mobility can be assessed.
RELIABILITY/SPECIFICITY/ SENSITIVITY	Unknown

GODFREY (GRAVITY) TEST[23]

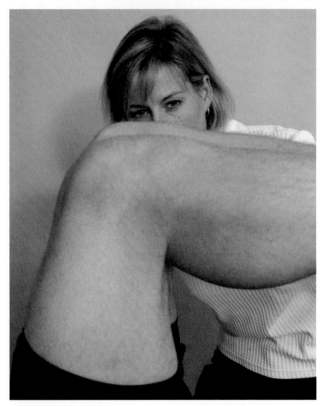

Figure 11–9
Godfrey test. The examiner watches for a posterior shift, which is not evident in this case.

PURPOSE	To assess for one-plane posterior instability.
SUSPECTED INJURY	Structures that may have been injured include: Posterior cruciate ligament Arcuate-popliteus complex Posterior oblique ligament Anterior cruciate ligament
PATIENT POSITION	The patient lies supine.
EXAMINER POSITION	The examiner is positioned adjacent to the patient's knees.
TEST PROCEDURE	The examiner holds/supports both legs at the ankles. The examiner flexes the patient's hips and knees to 90° and checks the levels of both tibia relative to each other.
INDICATIONS OF A POSITIVE TEST	A positive test result for posterior instability is indicated by a posterior sag of the tibia on the affected side.
CLINICAL NOTE	• If manual posterior pressure is applied to the tibia, posterior displacement may increase.
RELIABILITY/SPECIFICITY/ SENSITIVITY	Unknown

SPECIAL TESTS FOR ONE-PLANE ANTERIOR INSTABILITY

Relevant Special Tests

Lachman test
Drawer sign
Active drawer test

Definition

A sudden or violent shearing of the tibiofemoral joint can result in stretching or tearing of the anterior cruciate ligament and other, associated ligaments. The excessive shearing causes the tibia to translate anteriorly on a fixed tibia.

Suspected Injury

Structures that may have been injured include:
Anterior cruciate ligament (especially the posterolateral bundle)
Posterior oblique ligament
Arcuate-popliteus complex

Epidemiology and Demographics[6,7,9-11,14,15]

Anterior cruciate ligament injuries occur most commonly in individuals 4 to 29 years old. These years correspond to high levels of more vigorous activity. Epidemiologic studies estimate that approximately 1 in 3000 individuals have an ACL injury each year in the United States. This figure corresponds to an overall injury rate approaching 200,000 injuries annually. Female athletes are 2.4 to 9.5 times more likely to sustain an ACL injury than male athletes. Some studies have correlated menstruation with ACL tears in women. Studies have shown a twofold increase in female collegiate soccer players and a fourfold increase in female basketball players compared with their male counterparts.

Relevant History

The patient may report a previous history of a knee injury that has affected the mechanics of the knee. Previous injuries to the ankle or hip also may predispose the patient to increased stresses at the knee.

Relevant Signs and Symptoms

- Pain
- Feeling or hearing a pop
- Inability to continue activity
- Swelling or large hemarthrosis
- Instability and giving way (feeling the knee give out)
- Loss of knee motion

Mechanism of Injury

The ACL and PCL bridge the inside of the knee joint, forming an X pattern that stabilizes the knee against front to back and back to front forces. The ACL extends superiorly, posteriorly, and laterally, twisting on itself as it extends from the tibia to the femur. The main functions of the ACL are to prevent anterior movement of the tibia on the femur, to check lateral rotation of the tibia in flexion and, to a lesser extent, to check extension and hyperextension at the knee. The ACL helps control the normal rolling and gliding movement of the knee. The anteromedial bundle is tight in both flexion and extension, whereas the posterolateral bundle is tight on extension only. As a whole, the ligament has the least amount of stress on it between 30° and 60° flexion.

The ACL typically is sprained during one of the following knee movements: a sudden stop; a twist, pivot, or change in direction at the joint; extreme overstraightening (hyperextension); or a direct impact to the outside of the knee or lower leg. These injuries are seen among athletes in football, basketball, soccer, rugby, wrestling, gymnastics, and skiing.

The ACL provides 85% of the total restraining force to anterior translation of the tibia. This injury usually occurs during a sudden cut or deceleration; it typically is a noncontact injury. The patient states, "I planted, twisted, and then heard a pop."

Often the mechanism of injury results in injury to multiple structures. The most common structures to be injured in association with the ACL are the medial collateral ligament and the medial meniscus (the "terrible triad").

When performing the one-plane anterior instability tests, the examiner looks for abnormal (excessive) anterior translation of the tibia relative to the femur.

RELIABILITY/SPECIFICITY/SENSITIVITY/ODDS RATIO COMPARISON[24-47]

	Lachman Test	Drawer Sign	Active Anterior Drawer Test
Validity	*Predictive value:* Positive: 47% Negative: 64%	Unknown	Unknown
Interrater reliability	+/−: 0.19	Unknown	Unknown
Intrarater reliability	+/−: 0.51 End feel: K = 0.33	Unknown	Unknown
Specificity	46% to 100%	50% to 100%	Unknown
Sensitivity	48% to 100%	9% to 95%	Unknown
Positive likelihood ratio	1.31-102.1	1.2-87.9	Unknown
Negative likelihood ratio	0-0.63	0.1-0.8	Unknown

LACHMAN TEST[24-43,48-54]

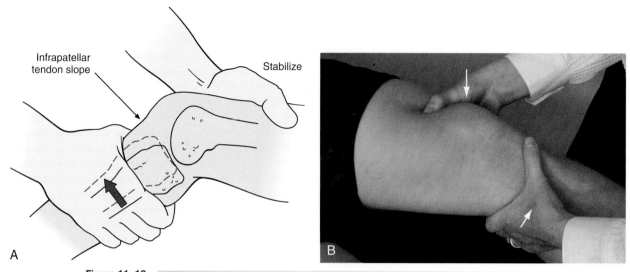

Figure 11–10
Hand position for the classic Lachman test (**A** and **B**).

PURPOSE	To test for one-plane anterior instability.
SUSPECTED INJURY	Structures that may have been injured include: Anterior cruciate ligament (especially the posterolateral bundle) Posterior oblique ligament Arcuate-popliteus complex
PATIENT POSITION	The patient lies supine.
EXAMINER POSITION	The examiner is positioned adjacent to the involved leg.
TEST PROCEDURE	The unaffected leg is tested first. One of the examiner's hands grasps the patient's tibia, and the other hand stabilizes the femur. The examiner holds the patient's knee between full extension and 30° of flexion. This position is close to the functional position of the knee, in which the ACL plays a major role. The patient's femur is stabilized with one of the examiner's hands (the "outside" hand) while the proximal aspect of the tibia is moved or translated forward with the other ("inside") hand. The two legs are compared.
INDICATIONS OF A POSITIVE TEST	A positive test result is indicated by a "mushy" or soft end feel when the tibia is moved forward on the femur (increased anterior translation with medial rotation of the tibia) and disappearance of the infrapatellar tendon slope. A false-negative test result may occur if the femur is not properly stabilized, if a meniscal lesion blocks translation, or if the tibia is medially rotated.
TEST MODIFICATION	The Stable Lachman test is recommended for examiners with small hands. The patient lies supine with the knee resting on the examiner's knee. One of the examiner's hands stabilizes the femur against the examiner's thigh, and the other hand applies an anterior stress. Adler and associates[54] described a modification of this method, which they called the "drop leg Lachman test." The patient lies supine. The test leg is abducted off the side of the examining table, and the knee is flexed to 25°. One of the examiner's hands

Continued

LACHMAN TEST[24-45,50-53]—cont'd

stabilizes the femur against the table while the patient's foot is held between the examiner's knees. The examiner's other hand then is free to apply the anterior translation force. These researchers found that greater anterior laxity was demonstrated by this version of the test than by the classic version. The two legs are compared.

CLINICAL NOTES/CAUTIONS

- Many contend that the Lachman test (also known as the *Ritchie, Trillat,* or *Lachman-Trillat test*), is the best indicator of injury to the anterior cruciate ligament, especially the posterolateral band, although this has been questioned.[26]
- The modification method that works for the examiner and that the examiner can use competently should be selected.
- Frank[52] reported that to achieve the best results, the tibia should be slightly laterally rotated and the anterior tibial translation force should be applied from the posteromedial aspect. The hand on the tibia should apply the translation force.
- The Lachman test can be done a number of ways. The key is to make sure the patient relaxes and the knee is held between full extension and 30° of flexion (see *Orthopedic Physical Assessment,* fifth edition, pages 767-770, for details).
- With acute trauma, swelling prevents the examiner from getting a true indication of the joint's mobility. The best time to assess joint laxity is immediately after the injury, before swelling occurs, or in the chronic state. The examiner may need to allow time for swelling to reduce before true joint mobility can be assessed.

RELIABILITY/SPECIFICITY/ SENSITIVITY[24-43]

Reliability range: Intrarater: k = 0.33-0.51
Interrater: k = 0.19-0.23
Specificity range: 46% to 100%
Sensitivity range: 48% to 100% (chronic)

DRAWER SIGN[12,23-25,27,28,30,33,34,37,39-47,55-59]

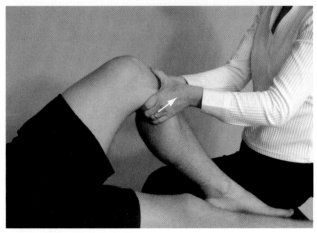

Figure 11-11
Position for drawer sign.

PURPOSE	To test for one-plane anterior and one-plane posterior instabilities.
Part 1	This part of the test assesses for one-plane anterior instability
SUSPECTED INJURY	Structures that may have been injured include: Anterior cruciate ligament (especially the anteromedial bundle) Posterolateral capsule Posteromedial capsule Medial collateral ligament (deep fibers) Iliotibial band Posterior oblique ligament Arcuate-popliteus complex
PATIENT POSITION	The patient's knee is flexed to 90°, and the hip is flexed to 45°. In this position, the anterior cruciate ligament is almost parallel with the tibial plateau.
EXAMINER POSITION	The examiner sits on the assessment table facing the patient.
TEST PROCEDURE	The unaffected leg is tested first. To hold the patient's foot on the table, the examiner gently sits on the forefoot with the foot in neutral rotation. The examiner's hands are placed around and behind the tibia with the examiner's fingers palpating the posterior aspect of the knee to ensure that the hamstring muscles are relaxed. The examiner draws the tibia forward on the femur. The two legs are compared. For an accurate anterior drawer test, the examiner must make sure the hamstrings are relaxed.
INDICATIONS OF A POSITIVE TEST	The normal amount of anterior movement that should be present is approximately 6 mm.
CLINICAL NOTES/CAUTIONS	• This examination must be performed with particular care, because the start position could result in a false-positive anterior drawer test result for the anterior cruciate ligament if a posterior sag (an indication of a posterior cruciate problem) goes unnoticed before the test is started. If minimal or no swelling is present, the sag is evident because of an obvious concavity distal to the patella.

Continued

DRAWER SIGN [12,23-25,27,28,30,33,34,37,39-47,55-59] —cont'd

- If only the anterior cruciate ligament is torn, the test result is negative, because other structures (posterior capsule and posterolateral and posteromedial structures) limit movement. In addition, hemarthrosis, a torn medial meniscus (posterior horn) wedged against the medial femoral condyle, or hamstring spasm may result in a false-negative test result. Hughston[12] points out that tearing of the coronary or menisco-tibial ligament can allow the tibia to translate forward more than normal, even with an intact anterior cruciate ligament. In this case, when the anterior drawer test is performed, anteromedial rotation (subluxation) of the tibia occurs.
- When the anterior drawer test is done, if an audible snap or palpable jerk (Finochietto jumping sign) occurs when the tibia is pulled forward, and the tibia moves forward excessively, a meniscal lesion is likely in addition to the torn anterior cruciate ligament.[23]
- Weatherwax[58] described a modified means of testing the anterior drawer (90-90 anterior drawer test). The patient lies supine. The examiner flexes the patient's hip and knee to 90° and supports the lower leg between the examiner's trunk and forearm. The examiner places the hands around the tibia, as with the standard test, and applies sufficient force to slowly lift the patient's buttock off the table.
- Feagin[59] recommended that the drawer test be done with the patient sitting with the leg hanging relaxed over the end of the examining table (sitting anterior drawer test). The examiner places the hands as with the standardized test and slowly draws the tibia first forward and then backward to test the anterior and posterior drawer. The examiner uses the thumbs to palpate the tibial plateau movement relative to the femur. The examiner also may note any rotational deformity. The advantage of doing the test this way is that the posterior sag is eliminated, because the effect of gravity is eliminated.

Part 2	This part of the test assesses one-plane posterior instability.
SUSPECTED INJURY	Structures that may have been injured include: Posterior cruciate ligament Arcuate-popliteus complex Posterior oblique ligament Anterior cruciate ligament
PATIENT POSITION	The patient's knee is flexed to 90°, and the hip is flexed to 45°.
EXAMINER POSITION	The examiner sits on the assessment table facing the patient.
TEST PROCEDURE	The unaffected leg is tested first. To hold the patient's foot on the table, the examiner gently sits on the forefoot with the foot in neutral rotation. The examiner's fingers are placed around and behind the tibia, palpating the posterior aspect of the knee to ensure that the hamstring muscles are relaxed. The position of the tibia relative to the femur should be noted before the test is done, in case the posterior sag sign is present. After the anterior movement of the tibia on the femur, the posterior movement of the tibia on the femur should be completed using the heels of the hand. In this part of the test, the tibia is pushed back on the femur.
INDICATIONS OF A POSITIVE TEST	If the PCL has been torn, the tibia will drop or slide back on the femur, and when the examiner pulls the tibia forward, a large amount of movement will occur, giving a false-positive sign (see Posterior Sag Sign). Therefore, this test result should be considered positive only if it is shown that the posterior sag is present. The two legs are compared.
CLINICAL NOTES/CAUTIONS	• The difficulty with this test is in determining the neutral starting position if the ligaments have been injured. • As with the Lachman test, swelling in the joint affects the examiner's ability to assess for joint laxity.

DRAWER SIGN[12,23-25,27,28,30,33,34,37,39-47,55-59]—cont'd

- If the arcuate-popliteus complex remains intact, a positive posterior drawer sign may not be elicited.
- When the tibia is pushed backward, if the examiner forcefully rotates it laterally and excessive movement occurs, the test result is positive for posterolateral instability. Warren[57] calls this maneuver the arcuate spin test.

RELIABILITY/SPECIFICITY/ SENSITIVITY*   Specificity range: 50% to 100%
Sensitivity range: 9% to 95%

---

*References 24, 25, 27, 28, 30, 33, 34, 37, 39-47

ACTIVE DRAWER TEST[22,23,60,61]

DVD

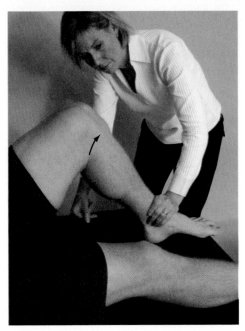

Figure 11–12
Active anterior drawer test. The examiner watches for an anterior shift.

PURPOSE	To test for one-plane anterior and one-plane posterior instabilities.
SUSPECTED INJURY	Structures that may have been injured include: Anterior cruciate ligament (especially the anteromedial bundle) Posterolateral capsule Posteromedial capsule Medial collateral ligament (deep fibers) Iliotibial band Posterior oblique ligament Arcuate-popliteus complex
PATIENT POSITION	The patient lies supine with the knee flexed to 90° and the hip flexed to 45°.
EXAMINER POSITION	The examiner stands directly adjacent to the test knee.
TEST PROCEDURE	One of the examiner's hands grasps the patient's ankle and anchors the foot to the assessment table. The patient is asked to try to straighten the leg while the examiner prevents this (isometric test). The two legs are compared.
INDICATIONS OF A POSITIVE TEST	If the ACL or PCL is torn, the anterior contour of the knee changes as the tibia is drawn forward. If the PCL is torn, a posterior sag is evident before the patient contracts the quadriceps. Contraction of the quadriceps causes the tibia to shift forward to its normal position, indicating a positive test result for a torn PCL. If posterior sag is absent and if the tibia shifts forward more on the affected side than on the unaffected side, this is a positive test result for ACL disruption.

ACTIVE DRAWER TEST[22,23,59,60]—cont'd

CLINICAL NOTES

- A second part of the test may be done by having the patient contract the hamstrings isometrically so that the tibial plateau moves posteriorly. This part of the test accentuates the posterior sag for posterior cruciate insufficiency, if present, and ensures maximum movement for anterior cruciate insufficiency if a quadriceps contraction is tried a second time.
- The active drawer test is a better expression of posterior cruciate insufficiency than of anterior cruciate insufficiency.
- With the drawer sign or test, if the anterior or posterior cruciate ligament is torn (third-degree sprain), some rotary instability is evident when the appropriate ligamentous tests are performed.

RELIABILITY/SPECIFICITY/ SENSITIVITY

Unknown

SPECIAL TESTS FOR ANTEROLATERAL ROTARY INSTABILITY

Relevant Special Tests

- Lateral pivot shift maneuver (test of MacIntosh)
- Jerk test of Hughston
- Slocum anterolateral rotary instability (ALRI) test
- Crossover test of Arnold

Definition

A sudden or violent twist or wrench of the tibiofemoral joint can result in stretching or tearing of the anterior cruciate ligament and other, associated ligaments. These injuries usually are seen with medial rotation of the femur on a fixed tibia or lateral rotation of the tibia on a fixed femur.

Suspected Injury

Structures that may have been injured include:
Anterior cruciate ligament
Posterolateral capsule
Arcuate-popliteus complex
Lateral collateral ligament
Iliotibial band
NOTE: The structures damaged and the degree of injury depend on the force applied. The more structures damaged, the more unstable the knee.

Epidemiology and Demographics[6,7,9-11,14,15]

The epidemiology and demographics of anterolateral instability are similar to those for the ACL; also, several ligaments in addition to the ACL are injured.

Relevant History

The patient may report a previous history of a knee injury that has affected the mechanics of the knee. Previous injuries to the ankle or hip also may predispose a person to increased stresses at the knee.

Relevant Signs and Symptoms

- Pain
- Feeling or hearing a pop
- Instability and giving way (feeling the knee give out)
- Inability to do activity
- Swelling or large hemarthrosis
- Loss of knee motion

Mechanism of Injury

See the anterior cruciate injury.

LATERAL PIVOT-SHIFT MANEUVER (TEST OF MACINTOSH)[26,32,34,37,38,62-64]

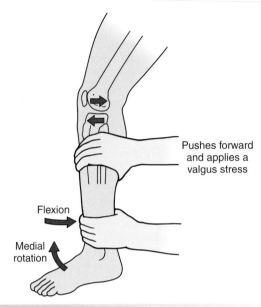

Pushes forward
and applies a
valgus stress

Flexion

Medial
rotation

Figure 11–13
Lateral pivot-shift test.

PURPOSE	To assess for anterolateral rotary instability of the knee. This is an excellent test for ruptures (third-degree sprains) of the anterior cruciate ligament as it mimics the "giving way" mechanism during the test.
SUSPECTED INJURY	Structures that may have been injured include: Anterior cruciate ligament Posterolateral capsule Arcuate-popliteus complex Lateral collateral ligament Iliotibial band
PATIENT POSITION	The patient lies supine. The hip is both flexed and abducted 30° and relaxed in slight medial rotation (20°) with the knee in extension.
EXAMINER POSITION	The examiner stands beside the patient.
TEST PROCEDURE	The test involves two phases: first subluxation (in extension) and then reduction (in flexion). The iliotibial band must be intact for the test to work. The unaffected knee is tested first. The examiner holds the patient's foot with one hand and places the other hand at the knee, holding the leg in slight medial rotation (i.e., the heel of the examiner's hand is placed behind the fibula and over the lateral head of the gastrocnemius muscle). The tibia then is medially rotated, causing it to subluxate anteriorly as the knee is taken into extension. The leg is flexed, and at approximately 30° to 40°, the tibia reduces, or "jogs," backward. The two legs are compared.
Note	This test does not work in cases of anterolateral instability in which the iliotibial band also has been torn; the subluxation will be evident, but the "jog" will not occur. A tear in either meniscus may limit or prevent the subluxation reduction motion seen in this test.

LATERAL PIVOT-SHIFT MANEUVER (TEST OF MACINTOSH)[26,32,34,37,38,62-64]—cont'd

INDICATIONS OF A POSITIVE TEST

A positive test result is indicated if the patient says that the jog is what the giving way sensation feels like. The reduction of the tibia on the femur is caused by the change in position of the iliotibial band when it switches from an extensor function to a flexor function, pulling the tibia back into its normal position.

CLINICAL NOTES

- During the test, the tibia moves away from the femur on the lateral side (but rotates medially) and moves anteriorly in relation to the femur.
- Normally, the knee's center of rotation changes constantly through its ROM because of the shape of the femoral condyles, ligamentous restraint, and muscle tension. The path of movement of the tibia on the femur is described as a combination of rolling and sliding, with rolling predominating when the instant center is near the joint line and sliding predominating when the instant center shifts distally from the contact area.
- The lateral pivot-shift maneuver (MacIntosh test) is a duplication of the anterior subluxation-reduction phenomenon that occurs during the normal gait cycle when the anterior cruciate ligament is torn. Therefore, the test illustrates a dynamic subluxation. This shift occurs between 20° and 40° of flexion (0° being full extension). This is the phenomenon that prompts patients to give the clinical description of feeling the knee "give way."
- Like most provocative tests, the lateral pivot-shift test (MacIntosh test) does have a disadvantage. Because of the forces applied during the test, in an apprehensive patient protective muscle contraction may lead to a false-negative test result.
- Hoher et al.[64] modified the original position (lateral pivot-shift test) to slight lateral rotation, because they believed that lateral tibial rotation gives a more pronounced pivot shift when the test result is positive. In slight flexion, the secondary restraints (i.e., hamstrings, lateral femoral condyle, lateral meniscus) are less efficient than in full flexion. It is important to realize that subluxation does not occur in full extension because of the "locking home" of the tibia on the femur. With slight flexion, however, the secondary restraints are less restrictive, and subluxation occurs. The examiner then applies a valgus stress to the knee while maintaining a medial rotation torque on the tibia at the ankle.

RELIABILITY/SPECIFICITY/ SENSITIVITY[63]

Sensitivity: Acute: 25%
Subacute: 40%
Chronic: 52%
Overall: 36%

JERK TEST OF HUGHSTON[42,63,65]   DVD

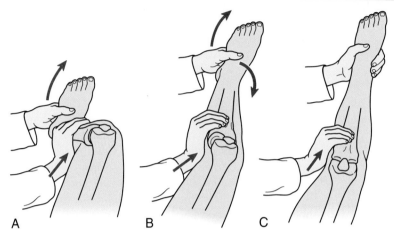

Figure 11–14

Jerk test of Hughston. **A,** The knee is flexed to 90°, and the heel of one hand is placed behind the fibular head to produce medial rotation of the tibia. **B,** At 20° to 30°, the lateral tibial plateau subluxes anteriorly. **C,** At full extension, the lateral tibial plateau is reduced. (Redrawn from Irrgang JJ, Safran MR, Fu FH: The knee: ligamentous and meniscal injuries. In Zachazewski JE, Magee DJ, Quillen WS [eds]: *Athletic injuries and rehabilitation*, p 644, Philadelphia, 1996, Saunders.)

PURPOSE	To assess for anterolateral rotary instability of the knee. This is an excellent test for ruptures (third-degree sprains) of the anterior cruciate ligament, because the test mimics the giving way mechanism often experienced by patients during function.
SUSPECTED INJURY	Structures that may have been injured include: Anterior cruciate ligament Posterolateral capsule Arcuate-popliteus complex Lateral collateral ligament Iliotibial band
PATIENT POSITION	The patient lies supine. The hip is both flexed and abducted 45° and relaxed in slight medial rotation (20°) with the knee flexed to 90°.
EXAMINER POSITION	The examiner stands beside the patient's knee, facing the patient.
TEST PROCEDURE	The unaffected leg is tested first., the examiner holds the patient's foot with one hand and places the other hand at the knee, holding the leg in slight medial rotation (i.e., the heel of the examiner's hand is behind the fibula and over the lateral head of the gastrocnemius muscle) with the tibia medially rotated. This will cause the tibia to sublux anteriorly when the knee is taken into extension. The examiner flexes the knee to 90° to begin. While holding the tibia medially rotated and applying an anterior force on the posterolateral aspect of the knee, the examiner slowly extends the lower leg, maintaining medial rotation and a valgus stress. The two legs are compared.
INDICATIONS OF A POSITIVE TEST	If the test result is positive, at approximately 20° to 30° of flexion, the tibia shifts forward, causing the lateral tibial plateau to sublux with a jerk. If the leg is carried into further extension, the tibia may spontaneously reduce.

JERK TEST OF HUGHSTON[42,63,65]—cont'd

CLINICAL NOTE   • This test is similar to the pivot-shift maneuver. However, instead of going from knee extension (start) to flexion, the examiner starts in knee flexion and goes to knee extension.

RELIABILITY/SPECIFICITY/   Sensitivity: Acute: 25%
SENSITIVITY[42,63]   Subacute: 33%
                                                  Chronic: 61%
                                                  Overall: 34%

SLOCUM ANTEROLATERAL ROTARY INSTABILITY (ALRI) TEST[66,67]

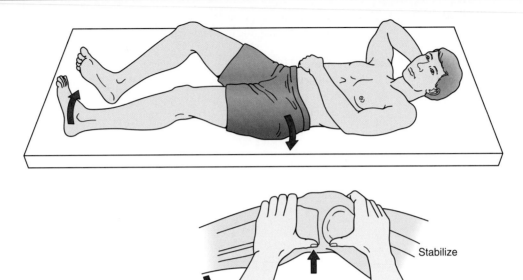

Figure 11–15
Slocum anterolateral rotary instability test.

PURPOSE	To assess for anterolateral rotary instability of the knee.
SUSPECTED INJURY	Structures that may have been injured include: Anterior cruciate ligament Posterolateral capsule Arcuate-popliteus complex Lateral collateral ligament Iliotibial band
PATIENT POSITION	The patient is in the side-lying position (approximately 30° from supine). The bottom leg is the uninvolved leg, and the knee of this leg is flexed to add stability.

SLOCUM ANTEROLATERAL ROTARY INSTABILITY (ALRI) TEST[66,67]—cont'd

EXAMINER POSITION   The examiner is positioned adjacent to the patient's knee.

TEST PROCEDURE   The unaffected leg, which is uppermost, is tested first. The patient's foot is stabilized on the examining table; the foot is in medial rotation, and the knee is in extension and valgus. This position helps eliminate hip rotation during the test. One of the examiner's hands grasps the lateral aspect of the femur, and the other hand grasps the lateral aspect of the tibia/fibula. To begin, the knee is extended, and the examiner attempts to sublux the tibia on the femur by pushing the lateral aspect of the tibia forward (in a normal knee, subluxation would not occur). The examiner then applies a valgus stress to the knee and flexes the knee. The test is repeated with the patient rolling onto the other side. The two legs are compared.

INDICATIONS OF A POSITIVE TEST   A positive test result is indicated if the subluxation of the knee reduces at 25° to 45° of flexion.

CLINICAL NOTES
- A positive test result indicates injury to the same structures identified in the pivot-shift maneuver.
- The main advantages of this test are that it helps relax the patient's hamstring muscles, and it is easier to perform on heavy or tense patients.

RELIABILITY/SPECIFICITY/ SENSITIVITY   Unknown

CROSSOVER TEST OF ARNOLD

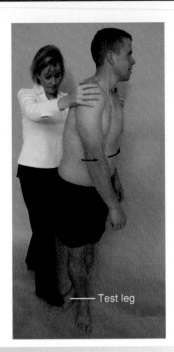

Figure 11–16
Crossover test.

PURPOSE	To assess for anterolateral rotary instability of the knee.
SUSPECTED INJURY	Structures that may have been injured include: Anterior cruciate ligament Posterolateral capsule Arcuate-popliteus complex Lateral collateral ligament Iliotibial band
PATIENT POSITION	The patient is standing.
EXAMINER POSITION	The examiner is positioned directly behind the patient.
TEST PROCEDURE	The test involves two phases: first subluxation and then reduction. The iliotibial band must be intact for the test to work. The examiner places a hand on each of the patient's shoulders to provide balance and to guide motion. The patient is asked to cross the uninvolved leg in front of the involved leg. The examiner then carefully steps on the patient's involved foot to stabilize it and instructs the patient to rotate the upper torso away from the involved leg approximately 90° from the fixed foot. When this position is achieved, the patient contracts the quadriceps muscles. The test is repeated with the uninvolved leg in front of the involved leg.
Note	In cases of anterolateral instability in which the iliotibial band has also been torn, the test may not work; the subluxation will be evident, but the "jog" will not occur.

CROSSOVER TEST OF ARNOLD—*cont'd*

INDICATIONS OF A POSITIVE TEST   A positive test result is indicated if the patient says that the test result on the affected leg is what the giving way sensation feels like.

CLINICAL NOTE   • A tear in either meniscus may limit or prevent the subluxation reduction motion seen in the test.

RELIABILITY/SPECIFICITY/ SENSITIVITY   Unknown

SPECIAL TEST FOR ANTEROMEDIAL ROTARY INSTABILITY

Relevant Special Test

Slocum test

Definition

A sudden or violent twist or wrench of the tibiofemoral joint can result in stretching or tearing of the ACL and other, associated ligaments. These injuries usually are seen with lateral rotation of the femur on a fixed tibia or medial rotation of the tibia on a fixed femur.

Suspected Injury

Structures that may have been injured include:
Anterior cruciate ligament
Posterolateral capsule
Arcuate-popliteus complex
Lateral collateral ligament
Posterior cruciate ligament
Iliotibial band
Medial collateral ligament (especially the superficial fibers, although the deep fibers may also be affected)
Posterior oblique ligament
Posteromedial capsule

Epidemiology and Demographics[6,7,9-11,14,15]

The epidemiology and demographics of anteromedial instability are similar to those for the ACL; also, several ligaments in addition to the ACL are injured.

Relevant History

The patient may report a previous history of a knee injury that has affected the mechanics of the knee. Previous injuries to the ankle or hip also may predispose a person to increased stresses at the knee.

Relevant Signs and Symptoms

- Pain
- Feeling or hearing a pop
- Instability and giving way (feeling the knee give out)
- Loss of knee motion
- Inability to do activity
- Swelling or large hemarthrosis

Mechanism of Injury

See anterior cruciate injury.

SLOCUM TEST[63,67,68]

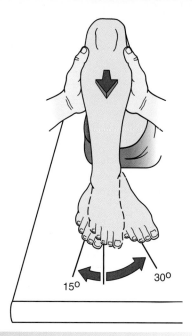

15° 30°

Figure 11–17
Slocum test.

PURPOSE To assess for both anteromedial and anterolateral rotary instabilities.

Part 1 (Anterolateral Rotary Instability)

SUSPECTED INJURY Structures that may have been injured include:
Anterior cruciate ligament
Posterolateral capsule
Arcuate-popliteus complex
Lateral collateral ligament
Posterior cruciate ligament
Iliotibial band

PATIENT POSITION The patient lies supine. The knee is flexed to 80° or 90°, and the hip is flexed to 45° with the foot in 30° of medial rotation.

EXAMINER POSITION The examiner is positioned directly in front of the test knee.

TEST PROCEDURE The unaffected leg is tested first. The examiner grasps behind the patient's knee with both hands, making sure the hamstrings are relaxed. The examiner then sits on the patient's forefoot to hold the foot in position and draws the tibia forward, similar to the anterior drawer test maneuver. The two legs are compared.

INDICATIONS OF A POSITIVE TEST A positive test result is indicated if movement (primarily rotary) occurs on the lateral side of the knee. If this movement is excessive compared to the unaffected side, this indicates anterolateral rotary instability. If the examiner finds anterolateral instability during this first position of the Slocum test, the second part of the test, which assesses anteromedial rotary instability in this position, is of less value.

Continued

SLOCUM TEST[63,67,68]—cont'd

Part 2 (Anteromedial Rotary Instability)

SUSPECTED INJURY Structures that may have been injured include:
Medial collateral ligament (especially the superficial fibers, although the deep fibers may also be affected)
Posterior oblique ligament
Posteromedial capsule
Anterior cruciate ligament

PATIENT POSITION In the second part of the test, the patient's foot is placed in 15° of lateral rotation

EXAMINER POSITION The examiner is positioned directly in front of the test knee.

TEST PROCEDURE Again, the unaffected leg is tested first. The examiner grasps behind the patient's knee with both hands, making sure the hamstrings are relaxed. The tibia is drawn forward, similar to an anterior drawer test. The two legs are compared. This part of the test sometimes is referred to as *Lemaire's T drawer test*.

INDICATIONS OF A POSITIVE TEST If the test result is positive, movement (primarily rotary) occurs on the medial side of the knee. If the movement is excessive compared to the unaffected side, this indicates anteromedial rotary instability.

CLINICAL NOTE • For the Slocum test, it is imperative that the examiner medially or laterally rotate the foot to the degrees noted. If the examiner rotates the tibia as far as it will go, the test result will be negative for movement, because this rotation action tightens all the remaining structures.

RELIABILITY/SPECIFICITY/ SENSITIVITY[42,63] Sensitivity: Acute: 40%
Subacute: 53%
Chronic: 64%
Overall: 50%

SPECIAL TESTS FOR POSTEROLATERAL ROTARY INSTABILITY

Relevant Special Tests

Hughston's posterolateral drawer sign (see Special Tests
  for Posteromedial Rotary Instability)
Jakob test (reverse pivot shift maneuver)
External rotation recurvatum test
Loomer's posterolateral rotary instability test

Definition

A sudden or violent twist or wrench of the tibiofemoral
joint can result in stretching or tearing of the posterior
cruciate ligament and other, associated ligaments. These
injuries usually are seen with lateral rotation of the femur
on a fixed tibia or medial rotation of the tibia on a fixed
femur.

Suspected Injury

Structures that may have been injured include:
Posterior cruciate ligament
Arcuate-popliteus complex
Lateral collateral ligament
Biceps femoris tendon
Posterolateral capsule
Anterior cruciate ligament

Epidemiology and Demographics

The PCL is the strongest of all the knee ligaments and the
least frequently injured (3% to 20% of all knee injuries).[6,7,10,11,14-17]

Relevant History

The patient may report a previous history of a knee injury
that has affected the mechanics of the knee. Previous injuries to the ankle or hip also may predispose a person to increased stresses at the knee.

Relevant Signs and Symptoms

- Mild knee pain
- Moderate swelling or hemarthrosis
- Instability and giving way
- Loss of knee motion and moderate stiffness
- Medial joint line pain (possible)
- Feeling or hearing a pop is rare (unlike with ACL injuries)
- Retropatellar pain symptoms

Mechanism of Injury

See posterior cruciate injury.

JAKOB TEST (REVERSE PIVOT SHIFT MANEUVER)[66,69,70]

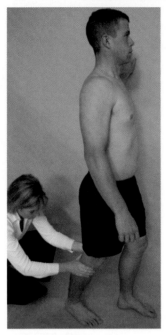

Figure 11–18
Jakob test: Method 1, showing valgus stress and flexion.

PURPOSE	To test for posterolateral rotary instability.
SUSPECTED INJURY	Structures that may have been injured include: Posterior cruciate ligament Arcuate-popliteus complex Lateral collateral ligament Biceps femoris tendon Posterolateral capsule Anterior cruciate ligament
PATIENT POSITION	The patient stands and leans against a wall. The unaffected side is adjacent to the wall, and the body weight is distributed equally over the two feet. The patient stands in a staggered or walk stance position.
EXAMINER POSITION	The examiner kneels directly behind the injured knee.
TEST PROCEDURE	The examiner's hands are placed above and below the affected knee. A valgus stress is exerted to the knee by the examiner while initiating flexion of the patient's knee. The two legs are compared.
INDICATIONS OF A POSITIVE TEST	Injury to the lateral collateral ligament, arcuate-popliteus complex, and middle third of the lateral capsule may be present if a jerk occurs in the knee or the tibia shifts posteriorly during this maneuver. The patient may describe that the maneuver produces the giving away sensation that occurs during function.
RELIABILITY/SPECIFICITY/ SENSITIVITY	Unknown

EXTERNAL ROTATION RECURVATUM TEST[71-73]

DVD

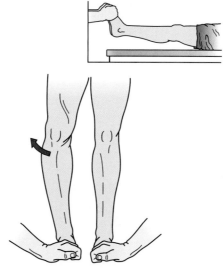

Figure 11–19
External rotational recurvatum test.

PURPOSE	To test for posterolateral rotary instability.
SUSPECTED INJURY	Structures that may have been injured include: Posterior cruciate ligament Arcuate-popliteus complex Lateral collateral ligament Biceps femoris tendon Posterolateral capsule Anterior cruciate ligament
PATIENT POSITION	The patient lies supine with the lower limbs relaxed.
EXAMINER POSITION	The examiner stands at the patient's feet, facing the patient.
TEST PROCEDURE	The examiner gently grasps the big toe of each foot and lifts both feet off the examining table. The patient is told to keep the quadriceps muscles relaxed (i.e., this is a passive test). While elevating the legs, the examiner observes the tibial tuberosities and the relative position of the tibias. The two legs are compared.
INDICATIONS OF A POSITIVE TEST	This is a test for posterolateral rotary instability in extension. With a positive test result, the affected knee goes into relative hyperextension on the lateral aspect because of the force of gravity, with the tibia and tibial tuberosity rotating laterally. The affected (injured) knee has the appearance of a relative genu varum.
RELIABILITY/SPECIFICITY/ SENSITIVITY	Unknown

LOOMER'S POSTEROLATERAL ROTARY INSTABILITY TEST[62,73,74]

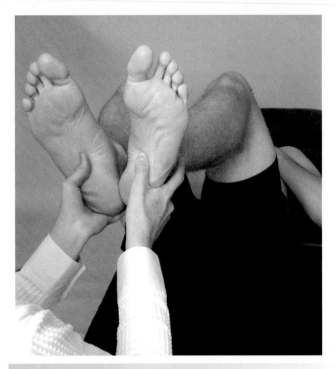

Figure 11–20
Loomer's test.

PURPOSE	To demonstrate loss of the posterolateral support structures of the knee.
SUSPECTED INJURY	Structures that may have been injured include: Posterior cruciate ligament Arcuate-popliteus complex Lateral collateral ligament Biceps femoris tendon Posterolateral capsule Anterior cruciate ligament
PATIENT POSITION	The patient lies supine.
EXAMINER POSITION	The examiner is positioned at the patient's feet.
TEST PROCEDURE	One of the examiner's hands supports the heel of each foot. The examiner flexes both of the hips and knees to 90°, holding the feet. The examiner then maximally laterally rotates both tibias. The amount of rotation of the two tibias is compared.
INDICATIONS OF A POSITIVE TEST	The test result is considered positive if the injured tibia laterally rotates excessively relative to the uninjured leg and if a posterior sag of the affected tibial tubercle is noted; both signs (sag and excessive rotation) must be present for a positive test result.

LOOMER'S POSTEROLATERAL ROTARY INSTABILITY TEST[62,73,74]—*cont'd*

CLINICAL NOTE   • Veltri et al.[75-77] described a modification of Loomer's test known as the *tibial lateral rotation test* or *dial test*. This test is designed to show loss of the posterolateral support structures of the knee. The patient may be positioned supine or prone. The examiner flexes the knee to 30°, extends the foot over the side of the examining table, and stabilizes the femur on the table.[78] The examiner then laterally rotates the tibia on the femur and compares the amount of rotation with that on the good side. If the test is done with the patient in the supine position, the examiner can observe the amount of tibial tubercle movement and compare the two sides. The test then is repeated with the knee flexed to 90° and the thigh still on the examining table. If the tibia rotates less at 90° than at 30°, an isolated posterolateral (popliteus corner) injury is more likely. If the knee rotates more at 90°, injury to both the popliteus corner and posterior cruciate ligament is more likely.[61,70,72,75,76]

RELIABILITY/SPECIFICITY/   Unknown
SENSITIVITY

SPECIAL TESTS FOR POSTEROMEDIAL ROTARY INSTABILITY

Relevant Special Tests

Hughston's posteromedial drawer sign
Posteromedial pivot-shift test

Definition

A sudden or violent twist or wrench of the tibiofemoral joint can result in stretching or tearing of the posterior cruciate ligament and other, associated ligaments. These injuries usually are seen with medial rotation of the femur on a fixed tibia or lateral rotation of the tibia on a fixed femur. The medial tubercle rotates posteriorly around the posterior cruciate ligament when the tibia is in mild medial rotation. If the posterior cruciate ligament is also torn, the posteromedial movement is greater, and the tibia subluxes posteriorly.

Suspected Injury

Structures that may have been injured include:
Posterior cruciate ligament
Posterior oblique ligament
Medial collateral ligament (superficial and deep fibers)
Semimembranosus tendon
Posteromedial capsule
Anterior cruciate ligament
Medial meniscus

Epidemiology and Demographics

The PCL is the strongest of all the knee ligaments and the least frequently injured (3% to 20% of all knee injuries).[5]

Relevant History

The patient may report a previous history of a knee injury that has affected the mechanics of the knee. Previous injuries to the ankle or hip also may predispose a person to increased stresses at the knee.

Relevant Signs and Symptoms

- Mild knee pain
- Moderate swelling or hemarthrosis
- Instability and giving way
- Loss of knee motion and moderate stiffness
- Medial joint line pain (possible)
- Feeling or hearing a pop is rare (unlike with ACL injuries)
- Retropatellar pain symptoms

Mechanism of Injury[6,7,10,11,14-17]

Most PCL injuries occur when passive external forces are applied to the knee. A posteriorly directed force on a flexed knee (i.e., the anterior aspect of the flexed knee strikes a dashboard) may cause PCL injury. A fall onto a flexed knee with the foot in plantar flexion and the tibial tubercle striking the ground first, directing a posterior force to the proximal tibia, may result in injury to the PCL. Hyperextension alone may lead to an avulsion injury of the PCL from the origin. This kind of injury may be amenable to repair.

An anterior force to the anterior tibia in a hyperextended knee with the foot planted results in combined injury to the knee ligaments, along with knee dislocation.

HUGHSTON'S POSTEROLATERAL AND POSTEROMEDIAL DRAWER SIGN[72,79,80]

DVD

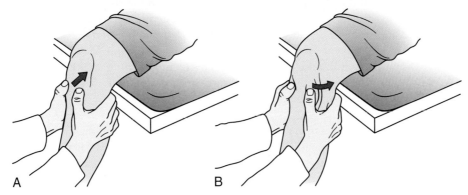

Figure 11–21
Hughston's posteromedial and posterolateral drawer test, anterior view. **A,** Starting position for postero-lateral drawer test. **B,** Positive result on the posterolateral drawer test with posterior and lateral rotation of the lateral tibial condyle.

PURPOSE	To assess for posteromedial and posterolateral rotary instability of the knee.
SUSPECTED INJURY	**Posterolateral Instability.** Structures that may have been injured include: Posterior cruciate ligament Arcuate popliteus complex Lateral collateral ligament Biceps femoris tendon Posterolateral capsule Anterior cruciate ligament **Posteromedial Instability.** Structures that may have been injured include: Posterior cruciate ligament Posterior oblique ligament Medial collateral ligament Semimembranosus tendon Posteromedial capsule Anterior cruciate ligament Medial meniscus
PATIENT POSITION	The patient lies supine or sits at the end of the examining table while the examiner holds the knee flexed to 80° to 90°.
EXAMINER POSITION	The examiner stands or sits in front of the patient's knee, facing the patient.
TEST PROCEDURE	The unaffected leg is tested first. The examiner medially rotates the patient's foot slightly and sits on or holds the foot to stabilize it. Both of the examiner's hands grasp the patient's tibia. The examiner then pushes the tibia posteriorly. The two legs are compared.

Continued

HUGHSTON'S POSTEROLATERAL AND POSTEROMEDIAL DRAWER SIGN[72,79,80]—*cont'd*

INDICATIONS OF A POSITIVE TEST   If the tibia moves or rotates posteriorly on the medial aspect an excessive amount compared to the unaffected knee, the test result is positive and indicates posteromedial rotary instability. The medial tubercle rotates posteriorly around the posterior cruciate ligament when the tibia is in mild medial rotation. If the posterior cruciate ligament is also torn, the posteromedial movement is greater, and the tibia subluxes posteriorly. If the test is done in supine lying, gravity is more likely to assist getting a positive result when the ligamentous structures are injured.

CLINICAL NOTES
- The examiner may palpate the fibula while doing the movement to feel for excessive movement. For posterolateral instability, the fibula will move backwards. For posteromedial instability, it may or may not move. If it does move, the fibula will appear to move anteriorly although in reality the medial tibial plateau moves posteriorly.
- The test may also be done with the patient sitting with the knee flexed over the edge of the examining table. The examiner pushes posteriorly while holding the patient's leg in medial rotation and watches for the same excessive movement.
- Posterolateral rotary instability may be tested in a similar fashion. The patient and examiner are in the same position, but the patient's foot is slightly laterally rotated. When the examiner pushes the tibia posteriorly, if the tibia rotates posteriorly on the lateral side excessively relative to the uninvolved leg, the test result is positive for posterolateral rotary instability. The test result is positive only if the posterior cruciate ligament and lateral collateral ligaments are torn.

RELIABILITY/SPECIFICITY/ SENSITIVITY   Unknown

POSTEROMEDIAL PIVOT-SHIFT TEST[81]

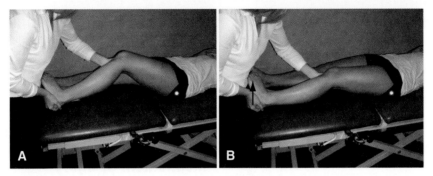

Figure 11–22
Posteromedial pivot-shift test. **A,** Starting position. Knee flexed with foot medially rotated, which puts the positive knee in a subluxed position. A varus stress and compression are applied as the knee is straightened. **B,** As the knee is extended, in a positive test, at between 20° and 40° of flexion, the tibia will jog into reduction.

PURPOSE	To assess for posteromedial rotary instability of the knee.
SUSPECTED INJURY	Structures that may have been injured include: Posterior cruciate ligament Posterior oblique ligament
PATIENT POSITION	The patient is in supine.
EXAMINER POSITION	The examiner is positioned adjacent to the test knee.
TEST PROCEDURE	The unaffected leg is tested first. One of the examiner's hands grasps the patient's ankle, and the other hand is placed on the medial aspect of the knee. The examiner passively flexes the knee more than 45° while applying a varus stress, compression, and medial rotation of the tibia. The two legs are compared.
INDICATIONS OF A POSITIVE TEST	In a positive test result, the varus stress, compression, and medial rotation of the tibia cause the medial tibial plateau to sublux posteriorly. The examiner then takes the knee into extension. At about 20° to 40° of flexion, the tibia shifts into the reduced or normal position. The two legs are compared.
RELIABILITY/SPECIFICITY/ SENSITIVITY	Unknown

SPECIAL TESTS FOR MENISCUS INJURY

Relevant Special Tests

McMurray test
Apley's test
Bounce home test

Definition

A meniscal injury may involve a tear or degeneration of the semilunar, fibrous piece of cartilage in the knee joint. These conditions are diagnosed arthroscopically (the gold standard) or by magnetic resonance imaging. Pathological conditions can be found in the medial or lateral meniscus or both. The medial meniscus is more commonly injured because of its attachment to the joint capsule, which makes it less mobile than the lateral meniscus.

Suspected Injury

Meniscal tear or derangement of the knee, medial or lateral

Epidemiology and Demographics

Age is a risk factor in older adults; 60% of individuals over age 65 have degenerative tears. Young, active, or athletic individuals are more susceptible to acute, traumatic meniscal tears secondary to sports or activities.[82-85]

Relevant History

The patient history may include knee joint osteoarthritis, a previous history of knee trauma or surgery, an ACL tear, or other ligament damage.

Relevant Signs and Symptoms

- Clicking, popping, locking, giving way, or catching
- Pain with weight bearing
- Joint line tenderness or pain
- Synovial swelling
- Decreased or painful knee ROM
- Meniscal injury does not have a referral pattern.

Mechanism of Injury

Meniscal tears can result from major or minor trauma to the knee or from degeneration of the meniscus.[82-85]

- *Traumatic tears.* Acute tears most commonly result from a sudden twisting motion or rapid change in direction. Compressive force coupled with rotation while the knee is in a flexed position is the most common mechanism of injury. Most tears occur from a noncontact event, such as landing from a jump, pivoting, decelerating, or cutting.
- *Degenerative tears.* Degenerative tears are age related or may result from repetitive activities over time, such as squatting and kneeling. They are most commonly observed in the elderly and often are nontraumatic. They frequently result from repetitive activities over time or from a previous history of trauma to the knee, such as an ACL tear or a previous history of knee surgery.

MCMURRAY TEST[86-89]

DVD

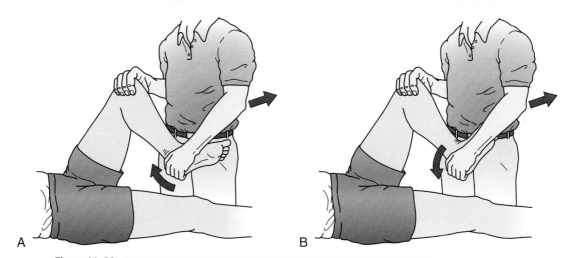

Figure 11–23
McMurray test. **A,** Medial meniscus test. **B,** Lateral meniscus test.

PURPOSE	To assess for meniscal injuries in the knee.
PATIENT POSITION	The patient lies supine.
EXAMINER POSITION	The examiner stands adjacent to the test knee.
TEST PROCEDURE	The unaffected leg is tested first. One of the examiner's hands grasps the patient's heel, and the other hand is placed on the knee to stabilize and support the lower extremity. The examiner completely flexes the patient's knee (the heel to the buttock). The examiner then laterally rotates the tibia (for the medial meniscus) and extends the knee while holding the rotation. The test is repeated in different amounts of flexion. The two legs are compared. The test is repeated in a similar fashion with the tibia medially rotated to test the lateral meniscus.
INDICATIONS OF A POSITIVE TEST	Indications of a positive test result include pain, a snap or grinding feeling, and limited rotation. The process of knee flexion and tibial lateral rotation (for the medial meniscus) or medial rotation (for the lateral meniscus) is repeated several times in different amounts of flexion.
CLINICAL NOTES/CAUTIONS	• The anterior half of the meniscus is not as easily tested, because the pressure on the meniscus is not as great. • Kim et al.[88] reported that meniscal lesions may be found on the medial side with medial rotation and on the lateral side with lateral rotation.

RELIABILITY/SPECIFICITY/ SENSITIVITY[87,89]	Specificity: Medial: 93%
	    Lateral: 93%
	Sensitivity: Medial: 65%
	    Lateral 52%

APLEY'S TEST[90]   DVD

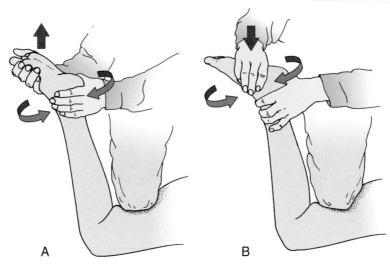

Figure 11–24
Apley's test. **A,** Distraction. **B,** Compression.

PURPOSE	To assess for meniscal and ligamentous injuries in the knee.
PATIENT POSITION	The patient lies prone with the knee flexed to 90°.
EXAMINER POSITION	The examiner is positioned adjacent to the test knee.
TEST PROCEDURE	The unaffected leg is tested first. Both of the examiner's hands grasp the patient's foot and/or ankle with the patient's knee flexed. The patient's thigh is anchored to the examining table by the examiner's knee. The examiner medially and laterally rotates the tibia, combined first with distraction (to test the ligaments), and notes any restriction, excessive movement, or discomfort. The process is repeated using compression (to test the meniscus) instead of distraction. The two legs are compared.
INDICATIONS OF A POSITIVE TEST	A positive test result for a meniscus is indicated by pain and decreased rotation, with or without a click or catch during compression. If rotation plus distraction is more painful or shows increased rotation relative to the unaffected side, the lesion is probably ligamentous.
CLINICAL NOTE	• The patient may feel a clicking or catching during compression with this test.
RELIABILITY/SPECIFICITY/ SENSITIVITY	Unknown

BOUNCE HOME TEST

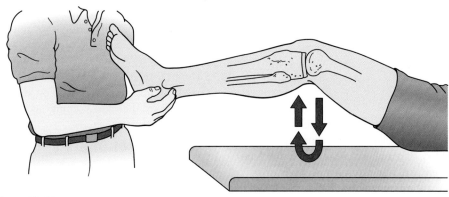

Figure 11–25
Bounce home test.

PURPOSE	To assess for meniscal injuries in the knee.
PATIENT POSITION	The patient lies supine.
EXAMINER POSITION	The examiner is positioned directly in front of the test foot.
TEST PROCEDURE	The unaffected leg is tested first. The examiner cups the heel of the patient's foot in both hands. The knee is completely flexed and then passively and slowly allowed to extend (or bounce) downward. The two legs are compared.
INDICATIONS OF A POSITIVE TEST	If extension is not complete or has a rubbery end feel ("springy block"), something is blocking full extension; the most likely cause is a torn meniscus.
CLINICAL NOTE	• Oni[91] reported that if the knee is allowed to extend quickly in one movement or jerk and the patient experiences a sharp pain on the joint line, which may radiate up or down the leg, the test result is positive for a meniscal lesion.
RELIABILITY/SPECIFICITY/ SENSITIVITY	Unknown

SPECIAL TESTS FOR SYNOVIAL PLICA

Relevant Special Tests

Mediopatellar plica test (Mital-Hayden test)
Hughston's plica test

Definition

Plica is an embryological extension of the synovial capsule of the knee. Synovial plica syndrome occurs when the plica becomes irritated or inflamed. Once an inflammatory process is established, the normal plical tissue may hypertrophy into a truly pathological structure.

Suspected Injury

Synovial plica syndrome

Epidemiology and Demographics

Plica are found embryologically in humans and during normal development they are absorbed and disappear. However, in some people, they remain and are vulnerable to trauma and repetitive stress activities. The exact prevalence of plica syndrome is unknown, but the signs and symptoms are similar to those of a meniscal injury.

Relevant History

The patient may or may not report a history of knee pain or trauma.

Relevant Signs and Symptoms

- A very diverse and broad range of symptoms makes this pathological condition difficult to diagnosis (it usually is a diagnosis of exclusion).
- Reported symptoms include anterior or anteromedial knee pain, especially on joint line, intermittent or episodic pain, clicking, high-pitched snapping, occasional giving way, locking (actually pseudolocking) and catching.
- Meniscal tears, patellar tendinitis, Osgood-Schlatter disease, Sinding-Larsen-Johansson disease, and patellar instability are the most common concomitant conditions.

Mechanism of Injury[5,8,92-94]

No specific mechanism of injury has ever been implicated for plica syndrome, but potential mechanisms include repetitive stress, blunt trauma, or inflammation secondary to other pathological conditions of the knee.

Potential causes of inflammation include repetitive stress, a single blunt trauma, loose bodies, osteochondritis dissecans, meniscal tears, or other aggravating pathological conditions of the knee. A popular theory for the initiation of inflammation is that the plica is converted to a bowstring, which causes it to contact the medial femoral condyle. During flexion of the knee, the plica causes an abrasion to the condyle, resulting in symptoms. An inflammatory process then leads to edema and thickening and decreased elasticity of the plica.

The plica may develop irregular edges and may snap over the femoral condyle, leading to a secondary synovitis and chondromalacia. Loose areolar fatty tissue appears to become gristlelike, and when plicae are soft, wavy, and vascular with synovial covered edges, they are not pathological.

MEDIOPATELLAR PLICA TEST (MITAL-HAYDEN TEST)[95]

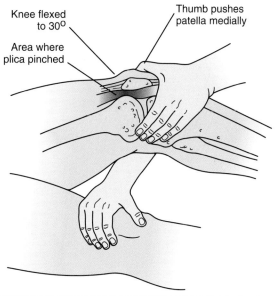

Knee flexed to 30°

Thumb pushes patella medially

Area where plica pinched

Figure 11–26
Test for mediopatellar plica.

PURPOSE	To assess for mediopatellar plica in the knee.
PATIENT POSITION	The patient lies supine with the affected knee flexed to 30° and resting on a support or the examiner's arm.
EXAMINER POSITION	The examiner is positioned adjacent to the patient's knee.
TEST PROCEDURE	The unaffected leg is tested first. The examiner places a thumb on the lateral aspect of the patella and pushes the patella medially. The two legs are compared.
INDICATIONS OF A POSITIVE TEST	A positive test result is indicated if the patient complains of pain or a click, which occurs because the edge of the plica is pinched between the medial femoral condyle and the patella. If the patient is asked to contract the quadriceps while the patella is held medially, the pain may be exacerbated.
CLINICAL NOTE/CAUTION	• Not all patients have a medial plica.
RELIABILITY/SPECIFICITY/ SENSITIVITY	Unknown

HUGHSTON'S PLICA TEST

DVD

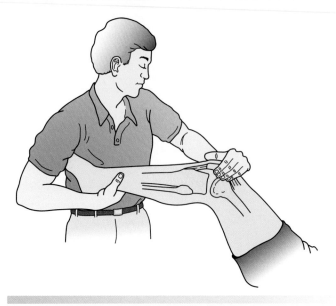

Figure 11–27
Examination for suprapatellar plica. The foot and tibia are held in medial rotation. The patella is displaced slightly medially with the fingers over the course of the plica. The knee is passively flexed and extended, eliciting a "pop" of the plica and associated tenderness. (Redrawn from Hughston JC, Walsh WM, Puddu G: *Patellar subluxation and dislocation,* p 29, Philadelphia, 1984, Saunders.)

PURPOSE	To assess for a plica in the knee.
PATIENT POSITION	The patient lies supine.
EXAMINER POSITION	The examiner stands adjacent to the test leg.
TEST PROCEDURE	The unaffected leg is tested first. The patient's foot is placed beneath the examiner's axilla and is held in this position. One of the examiner's hands cups and supports the patient's heel. The other hand is placed on the lateral aspect of the patella to support and guide patellar motion. The examiner flexes the patient's knee and medially rotates the tibia with one arm and hand while pressing the patella medially with the heel of the other hand and palpating the medial femoral condyle with the fingers of the same hand. The two legs are compared.
INDICATIONS OF A POSITIVE TEST	A popping of the plica band felt under the examiner's fingers may indicate a pathological condition of the plica.[65]
CLINICAL NOTE/CAUTION	• Not every patient has a medial plica.
RELIABILITY/SPECIFICITY/ SENSITIVITY	Unknown

SPECIAL TESTS FOR PATELLOFEMORAL DYSFUNCTION

Relevant Special Tests

Clarke's sign (patellar grind test)
McConnell test for chondromalacia patellae

Definition

Patellofemoral dysfunction (patellofemoral pain syndrome [PFPS]) implies a pathological condition affecting the patellofemoral joint, especially the patellar articular surface. This condition may be the result of biomechanical factors, pathophysiological processes, or loss of tissue homeostasis, and can include synovitis and an inflamed fat pad.

Suspected Injury

Patellofemoral pain syndrome
Patellofemoral dysfunction
Chondromalacia patellae

Epidemiology and Demographics[96-102]

PFPS is the most common problem involving the knee, accounting for 25% of knee injuries. The syndrome occurs most commonly in adolescents and young adults, especially active individuals. It affects females more often than males.

Relevant History

The patient may have a past history of patellar subluxation/dislocation or trauma, or a history of a recurrent change in activity levels. The patient also may report a long and chronic history of knee pain and may have had previous ACL surgery in which the patellar tendon was used as graft material.

Relevant Signs and Symptoms

- Commonly, patients with patellofemoral problems experience pain when climbing or descending stairs, when stepping up or down, with prolonged sitting (movie sign), when squatting, or when getting up from a chair.

- The examiner should consider assessing the whole lower kinetic chain and its effect on the patellofemoral joint when PFPS is suspected.
- In some cases, the pain may cause reflex inhibition, resulting in buckling or giving way of the knee.
- Patients may also report generalized knee pain, pain behind the patella, or peripatellar pain.
- Synovial swelling and crepitus may be present in the knee, and generally no referral pattern is seen for patellofemoral pain syndrome. Pain typically increases with prolonged or repeated activity.

Mechanism of Injury[96-102]

PFPS generally is insidious in nature and has no specific mechanism of injury. It can result from one or a combination of factors that produce abnormal patellofemoral joint mechanics. Patellofemoral joint pain occurs when increased or abnormal amounts of stress are placed on the articular surface of the patella as it tracks up and down in the trochlear groove during knee flexion and extension. Excessive joint loading secondary to abnormal patellofemoral joint mechanics during flexion-extension activities results in pain and inflammation. As the knee moves from extension to flexion, the quadriceps must increase force to counter the flexion moment. This leads to increased compressive loads at the patellofemoral joint as the knee moves into greater degrees of flexion. To minimize patellofemoral joint stress, the greatest amount of patellar contact surface area should ideally occur when compressive loads on the joint are at their highest.

Abnormal patellar tracking may increase stress to the patellofemoral joint if the articulating surface area of the patella changes or decreases as it glides up against the patellar articulating surface of the femur as the knee moves into flexion.

CLARKE'S SIGN (PATELLAR GRIND TEST)[103,104]

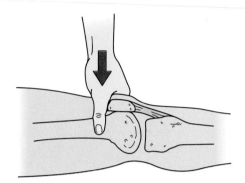

Figure 11–28
Clarke's sign.

PURPOSE	To assess for patellofemoral dysfunction.
PATIENT POSITION	The patient lies in supine with the knee extended.
EXAMINER POSITION	The examiner stands adjacent to the patient's knee.
TEST PROCEDURE	The unaffected leg is tested first. The thenar web space of one of the examiner's hands is placed slightly proximal to the upper pole or base of the patella. The examiner presses down several times with increasing force until pain is produced on the proximal aspect of the patella. The patient then is asked to contract the quadriceps muscles after the examiner pushes down. The test is repeated with the painful knee, and the amounts of pressure that cause pain are compared.
INDICATIONS OF A POSITIVE TEST	A positive test result is indicated if the test causes retropatellar pain and the patient cannot hold a contraction. If the patient can complete and maintain the contraction without pain, the test result is considered negative, as long as the same test on the unaffected leg does not cause pain.
CLINICAL NOTES/CAUTIONS	• Because a positive test result can be obtained on anyone if sufficient pressure is applied to the patella, the amount of pressure applied must be carefully controlled and compared with the opposite side. This is best done by repeating the procedure several times, increasing the pressure each time and comparing the results with those on the unaffected side. • To test different parts of the patella, the knee may be tested in 30°, 60°, and 90° of flexion and in full extension.
RELIABILITY/SPECIFICITY/ SENSITIVITY	Unknown

MCCONNELL TEST FOR CHONDROMALACIA PATELLAE[105,106]

DVD

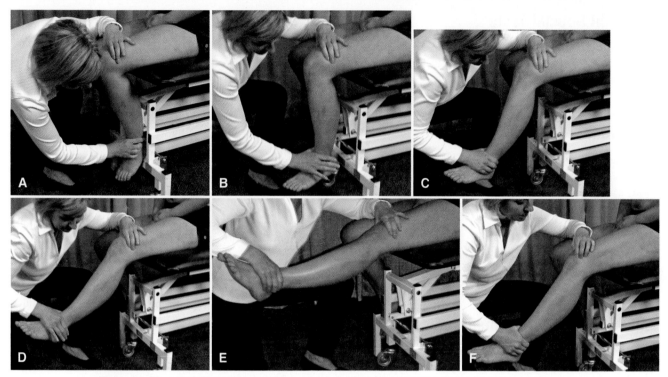

Figure 11–29
McConnell test for chondromalacia patellae. **A,** 120°. **B,** 90°. **C,** 60°. **D,** 30°. **E,** 0°. **F,** Testing at 60°, holding patella medially.

PURPOSE	To assess for patellofemoral dysfunction.
PATIENT POSITION	The patient is sitting.
EXAMINER POSITION	The examiner is positioned adjacent to the patient's knee.
TEST PROCEDURE	The unaffected leg is tested first. After the examiner has positioned the knee at 120°, 90°, 60°, 30°, and 0° (full extension), the patient performs isometric quadriceps contractions with the femur laterally rotated, with each contraction held for 10 seconds. If pain is produced during any of the contractions, the patient's leg is passively returned to full extension. The leg then is fully supported on the examiner's knee, and the examiner pushes the patella medially. The medial glide is maintained while the knee is returned to the painful angle, and the patient performs an isometric contraction again, with the patella held medially. The two legs are compared.
INDICATIONS OF A POSITIVE TEST	If the pain is decreased when the patella is held medially, the pain is patellofemoral in origin.
CLINICAL NOTE	• Each angle is tested in a similar fashion.
RELIABILITY/SPECIFICITY/ SENSITIVITY[106]	Reliability: Intrarater k = –0.6-0.35 Interrater k = –0.02-0.19

SPECIAL TESTS FOR SWELLING

Relevant Special Tests

Brush, stroke, or bulge test
Indentation test
Fluctuation test
Patellar tap test (ballotable patella)

Definition

Swelling or inflammation is a normal part of the healing process. It is the body's initial response to injury, and the body's attempt to maintain homeostasis in the injured area.

Suspected Injury

All injuries to the knee produce swelling in some form. The amount of swelling is largely determined by the types of tissue injured.

Epidemiology and Demographics

About 20% of the U.S. population has knee pain. Knee pain accounts for 1 million visits to the emergency department and 1.9 million primary care visits each year.[107]

Relevant History

The patient may or may not have a history of trauma to the knee. When arthritis is the source of inflammation, the patient may have a long history of knee pain that has progressively worsened. Autoimmune disorders, such as rheumatoid arthritis, also may be a source of inflammation.

Relevant Signs and Symptoms

The signs and symptoms of swelling are largely determined by the tissue injured. Some common traits of swelling are:
• Tenderness on palpation
• Pain with motion
• Redness
• Heat
• Bruising
• Knee in resting position (20° to 30° flexion)
• Tightness and stiffness with motion
• Restricted ROM

Mechanism of Injury

The pattern of swelling seen in the knee can help the examiner determine the structural source of the swelling. Swelling is largely the result of two factors: how fast inflammation is produced and how quickly is it removed or dissipates.

The production or generation of edema depends largely on the vascularity of the injured structures. Structures such as muscles are well-vascularized tissue; therefore, when injured, they produce a greater degree of inflammation and swelling. Conversely, the meniscus is poorly vascularized, and inflammation caused by meniscal injury generally is a slow process with minimal swelling.

If the body is able to remove the products of inflammation quickly, very little inflammation and swelling will be present in the injured area. If the body's removal of the products causing inflammation is poor, swelling remains in the region for a prolonged period. Extracapsular structures are well vascularized; therefore, swelling removal processes can adequately manage the production of swelling. On the other hand, intracapsular structures have difficulty removing the products causing inflammation and swelling; therefore, structures within the knee that are injured, such as the meniscus, have a difficult time removing swelling once it has been produced. If fluid removal exceeds fluid production, swelling is minimal. If fluid removal is less then fluid production, the knee joint will remain swollen for a prolonged period.

BRUSH, STROKE, OR BULGE TEST[103]

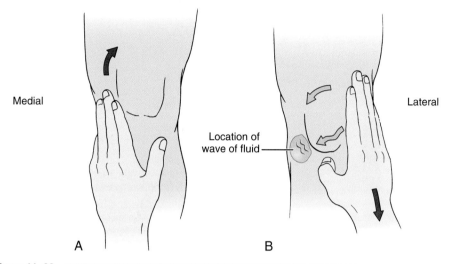

Figure 11–30
Brush test for swelling. **A,** Hand strokes up. **B,** Hand strokes down.

PURPOSE	To assess minimal effusion in the knee.
PATIENT POSITION	The patient lies supine.
EXAMINER POSITION	The examiner is positioned adjacent to the test knee.
TEST PROCEDURE	The examiner places one hand over the anteromedial tibia. Starting just below the joint line on the medial side of the patella and using the palm and fingers, the examiner strokes proximally toward the patient's hip, as far as the suprapatellar pouch, two or three times. With the opposite hand, the examiner strokes down the lateral side of the patella.
INDICATIONS OF A POSITIVE TEST	A positive test result is indicated when a wave of fluid passes along the medial side of the joint and bulges just below the medial distal portion or border of the patella during the down stroke. The wave of fluid may take up to 2 seconds to appear.
CLINICAL NOTES	• Also called the *wipe test,* this test assesses minimal effusion. • Normally, the knee contains 1 to 7 ml of synovial fluid. This test can show as little as 4 to 8 ml of extra fluid within the knee.
RELIABILITY/SPECIFICITY/ SENSITIVITY	Unknown

INDENTATION TEST[108]

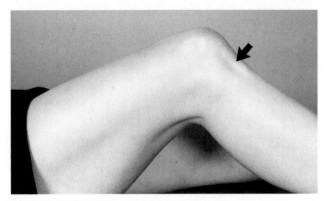

Figure 11–31
Indentation test. The arrow indicates where the examiner should watch for filling of the indentation.

PURPOSE	To assess for swelling in the knee.
PATIENT POSITION	The patient lies supine.
EXAMINER POSITION	The examiner is positioned adjacent to the test knee.
TEST PROCEDURE	The examiner passively flexes the unaffected leg, slowly keeping the patient's foot on the examining table, noting an indentation on the lateral side of the patellar tendon. Usually the unaffected knee can be almost fully flexed and the indentation will remain. The injured knee then is slowly flexed while the examiner watches for the disappearance of the indentation. At that point, knee flexion is stopped.
INDICATIONS OF A POSITIVE TEST	A positive test result is indicated by disappearance of the indentation (this disappearance is caused by the swelling) earlier than that found on the good leg. The angle at which the indentation disappears depends on the amount of swelling. The greater the swelling, the sooner the indentation disappears.
CLINICAL NOTE	• If the examiner's thumb and finger are placed on each side of the patellar tendon, the fluid can be made to fluctuate back and forth at the position where the indentation disappears. This method, like the brush test, can detect minimal levels of swelling.
RELIABILITY/SPECIFICITY/ SENSITIVITY	Unknown

FLUCTUATION TEST

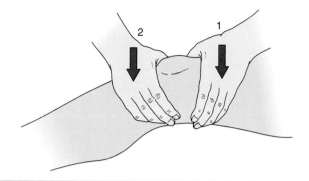

Figure 11–32

Hand positioning for fluctuation test. First one hand is pushed down *(arrow 1);* then the other hand is pushed down *(arrow 2).* With this test, fluid can be felt shifting back and forth under one hand and then the other.

PURPOSE	To assess for swelling in the knee.
PATIENT POSITION	The patient lies supine.
EXAMINER POSITION	The examiner is positioned adjacent to the test knee.
TEST PROCEDURE	The examiner places the palm of one hand over the suprapatellar pouch and the palm of the other hand anterior to the joint at the joint line, with the thumb and index finger just beyond the margins of the patella.
	Pressing down with one hand and then the other, the examiner may feel the synovial fluid fluctuate under the hands and move from one hand to the other.
INDICATIONS OF A POSITIVE TEST	Increased fluctuation of fluid in the knee compared to the contralateral knee indicates significant effusion.
CLINICAL NOTE	• The test assumes that the contralateral knee has no edema. If the contralateral knee also has edema, the examiner must compare to past experience with nonedematous knees.
RELIABILITY/SPECIFICITY/ SENSITIVITY	Unknown

PATELLAR TAP TEST (BALLOTABLE PATELLA)

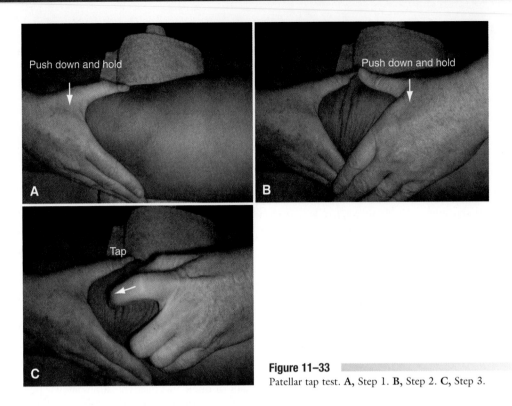

Figure 11–33
Patellar tap test. **A,** Step 1. **B,** Step 2. **C,** Step 3.

PURPOSE	To assess swelling in the knee.
PATIENT POSITION	The patient lies supine.
EXAMINER POSITION	The examiner is positioned adjacent to the test knee.
TEST PROCEDURE	With the patient's knee extended or flexed to discomfort, the examiner applies a slight tap or pressure over the patella.
INDICATIONS OF A POSITIVE TEST	When the tap is applied, the patella should be felt to float; this is sometimes called the "dancing patella" sign.
CLINICAL NOTE	• This test can detect a large amount of swelling (40 to 50 ml) in the knee, which can also be noted by simple observation.
RELIABILITY/SPECIFICITY/ SENSITIVITY	Unknown

OTHER SPECIAL TESTS

Q-ANGLE OR PATELLOFEMORAL ANGLE[1,36,65,109-112]

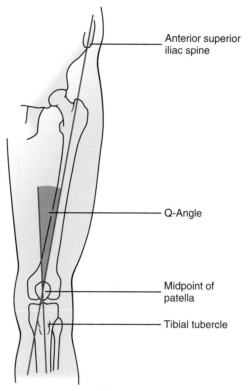

Anterior superior
iliac spine

Q-Angle

Midpoint of
patella

Tibial tubercle

Figure 11–34
Quadriceps angle (Q-angle).

PURPOSE	To assess the alignment (Q-angle) of the lower extremity.
SUSPECTED INJURY	Repetitive use/overuse pathological/or malalignment condition of the knee
PATIENT POSITION	The patient is assessed in supine (most commonly) or while sitting. Research has shown that different foot and hip positions alter the Q-angle; therefore, the foot should be in a neutral position with regard to supination and pronation, and the hip should be in a neutral position with regard to medial and lateral rotation.
EXAMINER POSITION	The examiner's position varies, but the examiner generally is located adjacent to the test knee.
TEST PROCEDURE	The unaffected leg is measured first. The examiner draws an imaginary line from the anterior superior iliac spine (ASIS) to the midpoint of the patella on the same side and a second line from the tibial tubercle to the midpoint of the patella. The angle formed by the crossing of these two lines is called the Q-angle. During the measurement, which may be done either using radiographs or physically on the patient, the quadriceps should be relaxed.
INDICATIONS OF A POSITIVE TEST	Normally, the Q-angle is 13° for males and 18° for females when the knee is straight (Grelsamer et al.[111] reported that male and female values are similar when the patient's height is considered). Any angle less than 13° may be associated with chondromalacia patellae or patella alta. An angle greater than 18° often is associated with chondromalacia patellae, subluxing patella, increased femoral anteversion, genu valgum, lateral displacement of the tibial tubercle, or increased lateral tibial torsion. If the Q-angle is measured with the patient in the sitting position, it should be 0°.

Continued

Q-ANGLE OR PATELLOFEMORAL ANGLE[1,36,65,109-112]—*cont'd*

CLINICAL NOTES

- The Q-angle is defined as the angle between the quadriceps muscles (primarily the rectus femoris) and the patellar tendon; it represents the angle of quadriceps muscle force or pull. The angle is obtained by first ensuring that the lower limbs are at a right angle to the line joining the two ASISs.
- Hughston et al.[65] recommend doing the test with the quadriceps contracted. If measured with the quadriceps contracted and the knee fully extended, the Q-angle should be 8° to 10°. Any angle greater than 10° is considered abnormal.
- The examiner must make sure that a standardized measurement procedure is used to ensure consistent values.
- While the patient is in a sitting position, the examiner may check for the bayonet sign, which indicates an abnormal alignment of the quadriceps musculature, patellar tendon, or tibial shaft. In this case, the tibial tuberosity is positioned laterally compared to the patella, resulting in a malalignment of the tendon and a tibial shaft that resembles a bayonet fixed to the end of a rifle.

RELIABILITY/SPECIFICITY/ SENSITIVITY[112]

Reliability: Interrater ICC: 0.20 (full extension)
Intrarater ICC: 0.22 (full extension)
Correlation with radiographs ICC: 0.32 (full extension)

FAIRBANK'S APPREHENSION TEST[65,113,114]

DVD

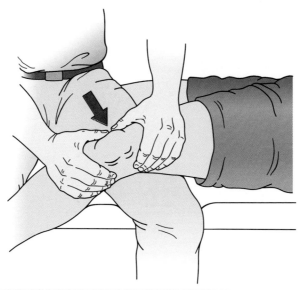

Figure 11–35

Apprehension test. (Redrawn from Hughston JC, Walsh WM, Puddu G: *Patellar subluxation and dislocation*, p 29, Philadelphia, 1984, Saunders.)

PURPOSE	To assess for dislocation of the patella.
SUSPECTED INJURY	Dislocation or subluxation of the patella
PATIENT POSITION	The patient lies supine with the quadriceps muscles relaxed and the knee flexed to 30° over the examiner's leg.
EXAMINER POSITION	The examiner sits directly adjacent to the test knee.
TEST PROCEDURE	The unaffected leg is tested first. The examiner's thumbs are placed on the medial border of the patella, and the fingers are placed on the lateral aspect of the patient's knee. The examiner carefully and slowly pushes the patella laterally with the thumbs. The two legs are compared.
INDICATIONS OF A POSITIVE TEST	If the patient feels that the patella is going to dislocate, he or she will contract the quadriceps muscles to bring the patella "back into line." This action indicates a positive test result. The patient also will have an apprehensive look.
CLINICAL NOTE	Tanner et al.[114] believed that the patella should be pushed laterally and distally to make the test more sensitive.
RELIABILITY/SPECIFICITY/ SENSITIVITY	Unknown

NOBLE COMPRESSION TEST[115]

DVD

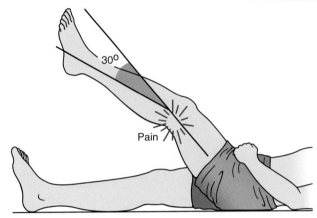

Figure 11–36
Noble compression test.

PURPOSE	To assess for iliotibial band friction syndrome.
SUSPECTED INJURY	Patellofemoral dysfunction or pathological condition
PATIENT POSITION	The patient lies supine.
EXAMINER POSITION	The examiner is positioned adjacent to the test limb.
TEST PROCEDURE	The unaffected leg is tested first. The examiner places a thumb of one hand on the lateral femoral epicondyle so the thumb is also over the distal end of the iliotibial band. The examiner's other hand helps stabilize the thigh. The examiner flexes the patient's knee to 90°, accompanied by hip flexion. The examiner then applies pressure to the lateral femoral epicondyle or 1 to 2 cm (0.4 to 0.8 inch) proximal to it with the thumb. While the pressure is maintained, the patient's knee is passively extended or the patient may extend the knee actively. The two legs are compared.
INDICATIONS OF A POSITIVE TEST	Pain indicates a positive test result. At approximately 30° of flexion (0° being a straight leg), the patient experiences severe pain over the lateral femoral epicondyle.
CLINICAL NOTE/CAUTION	• The patient states that it is the same pain that occurs with activity.
RELIABILITY/SPECIFICITY/ SENSITIVITY	Unknown

FUNCTIONAL LEG LENGTH[116]

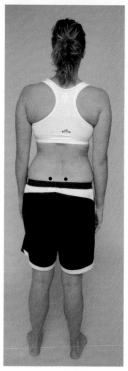

Figure 11–37
Functional leg length in standing position. The dots on the back indicate the posterior superior iliac spines.

PURPOSE	To assess for leg length discrepancies while the patient is in a weight-bearing position.
PATIENT POSITION	The patient is standing.
EXAMINER POSITION	The examiner is seated or kneeling directly in front of or behind the patient.
TEST PROCEDURE	The patient stands relaxed while the examiner palpates the level of the ASISs and posterior superior iliac spines (PSISs), noting any asymmetry. The patient then is placed in the "correct" stance (i.e., subtalar joints neutral, knees fully extended, and toes facing straight ahead). The ASISs and PSISs are palpated again, and the examiner notes any changes.
INDICATIONS OF A POSITIVE TEST	If the asymmetry is corrected by "correcting" the position of the limb, the leg is structurally normal (the bones have the proper length), but abnormal joint mechanics (a functional deficit) are producing a functional leg length difference (see Table 9-1). Therefore, if the asymmetry is corrected by proper positioning, the test result is positive for a functional leg length difference.
CLINICAL NOTE	• Functional limb length testing helps the clinician determine whether leg length discrepancies play a role in the patient's pain and dysfunction in weight-bearing positions.
RELIABILITY/SPECIFICITY/ SENSITIVITY	Unknown

JOINT PLAY MOVEMENTS

BACKWARD MOVEMENT OF THE TIBIA ON THE FEMUR

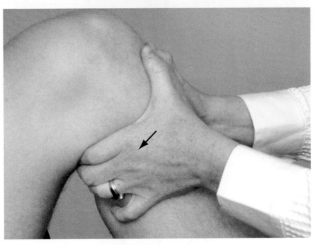

Figure 11–38
Posterior movement of the tibia on the femur.

PATIENT POSITION	The patient lies supine with the test knee flexed to 90° and the hip flexed to 45° (crook lying).
EXAMINER POSITION	The examiner is positioned adjacent to the test knee.
TEST PROCEDURE	Starting with the unaffected knee, the examiner places the heel of both hands around the knee with the thumbs on the anterior tibial plateau and the fingers are allowed to wrap laterally around the knee to the posterior aspect of the popliteal region (to ensure relaxation of the hamstrings). The examiner then pushes the tibia posteriorly, or backward, in relation to the femur. The examiner should direct the posterior force so that it parallels the plane of the tibiofemoral joint. The two legs are compared.
INDICATIONS OF A POSITIVE TEST	Both too little and too much motion are considered positive test results. The end feel of the movement normally is tissue stretch.
CLINICAL NOTES	• This test is similar to a posterior drawer test for the posterior cruciate ligament. • Alternatively, the examiner can place the heel of one hand on the tibial tuberosity and the other hand on the distal femur to stabilize the leg. The posterior force is delivered by the hand placed on the tibial tuberosity.

FORWARD MOVEMENT OF THE TIBIA ON THE FEMUR

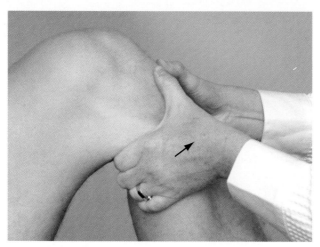

Figure 11–39
Anterior movement of the tibia on the femur.

PATIENT POSITION	The patient lies supine with the test knee flexed to 90° and the hip flexed to 45°.
EXAMINER POSITION	The examiner is positioned adjacent to the test knee.
TEST PROCEDURE	Starting with the unaffected knee, the examiner places both hands around the tibia with the thumbs on the tibial plateau and the fingers ensuring relaxation of the hamstrings. The tibia then is drawn forward (anteriorly) on the femur. The examiner should direct the anterior force so that it parallels the plane of the tibiofemoral joint.
INDICATIONS OF A POSITIVE TEST	Both too little and too much motion are considered positive test results. The end feel of the movement normally is tissue stretch.
CLINICAL NOTES/CAUTIONS	• This test is similar to the anterior drawer test for the anterior cruciate ligament. • The examiner also may place both thumbs across the tibiofemoral joint line to feel the movement of the tibia relative to the femur.

MEDIAL AND LATERAL TRANSLATION OF THE TIBIA ON THE FEMUR

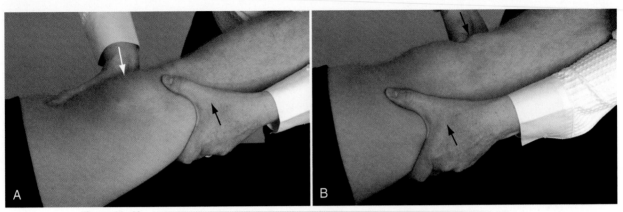

Figure 11–40
Medial and lateral shift of the tibia on the femur. **A,** Medial translation. **B,** Lateral translation.

PATIENT POSITION	The patient lies supine, and the leg is held (stabilized) between the examiner's trunk and forearm.
EXAMINER POSITION	The examiner is positioned adjacent to the test knee.
TEST PROCEDURE	For medial translation, the examiner puts one hand on the lateral side of the tibia and one hand on the medial side of the femur. The examiner then pushes, or translates, the tibia medially on the femur while the other hand stabilizes the femur. For lateral translation, the examiner pushes the tibia laterally on a stable femur. The other knee is tested for comparison.
INDICATIONS OF A POSITIVE TEST	Excessive movement may indicate a torn cruciate ligament (medial—anterior cruciate ligament; lateral—posterior cruciate ligament).
CLINICAL NOTES	• If the knee is held in full extension, joint motion is limited by joint congruency, because the joint is in a compressed (closed pack) position. • If the knee is flexed 15° to 30°, more motion is present, because the joint is in a more loose pack position.

MEDIAL AND LATERAL DISPLACEMENT OF THE PATELLA

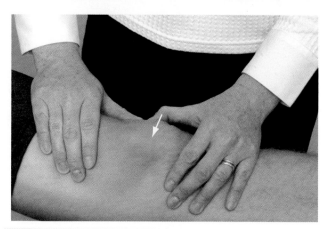

Figure 11–41
Patellar movement medially.

PATIENT POSITION	The patient is supine with the knee slightly flexed on a pillow or over the examiner's knee (30° flexion).
EXAMINER POSITION	The examiner is positioned adjacent to the test knee.
TEST PROCEDURE	Starting with the unaffected knee, the examiner's thumbs are placed against the lateral edge of the patella. The examiner's fingers are placed on the medial femur and tibia. The examiner applies a medially directed force to the lateral side of the patella. The fingers on the femur and tibia act as a counterforce to the pressure placed by the examiner's thumbs. For lateral displacement, the hands and thumbs are positioned on the opposite side of the knee and the patella. The two knees are compared.
INDICATIONS OF A POSITIVE TEST	Excessive movement or pain indicates a positive test result.
CLINICAL NOTES/CAUTIONS	• This joint play is similar to the passive movements of the patella; as in the passive test, the patella can be displaced by approximately half its width medially and laterally. • The examiner must do the movements slowly and carefully to make sure the patella is not prone to dislocation, especially when pushing the patella laterally.

DEPRESSION (DISTAL MOVEMENT) OF THE PATELLA

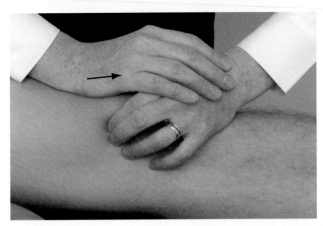

Figure 11–42
Patellar movement distally.

PATIENT POSITION	The patient is supine with the knee slightly flexed.
EXAMINER POSITION	The examiner is positioned adjacent to the test knee.
TEST PROCEDURE	Starting with the unaffected knee, the examiner places one hand over the patella so that the pisiform bone of that hand rests over the base of the patella. The examiner's other hand is placed so that the fingers and thumb of that hand can grasp the medial and lateral edges of the patella to direct its movement. The examiner then rests the first hand over the second hand and applies a caudal force to the base of the patella, directing the caudal movement with the second hand so that the patella does not grind against the femoral condyles. The two knees are compared.
INDICATIONS OF A POSITIVE TEST	Excessive movement or pain indicates a positive test result.
CLINICAL NOTES	• This joint play is similar to the passive movements of the patella; as in the passive test, the patella can be displaced by approximately half its width distally. • The medial and lateral edges of the patella can be squeezed to separate the patella from the femur beneath; this also allows for improved gliding of the patella distally.

ANTERIOR MOVEMENT OF THE FIBULA ON THE TIBIA

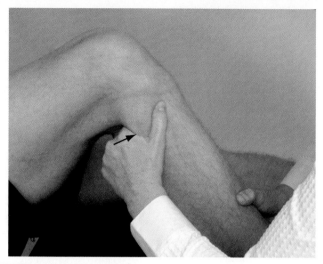

Figure 11–43
Anterior movement of the head of the fibula.

PATIENT POSITION The patient is supine with the knee flexed to 90° and the hip to 45°.

EXAMINER POSITION The examiner sits on the patient's foot.

TEST PROCEDURE The unaffected leg is tested first. The examiner's mobilizing hand is placed around the head of the fibula. The other hand grasps the tibia to stabilize the leg. The fibula is drawn forward on the tibia, and the movement and end feel are tested. The fibula then slides back to its resting position of its own accord. The movement is tested several times and compared with that of the other side.

INDICATIONS OF A POSITIVE TEST If the superior tibiofibular joint is stiff or hypomobile, the test itself will cause discomfort. The two sides must be compared for differential symptoms.

CLINICAL NOTES
- The examiner must take particular care in performing this test, because the common peroneal nerve, which winds around the head of the fibula, may be easily compressed by the examiner's fingers. Compression of the nerve may cause localized pain, tingling, or shooting pain down the leg.
- In most cases, foot dorsiflexion will have caused lateral knee pain if the superior tibiofibular joint is hypomobile.

References

1. Fulkerson JP: Patellofemoral pain disorders: evaluation and management, *J Am Acad Orthop Surg* 2:124-132, 1994.

2. Katchburian MV, Ball AM, Shih YF et al: Measurement of patellar tracking: assessment and analysis of the literature, *Clin Orthop Relat Res* 412:241-259, 2003.

3. McConnell J: Management of patellofemoral problems, *Man Ther* 1:60-66, 1996.

4. Jacobson KE, Flandry FC: Diagnosis of anterior knee pain, *Clin Sports Med* 8:179-195, 1989.

5. Li B: Synovial plica syndrome. In Sueki D, Brechter J (eds): *Orthopedic rehabilitation clinical advisor,* St Louis, 2010, Mosby.

6. Browner BD: *Skeletal trauma: fractures, dislocations, ligamentous injuries,* Philadelphia, 1998, Saunders.

7. Hastings DE: The non-operative management of collateral ligament injuries of the knee joint, *Clin Orthop* 147:22-28, 1980.

8. O'Dwyer KJ, Peace PK: The plica syndrome, *Injury* 19:350-352, 1988.

9. Quarles JD, Hosey RG: Medial and lateral collateral injuries: prognosis and treatment, *Prim Care* 31:957-975, ix, 2004.

10. Strayer RJ, Lang ES: Evidence-based emergency medicine/systematic review abstract: does this patient have a torn meniscus or ligament of the knee? *Ann Emerg Med* 47:499-501, 2006.

11. Wiener SL: *Differential diagnosis of acute pain by body region,* New York, 1993, McGraw-Hill.

12. Hughston JC: *Knee ligaments: injury and repair,* St Louis, 1993, Mosby.

13. McClure PW, Rothstein JM, Riddle DL: Intertester reliability of clinical judgments of medial knee ligament integrity, *Phys Ther* 69:268-275, 1989.

14. Dugan SA: Sports-related knee injuries in female athletes: what gives? *Arch Phys Med Rehabil* 84:122-130, 2005.

15. Maday MG, Harner CD, Fu FH: Evaluation and treatment. In Feagin JA (ed): *The crucial ligaments: diagnosis, treatment of ligamentous injuries about the knee,* ed 2, New York, 1994, Churchill Livingstone.

16. Dandy DJ, Pusey RJ: The long-term results of unrepaired tears of the posterior cruciate ligament, *J Bone Joint Surg Br* 64:92-94, 1982.

17. Tietjens BR: Posterior cruciate ligament injuries, *J Bone Joint Surg Br* 67:674, 1985.

18. Wind WM, Bergfeld JA, Parker RD: Evaluation and treatment of posterior cruciate ligament injuries revisited, *Am J Sports Med* 32:1765-1775, 2004.

19. Emparanza JI, Aginaga JR: Validation of the Ottawa knee rules, *Ann Emerg Med* 38:364-368, 2001.

20. Hawkins RJ: *Musculoskeletal examination,* St Louis, 1995, Mosby.

21. Hughston JC: Extensor mechanism examination. In Fox JM, Del Pizzo W: *The patellofemoral joint,* New York, 1993, McGraw-Hill.

22. De Lee JC: Ligamentous injury of the knee. In Stanitski CL, DeLee JC, Drez D (eds): *Pediatric and adolescent sports medicine,* Philadelphia, 1994, Saunders.

23. Strobel M, Stedtfeld HW: *Diagnostic evaluation of the knee,* Berlin, 1990, Springer-Verlag.

24. Jonsson T, Althoff B, Peterson L et al: Clinical diagnosis of ruptures of the anterior cruciate ligament: a comparative study of the Lachman test and the anterior drawer sign, *Am J Sports Med* 10:100-102, 1982.

25. Torg JS, Conrad W, Allen V: Clinical diagnosis of anterior cruciate ligament instability in the athlete, *Am J Sports Med* 4:84-93, 1976.

26. Cooperman JM, Riddle DL, Rothstein JM: Reliability and validity of judgments of the integrity of the anterior cruciate ligament of the knee using the Lachman's test, *Phys Ther* 70:225-233, 1990.

27. Lee LK, Yao L, Phelps CT et al: Anterior cruciate ligament tears: MR imaging compared with arthroscopy and clinical tests, *Radiology* 166:861-864, 1988.

28. Rubinstein RA, Shelbourne KD, McCarroll JR et al: The accuracy of the clinical examination in the setting of posterior cruciate ligament injuries, *Am J Sports Med* 22:550-557, 1994.

29. Dahlstedt LJ, Dalen N: Knee laxity in cruciate ligament injury: value of examination under anesthesia, *Acta Orthop Scand* 60:181-184, 1989.

30. Sandberg R, Balkfors B, Henricson A et al: Stability tests in knee ligament injuries, *Arch Orthop Trauma Surg* 106:5-7, 1986.

31. Johnson DS, Ryan WG, Smith RB: Does the Lachman testing method affect the reliability of the International Knee Documentation Committee (IKDC) Form? *Knee Surg Sports Traumatol Arthrosc* 12:225-228, 2004.

32. Steiner ME, Brown C, Zarins B et al: Measurement of anterior-posterior displacement of the knee, *J Bone Joint Surg Am* 72:1307-1315, 1990.

33. Boeree NR, Ackroyd CE: Assessment of the menisci and cruciate ligaments: an audit of clinical practice, *Injury* 22:291-294, 1991.

34. Bomberg BC, McGinty JB: Acute hemarthrosis of the knee: indications for diagnostic arthroscopy, *Arthroscopy* 6:221-225, 1990.

35. Leamouth DJ: Incidence and diagnosis of anterior cruciate injuries in the accident and emergency department, *Injury* 22:287-290, 1991.

36. Guerra JP, Arnold MJ, Gajdosik RL: Q-angle: effects of isometric quadriceps contraction and body position, *J Orthop Sports Phys Ther* 19:200-204, 1994.

37. Benjaminse A, Gokeler A, van der Schans CP: Clinical diagnosis of an anterior cruciate ligament rupture: a meta-analysis, *J Orthop Sports Phys Ther* 36:267-288, 2006.

38. Kim SJ, Kim HK: Reliability of the anterior drawer test, the pivot shift test, and the Lachman test, *Clin Orthop Relat Res* 317:237-242, 1995.

39. Anderson AF, Lipscomb AB: Preoperative instrumented testing of anterior and posterior knee laxity, *Am J Sports Med* 17:1299-1306, 1986.

40. DeHaven KE: Diagnosis of acute knee injuries with hemarthrosis, *Am J Sports Med* 8:9-14, 1980.

41. Donaldson WF, Warren RF, Wickiewicz T: A comparison of acute anterior cruciate ligament examinations: initial vs examination under anesthesia, *Am J Sports Med* 13:5-9, 1985.

42. Hardaker WT, Garrett WE, Bassett FH: Evaluation of acute traumatic hemarthrosis of the knee joint, *South Med J* 83:640-644, 1990.

43. Liu SH, Osti L, Henry M et al: The diagnosis of acute complete tears of the anterior cruciate ligament: comparison of MRI, arthrometry and clinical examination, *J Bone Joint Surg Br* 77:586-588, 1995.

44. Braunstein EM: Anterior cruciate ligament injuries: a comparison of arthrographic and physical diagnosis, *Am J Roentgenol* 138:423-425, 1982.

45. Hughston JC, Andrews JR, Cross MJ et al: Classification of knee ligament instabilities. I. The medial compartment and cruciate ligaments, *J Bone Joint Surg Am* 58:159-172, 1976.

46. Noyes FR, Paulos L, Mooar LA et al: Knee sprains and acute knee hemarthrosis: misdiagnosis of anterior cruciate ligament tears, *Phys Ther* 60:1596-1601, 1980.

47. Warren RF, Marshall JL: Injuries of the anterior cruciate and medial collateral ligaments of the knee: a retrospective analysis of clinical records. I, *Clin Orthop Relat Res* 136:191-197, 1978.

48. Paessler HH, Michel D: How new is the Lachman test? *Am J Sports Med* 20:95-98, 1992.

49. Jackson R: The torn ACL: natural history of untreated lesions and rationale for selective treatment. In Feagin JA (ed): *The crucial ligaments,* Edinburgh, 1988, Churchill Livingstone.

50. Rosenberg TD, Rasmussen GL: The function of the anterior cruciate ligament during anterior drawer and Lachman's testing, *Am J Sports Med* 12:318-322, 1984.

51. Logan MC, Williams A, Lavelle J et al: What really happens during the Lachman test: a dynamic MRI analysis of tibiofemoral motion, *Am J Sports Med* 32:369-375, 2004.

52. Frank C: Accurate interpretation of the Lachman test, *Clin Orthop* 213:163-166, 1986.

53. Bechtel SL, Ellman BR, Jordon JL: Skier's knee: the cruciate connection, *Phys Sports Med* 12:50-54, 1984.

54. Adler GG, Hoekman RA, Beach DM: Drop Leg Lachman test - A new test of anterior knee laxity. *Am J Sports Med* 23(3):320-323, 1995.

55. Butler DL, Noyes FR, Grood ES: Ligamentous restraints to anterior-posterior drawer in the human knee, *J Bone Joint Surg Am* 62:259-270, 1980.

56. Hughston JC: The absent posterior drawer test in some acute posterior cruciate ligament tears of the knee, *Am J Sports Med* 16:39-43, 1988.

57. Warren RF: Physical diagnosis of the knee. In Post M (ed): *Physical examination of the musculoskeletal system,* Chicago, 1987, Year Book Medical.

58. Weatherwax RJ: Anterior drawer sign, *Clin Orthop* 154:318-319, 1981.

59. Feagin JA: *The crucial ligaments,* Edinburgh, 1988, Churchill Livingstone.

60. Daniel DM, Stone ML, Barnett P et al: Use of the quadriceps active test to diagnose posterior cruciate ligament disruption and measure posterior laxity of the knee, *J Bone Joint Surg Am* 70:386-391, 1988.

61. Veltri DM, Warren RF: Isolated and combined posterior cruciate ligament injuries, *J Am Acad Orthop Surg* 1: 67-75, 1993.

62. Liorzou G: *Knee ligaments: clinical examination,* Berlin, 1991, Springer-Verlag.

63. Anderson AF, Rennirt GW, Standeffer WC: Clinical analysis of the pivot shift tests: description of the pivot drawer test, *Am J Knee Surg* 13:19-23, 2000.

64. Hoher J, Bach T, Munster A et al: Does the mode of data collection change results in a subjective knee score? Self administration vs interview, *Am J Sports Med* 25: 642-647, 1997.

65. Hughston JC, Walsh WM, Puddu G: *Patellar subluxation and dislocation,* Philadelphia, 1984, Saunders.

66. Muller W: *The knee: form, function and ligament reconstruction,* New York, 1983, Springer-Verlag.

67. Slocum DB, James SL, Larson RL et al: A clinical test for anterolateral rotary instability of the knee, *Clin Orthop* 118:63-69, 1976.

68. Slocum DB, Larson RL: Rotary instability of the knee, *J Bone Joint Surg Am* 50:211-225, 1968.

69. Jakob RP, Hassler H, Staeubli HU: Observations on rotary instability of the lateral compartment of the knee, *Acta Orthop Scand* 52(suppl 191):1-32, 1981.

70. LaPrade RF, Terry GC: Injuries to the posterolateral aspect of the knee: association of anatomic injury patterns with clinical instability, *Am J Sports Med* 25:433-438, 1997.

71. Hughston JC, Norwood LA: The posterolateral drawer test and external rotational recurvatum test for posterolateral rotary instability of the knee, *Clin Orthop* 147: 82-87, 1980.

72. Chen FS, Rokito AS, Pitman MI: Acute and chronic posterolateral rotary instability of the knee, *J Am Acad Orthop Surg* 8:97-110, 2000.

73. Swain RA, Wilson FD: Diagnosing posterolateral rotary knee instability: two clinical tests hold key, *Phys Sportsmed* 21:95-102, 1993.

74. Loomer RL: A test for knee posterolateral rotary instability, *Clin Orthop* 264:235-238, 1991.

75. Veltri DM, Warren RF: Posterolateral instability of the knee, *J Bone Joint Surg Am* 76:460-472, 1994.

76. Veltri DM, Warren RF: Anatomy, biomechanics and physical findings in posterolateral knee instability, *Clin Sports Med* 13:599-614, 1994.

77. Veltri DM, Deng X-H, Torzelli PA et al: The role of the cruciate and posterolateral ligaments in stability of the knee: a biomechanical study, *Am J Sports Med* 23: 436-443, 1995.

78. LaPrade RF, Wentorf F: Acute knee injuries: on the field and sideline evaluation, *Phys Sportsmed* 27:55-61, 1999.

79. Ferrari JD, Bach BR: Posterolateral instability of the knee: diagnosis and treatment of acute and chronic instability, *Sports Med Arthrosc Rev* 7:273-288, 1999.

80. Covey DC: Injuries of the posterolateral corner of the knee, *J Bone Joint Surg Am* 83:106-117, 2001.

81. Owens TC: Posteromedial pivot shift of the knee: a new test for rupture of the posterior cruciate ligament, *J Bone Joint Surg Am* 76:532-539, 1994.

82. Fritz JM, Irrgang JJ, Harner CD: Rehabilitation following allograft meniscal transplantation: a review of the literature and case study, *J Orthop Sports Phys Ther* 24: 98-107, 2006.

83. Heckmann TP, Barber-Westin SD, Noyes FR: Meniscal repair and transplantation: indications, techniques, rehabilitation, and clinical outcome, *J Orthop Sports Phys Ther* 36:795-815, 2006.

84. Hegedus EJ, Cook C, Hasselblad V et al: Physical examination tests for assessing a torn meniscus: a systematic review with meta-analysis, *J Orthop Sports Phys Ther* 37:541-550, 2007.

85. Lee D: Meniscal injury. In Sueki D, Brechter J (eds): *Orthopedic rehabilitation clinical advisor*, St Louis, 2010, Mosby.

86. McMurray TP: The semilunar cartilages, *Br J Surg* 29:407-414, 1942.

87. Evans PJ, Bell GD, Frank C: Prospective evaluation of the McMurray test, *Am J Sports Med* 21:604-608, 1993.

88. Kim SJ, Min BH, Han DY: Paradoxical phenomena of the McMurray test: an arthroscopic examination, *Am J Sports Med* 24:83-87, 1996.

89. Corea JR, Moussa M, Othman AA: McMurray's test tested, *Knee Surg Sports Traumatol Arthrosc* 2:70-72, 1994.

90. Apley AG: The diagnosis of meniscus injuries: some new clinical methods, *J Bone Joint Surg Br* 29:78-84, 1947.

91. Oni O: The knee jerk test for diagnosis of torn meniscus, *Clin Orthop* 193:309, 1985.

92. Broom MJ, Fulkerson JP: The plica syndrome: a new perspective, *Orthop Clin North Am* 17:279-281, 1986.

93. Dupont JY: Synovial plicae of the knee: controversies and review, *Clin Sports Med* 16:87-122, 1997.

94. Tindel NL, Nisonson B: The plica syndrome, *Orthop Clin North Am* 23:613-618, 1992.

95. Mital MA, Hayden J: Pain in the knee in children: the medial plica shelf syndrome, *Orthop Clin North Am* 10:713-722, 1979.

96. Boling MC, Bolgla LA, Mattacola CG et al: Outcomes of a weight-bearing rehabilitation program for patients diagnosed with patellofemoral pain syndrome, *Arch Phys Med Rehabil* 87:1428-1435, 2006.

97. Brushoj C, Holmich P, Nielsen MB, Albrecht-Beste E: Acute patellofemoral pain: aggravating activities, clinical examination, MRI and ultrasound findings, *Br J Sports Med* 42:64-67, 2008.

98. Fredericson M, Yoon K: Physical examination and patellofemoral pain syndrome, *Am J Phys Med Rehabil* 85:234-243, 2006.

99. Lee D: Patellofemoral dysfunction. In Sueki D, Brechter J (eds): *Orthopedic rehabilitation clinical advisor*, St Louis, 2010, Mosby.

100. Steinkamp LA, Dillingham MF, Markel MD et al: Biomechanical considerations in patellofemoral joint rehabilitation, *Am J Sports Med* 21:339-444, 1993.

101. MacIntyre NJ, Hill NA, Fellows RA et al: Patellofemoral joint kinematics in individuals with and without patellofemoral pain syndrome, *J Bone Joint Surg Am* 88:2596-2605, 2006.

102. Willson JD, Davis IS: Lower extremity mechanics of females with and without patellofemoral pain across activities with progressively greater task demands, *Clin Biomech* 23:203-211, 2008.

103. Reider B: *The orthopedic physical examination*, Philadelphia, 1999, Saunders.

104. Nijs J, VanGeel C, Vanderauwera C et al: Diagnostic value of five clinical tests in patellofemoral syndrome, *Man Ther* 11:69-77, 2006.

105. McConnell J: The management of chondromalacia patellae: a long term solution, *Aust J Physiother* 32:215-223, 1986.

106. Watson CJ, Prepps M, Galt W et al: Reliability of McConnell's classification of patellar orientation in symptomatic and asymptomatic subjects, *J Orthop Sports Phys Ther* 29:378-385, 1999.

107. Jackson JL, O'Malley PG, Kroenke K: Evaluation of acute knee pain in primary care, *Ann Intern Med* 139:575-588, 2003.

108. Sibley MB, Fu FH: Knee injuries. In Fu FH, Stone DA (eds): *Sports injuries: mechanisms, prevention, treatment*, Baltimore, 1994, Williams & Wilkins.

109. Schulthies SS, Francis RS, Fisher AG et al: Does the Q-angle reflect the force on the patella in the frontal plane? *Phys Ther* 75:24-30, 1995.

110. Olerud C, Berg P: The variation of the Q angle with different positions of the foot, *Clin Orthop* 191:162-165, 1984.

111. Grelsamer RP, Dubey A, Weinstein CH: Men and women have similar Q-angles: a clinical and trigonometric evaluation, *J Bone Joint Surg Br* 87:1498-1501, 2005.

112. Geene CC, Edwards TB, Wade MR et al: Reliability of the quadriceps angle measurement, *Am J Knee Surg* 14:98-103, 2001.

113. Fairbank HAT: Internal derangement of the knee in children and adolescents, *Proc R Soc Med* 30:427-432, 1937.

114. Tanner SM, Garth WP, Soileau R et al: A modified test for patellar instability: the biomechanical basis, *Clin J Sports Med* 13:327-338, 2003.

115. Noble HB, Hajek MR, Porter M: Diagnosis and treatment of iliotibial band tightness in runners, *Phys Sportsmed* 10:67-74, 1982.

116. Wallace LA: Limb length difference and back pain. In Grieve GP (ed): *Modern manual therapy of the vertebral column*, Edinburgh, 1986, Churchill Livingstone.

LOWER LEG, ANKLE, AND FOOT

Précis of the Lower Leg, Ankle, and Foot Assessment*

History
Observation
Examination

Active movements, weight-bearing (standing)
  Plantar flexion
  Dorsiflexion
  Supination
  Pronation
  Toe extension
  Toe flexion
Active movements, non-weight-bearing (sitting or supine lying)
  Plantar flexion
  Dorsiflexion
  Supination
  Pronation
  Toe extension
  Toe flexion
  Toe abduction
  Toe adduction
Special tests (sitting)
  Tibial torsion
  External rotation stress test
Passive movements (supine lying)
  Plantar flexion at the talocrural (ankle) joint
  Dorsiflexion at the talocrural joint
  Inversion at the subtalar joint
  Eversion at the subtalar joint
  Adduction at the midtarsal joints
  Abduction at the midtarsal joints
  Flexion of the toes
  Extension of the toes
  Adduction of the toes
  Abduction of the toes
Resisted isometric movements (supine lying)
  Knee flexion
  Plantar flexion
  Dorsiflexion

  Supination
  Pronation
  Toe extension
  Toe flexion
Special tests (supine lying)
  Neutral position of the talus
  Anterior drawer sign
  Talar tilt
  Leg length
Reflexes and cutaneous distribution (supine lying)
Joint play movements (supine and side lying)
  Long axis extension
  Anterior-posterior glide
  Talar rock
  Side tilt
  Rotation
  Side glide
  Tarsal bone mobility
Palpation (supine lying and prone lying)
Special tests (prone lying)
  Neutral position of the talus
  Leg-heel alignment
  Foot-heel alignment
  Tibial torsion
  Prone anterior drawer test
  Thompson's test
Functional assessment (standing)
Special tests (standing)
  Neutral position of the talus
  Functional leg length
Diagnostic imaging

---

*The précis is shown in an order that limits the amount of movement the patient must do but ensures that all necessary structures are tested; it does not follow the order of the text. After any assessment, the patient should be warned that symptoms may be exacerbated by the assessment.

SELECTED MOVEMENTS

ACTIVE MOVEMENTS

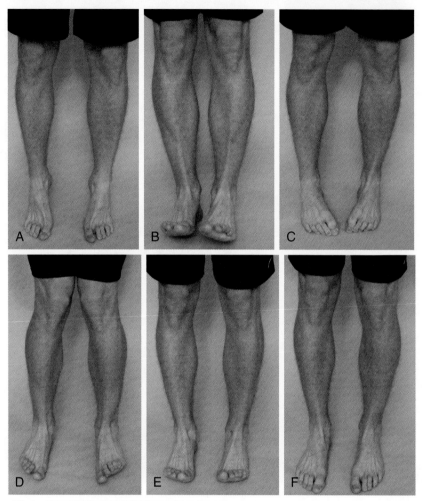

Figure 12–1
Active movements (weight-bearing posture). **A,** Plantar flexion. **B,** Dorsiflexion. **C,** Supination.
D, Pronation. **E,** Toe extension. **F,** Toe flexion.

GENERAL INFORMATION	Active movements of the lower leg, ankle, and foot should be done in both weight-bearing and non-weight-bearing positions (long leg sitting or supine lying), and the examiner should note any differences, because foot deformities and deviations, in addition to decreased range of motion (ROM), can lead to injury in other parts of the lower kinetic chain and spine.[1]
PATIENT POSITION	The patient is supine lying (non-weight bearing) or standing (weight bearing).
EXAMINER POSITION	The examiner stands to the side of the patient to instruct the person and to observe the available ROM.

Continued

ACTIVE MOVEMENTS—*cont'd*

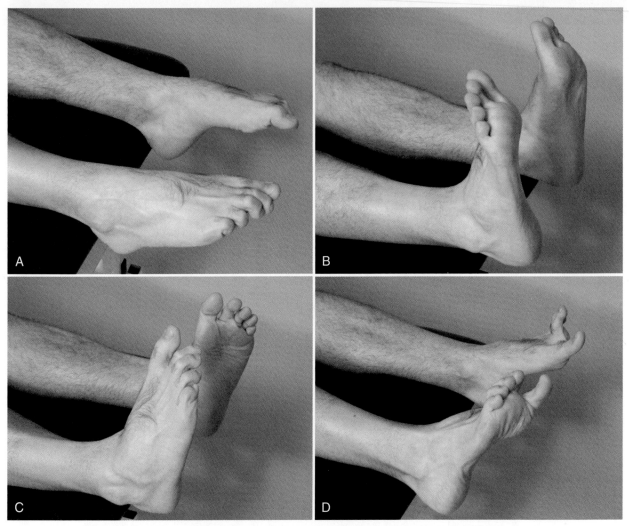

Figure 12–2
Active movements (non-weight-bearing posture). **A,** Plantar flexion. **B,** Dorsiflexion. **C,** Supination.
D, Pronation.

Continued

Plantar Flexion

TEST PROCEDURE   The patient is asked to plantar flex the foot as far as possible.

INDICATIONS OF A POSITIVE TEST   Plantar flexion of the ankle is approximately 50°. If the ROM is less than this or is less than for the unaffected leg, the movement is restricted for some reason. The patient's heel normally inverts when the movement is performed in weight bearing. If heel inversion does not occur, the foot is unstable, or tibialis posterior weakness or tightness is present.[2-4] The tibialis posterior muscle and tendon balance the pull of the peroneal muscles, protect the spring ligament, and invert and stabilize the hindfoot during toe-off.[5]

ACTIVE MOVEMENTS—*cont'd*

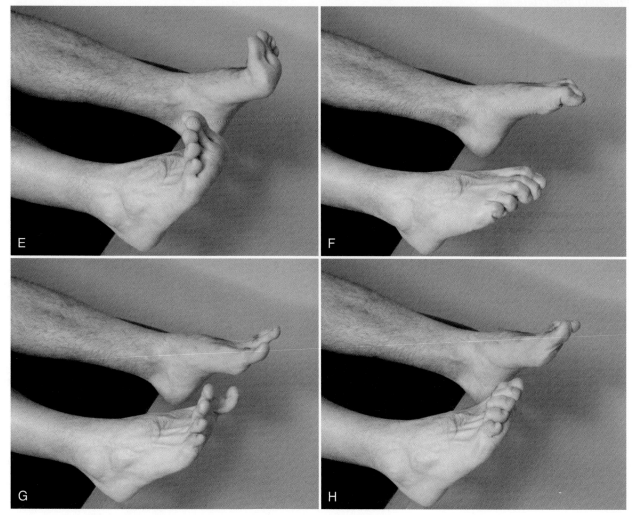

Figure 12–2 cont'd
E, Toe extension. **F,** Toe flexion. **G,** Toe abduction. **H,** Toe adduction.

Dorsiflexion

TEST PROCEDURE   The patient is asked to dorsiflex the foot as far as possible.

INDICATIONS OF A POSITIVE TEST   Dorsiflexion of the ankle is usually 20° past the anatomical position (plantigrade), which is with the foot at 90° to the bones of the leg. If the ROM is less than this or is less than for the unaffected leg, it is restricted for some reason.

CLINICAL NOTE   • For normal locomotion, 10° of dorsiflexion, and 20° to 25° of plantar flexion at the ankle are required.

Continued

ACTIVE MOVEMENTS—cont'd

Supination and Pronation

TEST PROCEDURE   The patient is asked to supinate both feet and then pronate both feet.

INDICATIONS OF A POSITIVE TEST   Supination is 45° to 60°, and pronation is 15° to 30°, although individuals vary. If the ROM is less than this or is less than for the unaffected leg, it is restricted for some reason. It is more important to compare the movement of the affected foot with that of the unaffected foot. Supination combines the movements of inversion, adduction, and plantar flexion; pronation combines the movements of eversion, abduction, and dorsiflexion of the foot and ankle.

Toe Flexion, Extension, Abduction, and Adduction

TEST PROCEDURE   The patient is asked to bilaterally flex the toes and then, in sequence, to extend, abduct, and adduct ("scrunch together") the toes.

INDICATIONS OF A POSITIVE TEST   Extension of the toes occurs at the metatarsophalangeal and proximal and distal interphalangeal joints. Extension of the great toe occurs primarily at the metatarsophalangeal joint (70°); minimal or no extension occurs at the interphalangeal joint. For the great toe, 45° flexion occurs at the metatarsophalangeal joint, and 90° occurs at the interphalangeal joint. For the lateral four toes, extension occurs primarily at the metatarsophalangeal (40°) and distal interphalangeal (30°) joints.

Extension at the proximal interphalangeal joins is negligible. For the lateral four toes, 40° flexion occurs at the metatarsophalangeal joints, 35° occurs at the proximal interphalangeal joints, and 60° occurs at the distal interphalangeal joints. If the ROM is less than this or is less than for the unaffected leg, it is restricted for some reason.

Abduction and adduction of the toes are measured with the second toe as midline. Although the ROM of abduction can be measured, this is not usually done. The common practice is to ask the patient to spread the toes and then bring them back together ("scrunching" the toes). The amount and quality of these movements are compared with those of the unaffected side.

SPECIAL TESTS FOR NEUTRAL POSITION OF THE TALUS

Relevant Special Tests

Neutral position of the talus (prone)
Neutral position of the talus (supine)
Neutral position of the talus (weight-bearing position)

Definition

The neutral position of the talus often is referred to as the *neutral* or *balanced* position of the foot. This so-called neutral position is an ideal position that, in reality, is not commonly found in people in normal weight bearing. For most patients, the subtalar joint and the calcaneus normally are in slight valgus, with the forefoot in slight varus. The tibia also is in slight varus, so each joint slightly compensates for the adjacent one. The neutral position is used as a starting position to determine foot and leg deviations. Functional asymmetry may occur in the lower limb in normal standing. If so, the examiner should put the talus in the neutral position to see whether the asymmetry remains. If it does, anatomical or structural asymmetry is a factor, as well as functional asymmetry. If the asymmetry disappears, only functional asymmetry is present, which often is easier to treat.

Suspected Injury

- Talar position tests are not designed to identify specifically any particular pathological condition; rather, they identify anatomical and biomechanical abnormalities that contribute to a pathological condition. That pathology may occur locally at the foot and ankle or remotely at areas such as the back, knee, or hip.
- Malalignment of the talus
- Talar dome injury

Epidemiology and Demographics

The overall prevalence of malalignment reported in the literature ranges from 10% in the Cheshire Foot Pain and Disability Survey in the United Kingdom to 28% in the Framingham Foot Study in the United States. Clinically, it has been hypothesized that abnormal talar alignment and mechanics can result in pathological conditions of the foot. Regardless of the prevalence of foot pain, the cause-and-effect relationship between talar position and pathological conditions has yet to be definitively determined.[6-10]

Relevant History

Patients with poor talar alignment or biomechanics may have a history of ankle sprains with or without talar dome osteochondral lesions. Ankle sprains may also result in talocrural instability or laxity, which could affect the position and mechanics of the talus in the ankle mortise.

Relevant Signs and Symptoms

The signs and symptoms depend on the pathological condition. Talar malalignment can manifest as pain in the foot, knee, hip, pelvis, or low back. Because talar malalignment results in compensations in other regions, most associated pathological conditions become problematic gradually. Generally, the patient cannot identify a specific mechanism of injury. Symptoms increase with use and lessen with rest. Positions or activities that require end-range dorsiflexion are the most problematic, because biomechanically, altered talus mechanics affect this most significantly. The ankle mortise must spread to accommodate the wider anterior aspect of the talus. If the talus is malpositioned, the talus may not be able to track through the mortise as efficiently or completely.

A sharp pain or pinching may be noted with end-range dorsiflexion. Hip lateral rotation or increased foot pronation may be noted during the middle to late stages of the stance phase of gait as a compensation for the lack of ankle dorsiflexion.

Mechanism of Injury

Malalignments may or may not be the result of previous injuries. Because of this, a mechanism of injury may or may not exist. Talar malalignment may be the result of previous injuries, repetitive use, leg length discrepancies, or genetics. Inversion ankle sprains may result in an osteochondral lesion, or bone bruise, on the medial aspect of the talus. Conversely, eversion ankle sprains can result in lesions or bruising on the lateral aspect of the talus. Either of these lesions, medial or lateral, could prevent proper tracking and alignment of the talus as it moves through the ankle mortise.

RELIABILITY/SPECIFICITY/SENSITIVITY COMPARISON[11-16]

	Validity	Interrater Reliability	Intrarater Reliability
Neutral position of the talus (weight-bearing position)	Unknown	0.15-0.79	0.14-0.85
Neutral position of the talus (supine)	Unknown	Unknown	Unknown
Neutral position of the talus (prone)	Unknown	0.25	0.06-0.77

NEUTRAL POSITION OF THE TALUS (PRONE)[11-13,17-20]

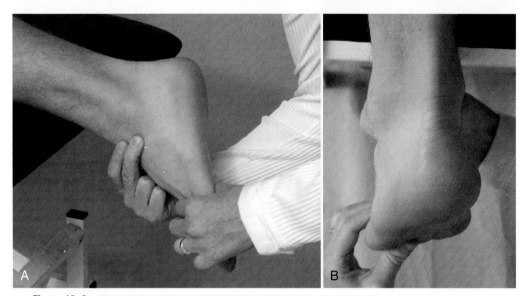

Figure 12–3
Determining the neutral position of the subtalar joints in the prone position. **A,** Side view. **B,** Superior view.

PURPOSE	To determine the neutral position of the talus, which often is referred to as the *neutral (subtalar neutral)* or *balanced* position of the foot.
PATIENT POSITION	The patient lies prone with the foot extended over the end of the examining table.
EXAMINER POSITION	The examiner is seated or stands at the patient's feet.
TEST PROCEDURE	Starting with the unaffected foot, the examiner grasps the foot over the fourth and fifth metatarsal heads with the index finger and thumb of one hand. The examiner palpates both sides of the talus on the dorsum of the foot, using the thumb and index finger of the other hand. The examiner then passively and gently dorsiflexes the foot until resistance is felt. Maintaining the dorsiflexed position, the examiner moves the foot back and forth through an arc of supination (the talar head bulges laterally) and pronation (the talar head bulges medially). The two feet are compared.
INDICATIONS OF A POSITIVE TEST	As the arc of movement is performed, there is a point in the arc at which the foot appears to fall off to one side or the other more easily. At this point, the talus should feel equally prominent on both sides (medial and lateral) of the talus. This point is the neutral, non-weight-bearing position of the subtalar joint. While holding this position, the examiner can observe the alignment of the leg relative to the calcaneus.
CLINICAL NOTE	• This prone test position is best for determining the relation of the hindfoot (rearfoot) to the leg.
RELIABILITY/SPECIFICITY/ SENSITIVITY[11-13]	Reliability intrarater range ICC: 0.06-0.77 Reliability nterrater range ICC: 0-0.25

NEUTRAL POSITION OF THE TALUS (SUPINE)[14,15,17-20]

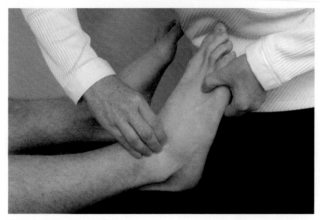

Figure 12–4
Determining the neutral position of the subtalar joint in the supine position.

PURPOSE	To determine the neutral position of the talus, which often is referred to as the *neutral (subtalar neutral)* or *balanced* position of the foot.
PATIENT POSITION	The patient lies supine with the feet extended over the end of the examining table.
EXAMINER POSITION	The examiner sits or stands at the patient's feet.
TEST PROCEDURE	Starting with the unaffected leg, the examiner grasps the foot over the fourth and fifth metatarsal heads, using the thumb and index finger of one hand. The examiner palpates both sides of the head of the talus on the dorsum of the foot with the thumb and index finger of the other hand. The examiner then gently and passively dorsiflexes the foot until resistance is felt. Maintaining the dorsiflexion, the examiner passively moves the foot through an arc of supination (the talar head bulges laterally) and pronation (the talar head bulges medially). The two sides are compared.
INDICATIONS OF A POSITIVE TEST	If the foot is positioned so that the talar head does not appear to bulge to either side (medial or lateral), the subtalar joint is in its neutral non-weight-bearing position.
CLINICAL NOTE	• This supine test position is best for determining the relation of the forefoot to the hindfoot.
RELIABILITY/SPECIFICITY/ SENSITIVITY[14,15]	Reliability intrarater ICC: 0.76 Reliability interrater ICC: 0.60

NEUTRAL POSITION OF THE TALUS (WEIGHT-BEARING POSITION)[11,13,16,18,21,22]

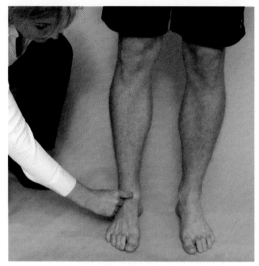

Figure 12–5
Determining the neutral position of the subtalar joint in standing (weight bearing).

PURPOSE	To determine the neutral position of the talus, which often is referred to as the *neutral (subtalar neutral)* or *balanced* position of the foot.
PATIENT POSITION	The patient stands with the feet in a relaxed standing position so that the base width and Fick angle (normally, the patella faces straight ahead while the foot faces slightly laterally) are normal for the patient.
EXAMINER POSITION	The examiner kneels at the patient's feet.
TEST PROCEDURE	The unaffected leg is tested first. The examiner palpates the head of the talus on the dorsal aspect of the foot with the thumb and forefinger of one hand (the thumb is placed on the lateral aspect of the talus and the forefinger is placed on the medial aspect of the talus). The patient then actively (or the examiner passively) slowly rotates the trunk to the right and then to the left, which causes the tibia to medially and laterally rotate so that the talus supinates and pronates. The two sides are compared.
INDICATIONS OF A POSITIVE TEST	If the foot is positioned so that the talar head does not appear to bulge to either side (medial or lateral), the subtalar joint is in its neutral position in weight bearing.
CLINICAL NOTE/CAUTION	• Mueller et al.[13] described a progression of neutral talus positions in standing (i.e., the navicular drop test) to quantify midfoot mobility and its effect on other parts of the kinetic chain. With a small, rigid ruler, the examiner first measures the height of the navicular from the floor in the neutral talus position, using the most prominent part of the navicular tuberosity; the height of the navicular in normal relaxed standing then is measured. The difference, called the *navicular drop*, indicates the amount of foot pronation or flattening of the medial longitudinal arch during standing. Any measurement greater than 10 mm is considered abnormal.
RELIABILITY/SPECIFICITY/ SENSITIVITY[11,16]	Reliability intrarater range ICC: 0.14-0.85 Reliability interrater range ICC: 0.15-0.79

SPECIAL TESTS FOR ALIGNMENT

Relevant Special Tests

Leg-rearfoot (heel) alignment
Rearfoot-forefoot alignment

Definition

Alignment tests are used to determine the relation of the leg to the hindfoot (heel) and the relation of the hindfoot to the forefoot. These tests are used to differentiate functional from anatomical (structural) deformities or asymmetries in the lower leg, ankle, and foot.

Suspected Injury

Alignment tests are not designed to identify specifically any particular pathological condition; rather, they identify lower leg, ankle, and/or foot anatomical and biomechanical abnormalities that may contribute to a pathological condition. That pathology may occur locally, at the foot or ankle, or remotely, at areas such as the back, pelvis, hip, or knee.

Epidemiology and Demographics

Few population-based studies have examined the prevalence of foot pain in the general population. Causal relationships between specific malalignments and injuries have been difficult to verify. In a random sampling of people in Australia, foot pain affected nearly 1 in 5 individuals. The pain was associated with increased age, female gender, obesity, and pain in other body regions, and it had a significant detrimental impact on health-related quality of life. The overall prevalence reported in this study was higher than that reported in the Cheshire Foot Pain and Disability Survey in the United Kingdom (10%). However, it was lower than the prevalence rates reported in two studies in the United States: the National Health Interview Survey in the United States (24%) and the Framingham Foot Study (28%).[6-10]

Relevant History

Often anatomical and biomechanical abnormalities can produce injury and pathological conditions in other regions of the body. Similarly, abnormalities in other regions may produce compensation in the body at the foot and ankle. Therefore, patients may have a history of injury or a pathological condition in other regions. Examination of the patient should include screening of the pelvis, hip, back, and knee, because a previous injury to these regions may produce foot and ankle malalignments. Injuries directly to the foot and ankle also may be present in many patients with malalignments.

Relevant Signs and Symptoms

The signs and symptoms depend on the pathological condition. Malalignment of the lower leg and foot generally results in overuse injuries. These may manifest as pain in the foot, knee, hip, pelvis, or low back. With most overuse injuries, the symptoms become gradually problematic. Generally the patient cannot identify a specific mechanism of injury. Symptoms increase with use and lessen with rest. Positions or activities that place the foot and lower leg at the end ranges of motion may produce a sharper, more localized pain in the affected area. Often, positional malalignments may be the result of protection and guarding by the muscles in the region. If the alignment is due to protection of neural or vascular structures, neural or vascular symptoms (or both), such as numbness, tingling, coldness, or weakness, may be present with overuse.

Mechanism of Injury

Malalignments may or may not be the result of previous injuries. Consequently, there may or may not be a mechanism of injury. Leg and heel alignment and forefoot to heel alignment issues may be the result of previous injuries, repetitive use, leg length discrepancies, or genetics. Injuries to the lower extremity in childhood often can result in structural abnormalities in the lower extremity; over time, the foot and ankle adapt to compensate for the structural changes.

RELIABILITY/SPECIFICITY/SENSITIVITY COMPARISON[23,24]

	Leg-Rearfoot (Heel) Alignment	Forefoot-Rearfoot (Heel) Alignment
Validity	Unknown	Unknown
Interrater reliability	Unknown	0.86
Intrarater reliability	0.86	0.88
Specificity	Unknown	Unknown
Sensitivity	Unknown	Unknown

LEG-REARFOOT (HEEL) ALIGNMENT[20,23]

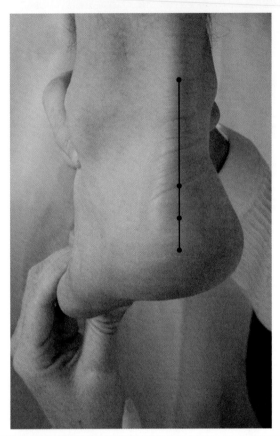

Figure 12–6
Alignment of the leg and heel (rearfoot).

PURPOSE	To assess for hindfoot (rearfoot) varus or valgus.
PATIENT POSITION	The patient lies prone with the foot extending over the end of the examining table.
EXAMINER POSITION	The examiner sits or stands at the patient's feet.
TEST PROCEDURE	Starting with the unaffected leg, the examiner places a mark over the midline of the calcaneus at the insertion of the Achilles tendon. The examiner makes a second mark approximately 1 cm distal to the first mark and as close to the midline of the calcaneus as possible. A calcaneal line then is made to join the two marks. Next, the examiner makes two marks on the lower third of the leg in the midline along the Achilles tendon. These two marks are joined, forming the tibial line, which represents the longitudinal axis of the tibia.
The examiner then places the subtalar joint in the prone neutral position (see the previous test). While the subtalar joint is held in neutral, the examiner looks at the two lines to see whether they form a single straight line or an angle, and if the latter, how much of an angle.
INDICATIONS OF A POSITIVE TEST	If the lines are parallel or in slight varus (2° to 8°), the leg to rearfoot (heel) alignment is considered normal. If the heel is inverted, the patient has hindfoot varus; if the heel is everted, the patient has hindfoot valgus.
CLINICAL NOTE	• The patient may be prepositioned in prone lying with the legs in figure-four position. This position should allow the examiner to place the test leg in the required position.
RELIABILITY/SPECIFICITY/ SENSITIVITY[23]	Reliability ICC: 0.86

REARFOOT-FOREFOOT ALIGNMENT[17,20,24]

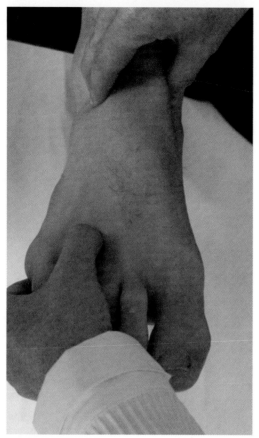

Figure 12–7
Alignment of the forefoot and heel (superior view).

PURPOSE	To assess for forefoot varus and valgus.
PATIENT POSITION	The patient lies supine with the feet extending over the end of the examining table.
EXAMINER POSITION	The examiner sits or stands at the patient's feet.
TEST PROCEDURE	Starting with the unaffected foot, the examiner positions the subtalar joint in supine neutral position (see the previous test). While maintaining this neutral position, the examiner pronates the midtarsal joints maximally and observes the relation between the vertical axis of the heel and the plane of the second through fourth metatarsal heads. The two sides are compared.
INDICATIONS OF A POSITIVE TEST	Normally, the plane is perpendicular to the vertical axis. If the medial side of the foot is raised, the patient has a forefoot varus; if the lateral side of the foot is raised, the patient has a forefoot valgus.
CLINICAL NOTES	• If the patient lacks hip medial rotation, it may be difficult to measure the alignment, because the lower limb is laterally rotated. • The test also may be performed in the prone position.
RELIABILITY/SPECIFICITY/ SENSITIVITY[24]	Reliability intrarater ICC: 0.88 Reliability interrater ICC: 0.86

SPECIAL TEST FOR TIBIAL TORSION

Relevant Special Test

Tibial torsion test

Definition

Tibial torsion refers to twisting of the tibia; it is a common cause of the in-toeing or out-toeing seen in adults and children.

Suspected Injury

Tibial torsion is not a pathological condition. It can result in a pathological condition in other regions, or it may be developmental.

Epidemiology and Demographics

Tibial torsion usually is first noticed in children as they approach 2 years of age. Some tibial medial rotation is normal in newborns. This medial rotation usually straightens during the first year of life. In the case of excessive tibial torsion, the tibial rotation fails to straighten or the amount of rotation is too great to correct totally. It becomes more apparent as the child begins to walk, although it usually is present before then. No gender preference is apparent; males and females are equally affected. It is more common for patients to be affected bilaterally. Two-thirds of patients with tibial torsion are affected in both tibias.[25-27]

Relevant History

The exact physiological mechanism that causes tibial torsion is unknown. It has been hypothesized that tibial malformations are the result of genetics, the positioning of the fetus in the uterus, or postures during early development.

Relevant Signs and Symptoms

Tibial torsions usually are painless. Functionally, severe in-toeing or out-toeing may result in abnormal gait mechanics. Patients may appear "knock-kneed," "pigeon-toed," or "bow-legged." Over time, the abnormal mechanics alter the forces placed on associated joints and structures, resulting in a pathological condition. At this point, the patient's signs and symptoms reflect the resultant condition.[28,29]

Mechanism of Injury

The lower extremity commonly compensates for tibial torsions. Internal or medial torsion causes the foot to adduct. In response, the patient attempts to compensate by everting the foot or by laterally rotating at the hip. Similarly, individuals with external or lateral tibial torsion invert at the foot and medially rotate at the hip as a method of compensation. These compensations produce abnormal stresses in the knee, foot, hip, pelvis, and low back. Over time, these regions begin to "break down," and a pathological condition ensues. Medial torsion often improves as a child matures. Conversely, lateral torsion often worsens.

When testing for tibial torsion, the examiner must realize that some lateral tibial torsion is normally present (13° to 18° in adults, less in children). If tibial torsion is more than 18°, it is referred to as a *toe-out* position. If tibial torsion is less than 13°, it is referred to as a *toe-in* position. A person with excessive toeing-in sometimes is referred to as "pigeon toed," a condition that may be caused by medial tibial torsion, medial femoral torsion, or excessive femoral anteversion.

TIBIAL TORSION TEST[30,31]

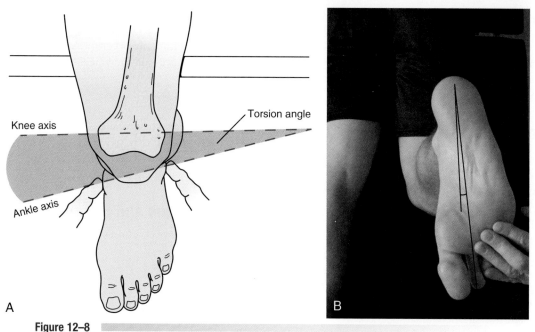

A

Figure 12–8

A, Determination of tibial torsion in sitting (superior view). The torsion angle determined by the intersection of the knee axis and the ankle axis. (**A** Modified from Hunt GC (ed): *Physical therapy of the foot and ankle*, p 80, New York, 1988, Churchill Livingstone.) **B,** Measurement of tibial torsion in the prone position.

PURPOSE	To determine the torsion of the tibial bone.
PATIENT POSITION	The patient sits with the knees flexed to 90° over the edge of the examining table.
EXAMINER POSITION	The examiner stands adjacent to the test foot.
TEST PROCEDURE	The examiner places the thumb of one hand over the apex of one malleolus and the index finger of the same hand over the apex of the other malleolus. The examiner visualizes the axes of the knee and the ankle.
INDICATIONS OF A POSITIVE TEST	The lines of the knee and ankle axes are not normally parallel, but rather form an angle of 12° to 18° because of lateral rotation of the tibia.
CLINICAL NOTES	• Tibial torsion may also be tested with the patient in the prone position. The patient lies prone with the knee flexed to 90°. The examiner views from above the angle formed by the foot and thigh after the subtalar joint has been placed in the neutral position, noting the angle the foot makes with the tibia. This method most often is used in children, because it is easier to observe the feet from above. • The examiner must remember the midline of the foot is considered, by convention, to go through the second toe.
RELIABILITY/SPECIFICITY/ SENSITIVITY	Unknown

SPECIAL TESTS FOR LIGAMENTOUS INSTABILITY

Relevant Special Tests

Anterior drawer test
Prone anterior drawer test
Talar tilt test
External rotational stress test (Kleiger test)

Definition

Ligamentous instability in the foot and ankle generally occurs in association with an ankle or foot sprain. Sprains occur when the ligament is tensioned beyond its physiological capacity; this results in a partial or complete tear of the ligament. When this occurs, structural integrity in the associated joint is lost.

Ankle sprains are classified into three categories:[32-35]

- *Lateral (low ankle) sprains* occur when the ligaments on the lateral portion of the ankle are injured. The most common ligaments injured are the anterior talofibular ligament and the calcaneofibular ligament.
- *Syndesmotic (high ankle) sprains* are synonymous with anterior tibiofibular ligaments sprains. These sprains occur when the ligaments between the two major bones of the lower leg (the tibia and the fibula) are injured at the level of the ankle.
- *Medial ankle sprains* are the rarest and occur when the deltoid ligament is injured.

Suspected Injury

Anterior talofibular ligament sprain (low or lateral ankle sprain)
Calcaneofibular ligament sprain (lateral ankle sprain)
Syndesmotic sprain (high ankle sprain)
Deltoid ligament sprain (medial ankle sprain)

Epidemiology and Demographics[32-35]

Approximately 1 to 10,000 people a day experience an ankle sprain (5000 to 27,000 daily occurrences). Lateral ankle sprains account for 10% to 15% of all sports-related injuries. Of these sprains, the anterior talofibular ligament is injured in about 65% of cases. Syndesmotic sprains are responsible for approximately 10% of ankle sprains, and medial ankle sprains are reported to be responsible for 5% to 10%. Ankle sprains most commonly occur in patients under age 35; the highest occurrence is in individuals 15 to 19 years old.

Relevant History

Patients frequently have recurrent ankle sprains of the same ankle, particularly if they did not participate in a rehabilitation program. Patients commonly report that they have had an ankle injury in the past.

Relevant Signs and Symptoms

- Ecchymosis
- Bruising
- Tenderness
- Instability
- Loss of ROM
- Inability to bear full weight
- Pain in the region of the ligament

In the case of acute trauma, swelling prevents the examiner from getting a true measurement of joint mobility. The best time to assess the laxity of the joint is immediately after the injury and before swelling occurs. The examiner may need to allow time for the swelling to reduce before true joint mobility can be assessed.

Mechanism of Injury

Lateral (low ankle) sprain: Lateral ankle ligament injuries usually are the result of a rapid inversion movement at the ankle. The patient commonly reports that the ankle "rolled," or the person states that a pop was heard during activities such as planting the foot when running, stepping up or down, or stepping or landing on an uneven surface.

Syndesmosis (high ankle) sprain: Syndesmotic sprains are believed to occur when the ankle is planted in dorsiflexion with lateral rotation of the lower leg. Most syndesmotic ankle sprains are believed to be the result of direct contact between individuals.

Medial ankle sprain: Medial ankle sprains occur with plantar flexion with eversion.

ANTERIOR DRAWER TEST[36-48]

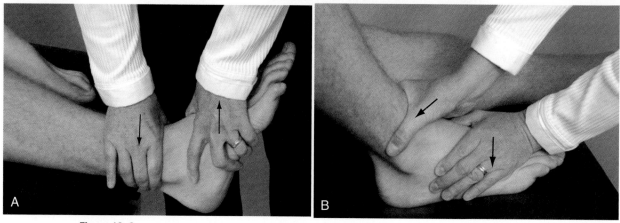

Figure 12–9
Anterior drawer test. **A,** Method 1: Pulling the foot forward. **B,** Method 2: Pushing the leg back.

PURPOSE To test for injuries to the anterior talofibular ligament, the most frequently injured ligament in the ankle.

SUSPECTED INJURY • Anterior talofibular ligament or low ankle sprain

PATIENT POSITION The patient lies supine with the foot relaxed. The patient's foot should be hanging over the edge of the table.

EXAMINER POSITION The examiner stands adjacent to the test foot.

TEST PROCEDURE The unaffected ankle is tested first. One of the examiner's hands stabilizes the distal tibia and fibula. The thenar web space of the examiner's other hand is placed over the patient's anterior talus. The examiner stabilizes the tibia and fibula, holds the patient's foot in 20° of plantar flexion, and draws the talus forward in the ankle mortise with the second hand. Normally, there is some anterior movement when the test is performed, so the examiner should ensure that the movement on the injured side is compared with the uninjured side.

INDICATIONS OF A POSITIVE TEST A positive result may be obtained on the anterior drawer test if only the anterior talofibular ligament is torn; however, anterior translation is greater if both the anterior talofibular and calcaneofibular ligaments are torn, especially if the foot is tested in dorsiflexion. Sometimes, a dimple appears over the area of the anterior talofibular ligament on anterior translation (dimple, or suction, sign) if pain, muscle spasm, and swelling are minimal. If straight anterior movement or translation occurs, the test result indicates both medial and lateral ligament insufficiencies. This bilateral finding, which often is more evident in dorsiflexion, means that the superficial and deep deltoid ligaments, as well as the anterior talofibular ligament and anterolateral capsule, have been torn. If the tear is on only one side, only that side translates forward more than normal. For example, with a lateral tear, the lateral side translates forward, causing medial rotation of the talus and resulting in anterolateral rotary instability, which is increasingly evident with increased plantar flexion of the foot.

Continued

ANTERIOR DRAWER TEST[36-48]—cont'd

CLINICAL NOTES

- In the plantar flexed position, the anterior talofibular ligament is perpendicular to the long axis of the tibia. By adding inversion, which gives an anterolateral stress, the examiner can increase the stress on the anterior talofibular ligament and the calcaneofibular ligament.
- Ideally, the knee should be placed in 90° of flexion to alleviate tension on the Achilles tendon. The test should be performed in plantar flexion and in dorsiflexion to test for straight and rotational instabilities.
- The test also may be performed by stabilizing the foot and talus and pushing the tibia and fibula posteriorly on the talus (method 2). In this case, excessive posterior movement of the tibia and fibula on the talus indicates a positive test result.

RELIABILITY/SPECIFICITY/ SENSITIVITY

Unknown

PRONE ANTERIOR DRAWER TEST[49]

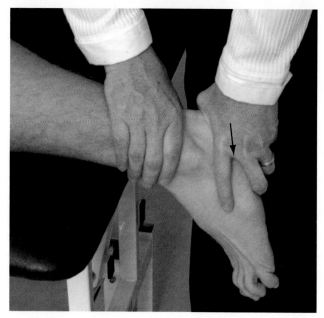

Figure 12–10
Prone anterior drawer test.

PURPOSE	To test for injuries to the anterior talofibular ligament.
SUSPECTED INJURY	Anterior talofibular ligament or low ankle sprain
PATIENT POSITION	The patient lies prone with the foot extending over the end of the examining table.
EXAMINER POSITION	The examiner stands adjacent to the test foot.
TEST PROCEDURE	The unaffected ankle is tested first. One of the examiner's hands stabilizes the distal tibia and fibula. The thenar web space of the examiner's other hand is placed over the posterior aspect of the talus and calcaneus. The examiner pushes the heel steadily forward, while the other hand stabilizes the distal tibia and fibula. The two sides are compared.
INDICATIONS OF A POSITIVE TEST	Excessive anterior movement and a sucking in of the skin on both sides of the Achilles tendon indicate a positive test result. This test, like the previous one, indicates ligamentous instability, primarily of the anterior talofibular ligament.
CLINICAL NOTE	• The patient may be prepositioned in prone lying with the legs in figure-four position. This position should allow the examiner to place the test leg in the required position.
RELIABILITY/SPECIFICITY/ SENSITIVITY	Unknown

TALAR TILT TEST[37,44,45,47,50,51]

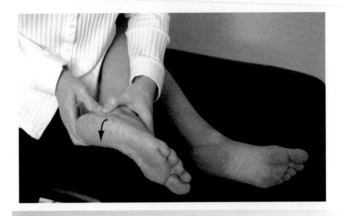

Figure 12–11
Talar tilt test.

PURPOSE	To determine whether the calcaneofibular ligament is torn.
SUSPECTED INJURY	Calcaneofibular ligament sprain
PATIENT POSITION	The patient lies supine or in the side-lying position with the foot relaxed. If the patient is tested in side lying, the test foot is positioned upward.
EXAMINER POSITION	The examiner stands adjacent to the test foot.
TEST PROCEDURE	The unaffected ankle is tested first. One of the examiner's hands is placed anterior to the tibia on top of the navicular, and the other hand is positioned posterior to the tibia over the calcaneus. The two thumbs are placed on the lateral aspect of the calcaneus. The foot is held in the anatomical position (90°), which brings the calcaneofibular ligament perpendicular to the long axis of the talus. The talus then is tilted first into adduction and then into abduction. Adduction tests the calcaneofibular ligament and, to some degree, the anterior talofibular ligament, by increasing the stress on the individual ligaments. Abduction stresses the deltoid ligament, primarily the tibionavicular, tibiocalcaneal, and posterior tibiotalar ligaments, which are components of the deltoid ligament. The two sides are compared.
INDICATIONS OF A POSITIVE TEST	Excessive motion or pain (or both) compared to the unaffected side indicates a positive test result.
CLINICAL NOTES	• The patient's gastrocnemius muscle may be relaxed by flexion of the knee. • If the foot is plantar flexed, the anterior talofibular ligament is more likely to be tested (inversion stress test). • On a radiograph, the talar tilt may be measured by obtaining the angle between the distal aspect of the tibia and the proximal surface of the talus.
RELIABILITY/SPECIFICITY/ SENSITIVITY	Unknown

EXTERNAL ROTATION STRESS TEST (KLEIGER TEST)[38,44,52-58]

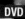

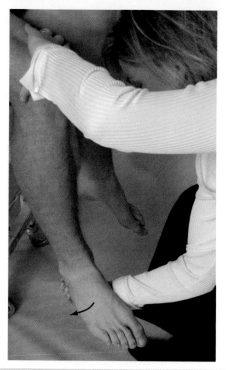

Figure 12–12
External rotation stress test.

PURPOSE	To test for injury to the syndesmosis of the ankle or a high ankle sprain.
SUSPECTED INJURY	Syndesmosis or high ankle sprain
PATIENT POSITION	The patient sits with the leg hanging over the examining table and the knee at 90°.
EXAMINER POSITION	The examiner kneels adjacent to the test foot.
TEST PROCEDURE	Starting with the unaffected ankle, the examiner stabilizes the leg with one hand. The other hand grasps the plantar aspect of the calcaneus. The examiner holds the foot in plantigrade (90°) and applies a passive lateral rotation stress to the foot and ankle. Care must be taken to stabilize the knee with the contralateral hand. The two sides are compared.
INDICATIONS OF A POSITIVE TEST	The test result is positive for a syndesmotic (high ankle) injury if pain is produced over the anterior or posterior tibiofibular ligaments and the interosseous membrane. If the patient has pain medially and the examiner feels the talus displace from the medial malleolus, this may indicate a tear of the deltoid ligament.
CLINICAL NOTES	• On a stress radiograph, if the lateral malleolus is intact, an increase in the medial clear space suggests rupture of the ligament. • The test also may be performed with the patient lying prone and the knee flexed to 90°. The examiner holds the foot in plantigrade and applies a passive lateral rotation stress to the foot and ankle.
RELIABILITY/SPECIFICITY/ SENSITIVITY[52]	Reliability interrater: k = 0.75

OTHER SPECIAL TESTS

FUNCTIONAL LEG LENGTH[59]

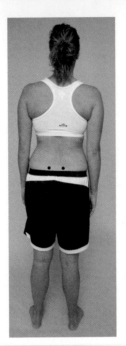

Figure 12–13
Functional leg length in standing (subtalar joint in neutral). The dots on the back indicate the posterior superior iliac spines.

PURPOSE	To assess for leg length discrepancies while the patient is in a weight-bearing position.
PATIENT POSITION	The patient is standing.
EXAMINER POSITION	The examiner sits or kneels directly in front of or behind the patient.
TEST PROCEDURE	The patient stands relaxed while the examiner palpates the level of the anterior superior iliac spines (ASISs) and posterior superior iliac spines (PSISs), noting any asymmetry. The patient then is placed in the "correct" stance (i.e., subtalar joints neutral, knees fully extended, and toes facing straight ahead). The ASISs and PSISs are palpated again, and the examiner notes any changes.
INDICATIONS OF A POSITIVE TEST	If the asymmetry is corrected by "correcting" the position of the limb, the leg is structurally normal (the bones have the proper length), but abnormal joint mechanics (a functional deficit) are producing a functional leg length difference (see Table 9-1). Therefore, if the asymmetry is corrected by proper positioning, the test result is positive for a functional leg length difference.
CLINICAL NOTE	• Functional limb length testing helps the clinician determine whether leg length discrepancies play a role in the patient's pain and dysfunction in weight-bearing positions.
RELIABILITY/SPECIFICITY/ SENSITIVITY	Unknown

THOMPSON'S (SIMMONDS') TEST (SIGN FOR ACHILLES TENDON RUPTURE)[60-63]

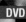

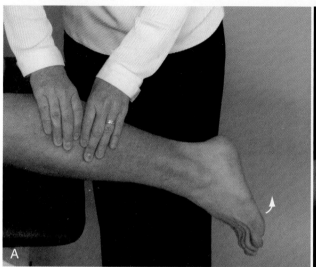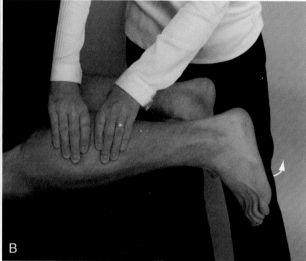

Figure 12–14

Thompson's test for Achilles tendon rupture. **A,** Prone-lying position. **B,** Kneeling position. In each case, the foot plantar-flexes *(arrow)* if the test result is negative.

PURPOSE	To assess for tears (third-degree strain) of the Achilles tendon.
PATIENT POSITION	The patient lies prone or kneels on a chair with the feet over the edge of the table or chair.
EXAMINER POSITION	The examiner stands by the test leg.
TEST PROCEDURE	Starting with the unaffected leg, the examiner squeezes each calf muscle in turn while the patient remains relaxed.
INDICATIONS OF A POSITIVE TEST	A positive test result for a ruptured Achilles tendon (third-degree strain) is indicated by the absence of plantar flexion when the muscle is squeezed.
CLINICAL NOTE	• The examiner should be careful not to assume that the Achilles tendon is not ruptured if the patient can actively plantar flex the foot while non-weight bearing. The long flexor muscles can perform this function in the non-weight bearing stance, even with a rupture of the Achilles tendon.
RELIABILITY/SPECIFICITY/ SENSITIVITY	Unknown

JOINT PLAY MOVEMENTS

LONG AXIS EXTENSION AT THE ANKLE (TALOCRURAL AND SUBTALAR JOINTS)

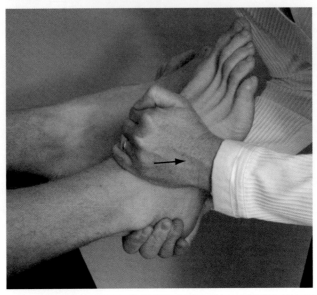

Figure 12–15
Long axis extension at the ankle.

PATIENT POSITION	The patient is supine.
EXAMINER POSITION	The examiner stands at the test foot, facing the patient.
TEST PROCEDURE	Both of the examiner's hands are placed around the ankle, distal to the malleoli, holding the calcaneus posteriorly and the navicular anteriorly. The examiner achieves long-axis extension by applying longitudinal traction to the foot and ankle. The two feet are compared.
INDICATIONS OF A POSITIVE TEST	A positive test result is indicated by too much or too little motion compared to the contralateral side.
CLINICAL NOTES	• A strap may be used at the tibia and fibula to stabilize the leg against the table. • The ankle should be placed in slight plantar flexion for testing. If the ankle is dorsiflexed, which locks the talocrural joint, or if tension is placed on the Achilles tendon, joint play will be restricted.

LONG AXIS EXTENSION AT THE METATARSOPHALANGEAL AND INTERPHALANGEAL JOINTS

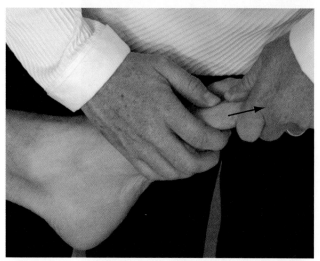

Figure 12–16
Long axis extension at the metatarsophalangeal and interphalangeal joints.

PATIENT POSITION   The patient is supine.

EXAMINER POSITION   The examiner stands by the test foot.

TEST PROCEDURE   The examiner stabilizes the metatarsal bone with the fingers of one hand and grasps the proximal phalanx with the fingers of the other hand, which will move the joint. The examiner stabilizes the metatarsal bone and applies a longitudinal distractive force to the proximal phalanx for the metacarpophalangeal joint. Similarly, by stabilizing the proximal phalanx and distracting the distal phalanx for the proximal and distal interphalangeal joints, traction can be applied. All metatarsophalangeal and interphalangeal joints are tested.

INDICATIONS OF A POSITIVE TEST   A positive test result is indicated by too much or too little motion compared to the contralateral side.

CLINICAL NOTE   • Complete stabilization of the metatarsal bone or proximal phalanx is difficult to achieve. Therefore, while providing the longitudinal force, the examiner should assess when the stabilized segment begins to move. This is also an indication of the end range of the joint.

ANTERIOR-POSTERIOR GLIDE AT THE ANKLE JOINT

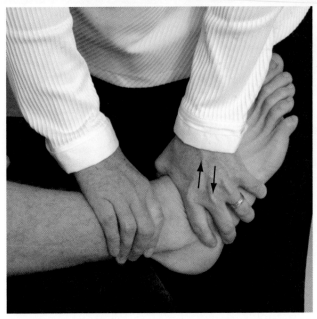

Figure 12–17
Anterior-posterior glide at the ankle joint.

PATIENT POSITION	The patient is supine.
EXAMINER POSITION	The examiner stands by the test foot.
TEST PROCEDURE	The examiner stabilizes the distal tibia and fibula with one hand and grasps the anterior aspect of the foot with the other hand around the navicular. To test posterior glide, the examiner stabilizes the tibia and fibula and pushes the foot posteriorly. To test anterior glide, the examiner pulls the foot forward. The two feet are compared.
INDICATIONS OF A POSITIVE TEST	A positive test result is indicated by too much or too little motion compared to the contralateral side.
CLINICAL NOTES	• During the anterior movement, the foot should move in an arc into plantar flexion. • During the posterior movement, the foot should move in an arc into dorsiflexion. • Although this test is similar to the anterior drawer test, the movements are not the same, because the joint play involves an arc of movement. • The ankle should be placed in slight plantar flexion for testing. If the ankle is dorsiflexed, which locks the talocrural joint, or if tension is placed upon the Achilles tendon, joint play will be restricted.

ANTERIOR-POSTERIOR GLIDE AT THE MIDTARSAL AND TARSOMETATARSAL JOINTS

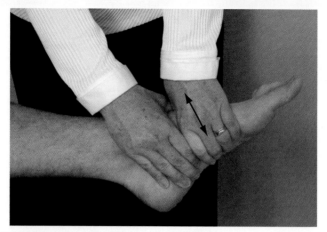

Figure 12–18
Anterior-posterior glide at the midtarsal and tarsometatarsal joints.

PATIENT POSITION The patient is supine.

EXAMINER POSITION The examiner stands by the test foot.

TEST PROCEDURE
- *Step 1:* The examiner stabilizes the navicular, talus, and calcaneus with one hand by grasping the bones in the web space, thumb, and fingers of the examiner's hand. The examiner's other hand is placed around the distal row of tarsal bones (cuneiforms and cuboid). If the hands are positioned properly, they should touch. An anteroposterior gliding movement of the distal row of tarsal bones is applied while the proximal row of tarsal bones is stabilized. The two feet are compared.
- *Step 2:* The examiner's hands then are moved distally so that the stabilizing hand rests over the distal row of tarsal bones and the mobilizing hand rests over the proximal aspect of the metatarsal bones. Again, the hands should be positioned so that they touch. An anteroposterior gliding movement of the metatarsal bones is applied while the distal row of tarsal bones is stabilized. The two feet are compared.

INDICATIONS OF A POSITIVE TEST A positive test result is indicated by too much or too little motion compared to the contralateral side.

CLINICAL NOTES
- Anterior-posterior glide at the midtarsal and tarsometatarsal joints is performed in a fashion similar to that used to test the carpal bones at the wrist stabilizing one bone and moving the adjacent bone.
- Minimal movement is felt when the midtarsal and tarsometatarsal joints are tested.

ANTERIOR-POSTERIOR GLIDE AT THE METATARSOPHALANGEAL AND INTERPHALANGEAL JOINTS

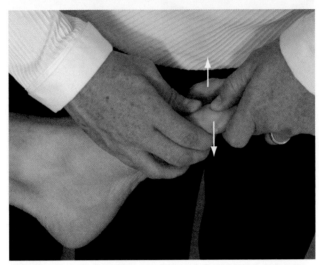

Figure 12–19

Anterior-posterior glide at the metatarsophalangeal and interphalangeal joints

PATIENT POSITION	The patient is supine.
EXAMINER POSITION	The examiner stands by the test foot.
TEST PROCEDURE	The examiner stabilizes the proximal bone (metatarsal or phalanx) and moves the distal bone (phalanx) in an anterior or posterior direction in relation to the stabilized bone. All metatarsophalangeal and interphalangeal joints can be tested in a similar fashion. The two feet are compared.
INDICATIONS OF A POSITIVE TEST	A positive test result is indicated by too much or too little motion compared to the contralateral side.
CLINICAL NOTE	• While applying the anterior or posterior gliding motion, the examiner should note when the stabilized segment begins to move; this indicates the end range of the gliding motion in that direction.

TALAR ROCK

DVD

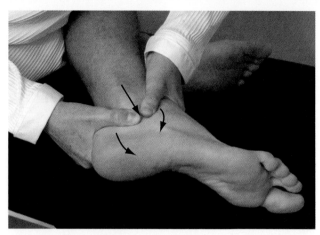

Figure 12–20
Talar rock with slight traction applied. The talus is rocked anteriorly and posteriorly.

PATIENT POSITION	The patient is in the side-lying position. Both the lower hip and knee are flexed for stabilization. The lateral aspect of the test ankle should be facing upward.
EXAMINER POSITION	The examiner sits with his or her back to the test foot so that the examiner's back is against the back of the patient's thigh.
TEST PROCEDURE	The examiner places both hands around the ankle just distal to the malleoli with one hand above the calcaneus and one hand on top of the navicular. The examiner's thumbs are positioned over the lateral calcaneus, and the examiner's fingers wrap around the ankle to the medial aspect of the calcaneus. The examiner applies a slight distractive force to the ankle and a rocking movement, forward and backward (plantar flexion–dorsiflexion), to the foot. The two feet are compared.
INDICATIONS OF A POSITIVE TEST	A positive test result is indicated by too much or too little motion compared to the opposite foot. Normally, the examiner would feel a clunk at the extreme of each movement.

SIDE TILT OF THE CALCANEUS ON THE TALUS

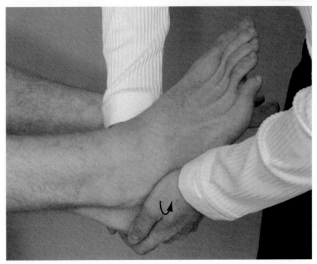

Figure 12–21
Side tilt of the calcaneus on the talus.

PATIENT POSITION	The patient is supine.
EXAMINER POSITION	The examiner stands in front of the test foot.
TEST PROCEDURE	The examiner places the heels of both hands around the calcaneus. The examiner's wrists are flexed and extended, tilting the calcaneus medially and laterally on the talus. The examiner keeps the patient's foot in the anatomical position (90°) while performing the movement. The two feet are compared.
INDICATIONS OF A POSITIVE TEST	A positive test result is indicated by too much or too little motion compared to the contralateral side.
CLINICAL NOTE	• The movement is identical to that used to test the calcaneofibular ligament in the talar tilt test.

ROTATION AT THE MIDTARSAL, TARSOMETATARSAL, METATARSOPHALANGEAL AND PHALANGEAL JOINTS

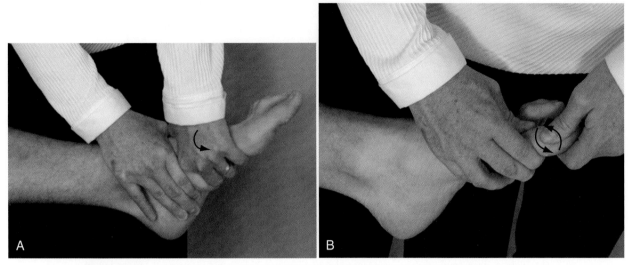

Figure 12–22
Rotation at the **(A)** midtarsal and tarsometatarsal joints and **(B)** metatarsophalangeal and phalangeal joints.

PATIENT POSITION	The patient is supine.
EXAMINER POSITION	The examiner stands beside the test foot.
TEST PROCEDURE	The examiner stabilizes the proximal row of tarsal bones (navicular, calcaneus, and talus) with one hand. The examiner's other (mobilizing) hand is placed around the distal tarsal bones (cuneiforms and cuboid). If the hands are positioned properly, they should touch. A slight distractive force is applied to the joint, and the distal row of bones is rotated on the proximal row of bones. The examiner then moves the hands down to the distal tarsal and metatarsal joints and repeats the rotation. Similarly, the examiner moves the hands down to the metatarsal and proximal phalanx joints and repeats the rotation, followed by the interphalangeal joints. The two feet are compared.
INDICATIONS OF A POSITIVE TEST	A positive test result is indicated by too much or too little motion compared to the contralateral side. Normally, movement is minimal and pain free.
CLINICAL NOTE	• Rotation at the metatarsophalangeal and interphalangeal joints is performed by stabilizing the proximal bone with one hand, applying slight traction, and rotating the distal bone with the other hand.

SIDE GLIDE AT THE METATARSOPHALANGEAL AND INTERPHALANGEAL JOINTS

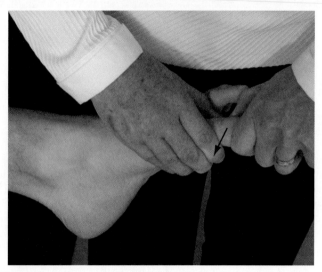

Figure 12–23
Side glide at the metatarsophalangeal and interphalangeal joints.

PATIENT POSITION	The patient is supine.
EXAMINER POSITION	The examiner stands beside the test foot.
TEST PROCEDURE	The examiner stabilizes the proximal bone with one hand and places the other (mobilizing) hand around the distal bone. The examiner then uses the mobilizing hand to apply a slight distractive force to the distal bone and moves the distal bone sideways (right and left) in relation to the stabilized bone. The two feet are compared.
INDICATIONS OF A POSITIVE TEST	A positive test result is indicated by too much or too little motion compared to the contralateral side. Normally, the amount of movement is small, and movement is pain free.
CLINICAL NOTE	• The examiner should avoid torsion motion at the joint.

References

1. Kaufman KR, Brodine SK, Schaffer RA et al: The effect of foot structure and range of motion on musculoskeletal overuse injuries, *Am J Sports Med* 27:585-593, 1999.

2. Mizel MS, Hecht PJ, Marymount JV et al: Evaluation and treatment of chronic ankle pain, *J Bone Joint Surg Am* 86:622-632, 2004.

3. Patla CE, Abbott JH: Tibialis posterior myofascial tightness as a source of heel pain: diagnosis and treatment, *J Orthop Sports Phys Ther* 30:624-632, 2000.

4. Stovitz SD, Coetzee JC: Hyperpronation and foot pain: steps toward pain-free feet, *Phys Sportsmed* 32:19-26, 2004.

5. McCrory P, Bladin C: Fractures of the lateral process of the talus: a clinical review—"snowboarder's ankle," *Clin J Sports Med* 6:124-128, 1996.

6. Garrow AP, Silman AJ, Macfarlane GJ: The Cheshire foot pain and disability survey: a population survey assessing prevalence and associations, *Pain* 110:378-384, 2004.

7. Greenberg L, Davis H: Foot problems in the US: the 1990 National Health Interview Survey, *J Am Podiatr Med Assoc* 83:475-483, 1993.

8. Hannan MT, McLennan CE, Rivinus MC et al: Population-based study of foot disorders in men and women from the Framingham Study, *Arthritis Rheum* 54(Suppl): S497, 2006.

9. Hill C, Gill T, Menz H, Taylor A: Prevalence and correlates of foot pain in a population-based study: the North West Adelaide Health Study, *J Foot Ankle Res* 1:1-7, 2008.

10. Kannus V: Evaluation of abnormal biomechanics of the foot and ankle in athletes, *Br J Sports Med* 26:83-89, 1992.

11. Picciano AM, Rowlands MS, Worrel T: Reliability of open and closed kinetic chain subtalar joint neutral positions and navicular drop test, *J Orthop Sports Phys Ther* 18: 553-558, 1993.

12. Elveru RA, Rothstein JM, Lamb RL: Goniometric reliability in a clinical setting: subtalar and ankle joint measurements, *Phys Ther* 68:672-677, 1988.

13. Mueller MJ, Host JV, Norton BJ: Navicular drop as a composite measure of excessive pronation, *J Am Podiatr Med Assoc* 83:198-202, 1993.

14. Torbum L, Perry J, Gronley JK: Assessment of rearfoot motion: passive positioning, one-legged standing gait, *Foot Ankle Int* 19:688-693, 1998.

15. Smith-Oricchio K, Harris BA: Interrater reliability of subtalar neutral calcaneal inversion and eversion, *J Orthop Sports Phys Ther* 12:10-15, 1990.

16. Sell KE, Verity TM, Worrell TW et al: Two measurement techniques for assessing subtalar joint position: a reliability study, *J Orthop Sports Phys Ther* 19:162-167, 1994.

17. Palmer ML, Epler M: *Clinical assessment procedures in physical therapy,* Philadelphia, 1990, JB Lippincott.

18. McPoil TG, Brocato RS: The foot and ankle: biomechanical evaluation and treatment. In Gould JA (ed): *Orthopedic and sports physical therapy,* St Louis, 1990, Mosby.

19. Root ML, Orien WP, Weed JH: *Normal and abnormal function of the foot,* Los Angeles, 1977, Clinical Biomechanics.

20. Roy S, Irvin R: *Sports medicine: prevention, evaluation, management and rehabilitation,* Englewood Cliffs, NJ, 1983, Prentice-Hall.

21. Shrader JA, Poporich JM, Gracey GC et al: Navicular drop measurement in people with rheumatoid arthritis: interrater and intrarater reliability, *Phys Ther* 85:656-664, 2005.

22. Loudon JK, Jenkins W, Loudon KL: The relationships between static posture and ACL injury in female athletes, *J Orthop Sports Phys Ther* 24:91-97, 1996.

23. Power CM, Maffucci R, Hampton S: Rearfoot posture in subjects with patellofemoral pain, *J Orthop Sports Phys Ther* 22:155-160, 1995.

24. Jonson SR, Gross MT: Intraexaminer reliability, interexaminer reliability, and mean values for nine lower extremity skeletal measures in healthy naval midshipmen, *J Orthop Sports Phys Ther* 25:253-263, 1997.

25. Davids JR, Davis RB: Tibial torsion: significance and measurement, *Gait Posture* 26:169-171, 2007.

26. Karol LA: Rotational deformities in the lower extremities, *Curr Opin Pediatr* 9:77-80, 1997.

27. Kling TF Jr, Hensinger RN: Angular and torsional deformities of the lower limbs in children, *Clin Orthop* 176: 136-147, 1983.

28. Nagamine R, Miyanishi K, Miura H et al: Medial torsion of the tibia in Japanese patients with osteoarthritis of the knee, *Clin Orthop Relat Res* 408:218-224, 2003.

29. Turner M: The association between tibial torsion and knee joint pathology, *Clin Orthop Relat Res* 302:47-51, 1994.

30. Staheli LT, Corbett M, Wyss C et al: Lower extremity rotational problems in children: normal values to guide management, *J Bone Joint Surg Am* 67:39-47, 1985.

31. Hunt GC, Brocato RS: Gait and foot pathomechanics. In Hunt GC (ed): *Physical therapy of the foot and ankle: clinics in physical therapy,* Edinburgh, 1988, Churchill Livingstone.

32. Reisch SF, Noceti-Dewit LM: The foot and ankle: physical therapy patient management utilizing current evidence. In *Current concepts of orthopaedic physical therapy,* ed 2, La Crosse, WI, 2006, Orthopedic Section, American Physical Therapy Association.

33. Strauss JE, Forsberg JA, Lippert FG: Chronic lateral ankle instability and associated conditions: a rationale for treatment, *Foot Ankle Int* 28:1041-1044, 2007.

34. Wolfe MW, Uhl ML, Mccluskey LC: Management of ankle sprains, *Am Fam Physician* 63:93-104, 2001.

35. Young CC: Ankle sprain, *EMedicine Journal* (1)3, 2002.

36. Lindstrand A: New aspects in the diagnosis of lateral ankle sprains, *Orthop Clin North Am* 7:247-249, 1976.

37. Hollis JM, Blasier RD, Flahiff CM: Simulated ankle ligamentous injury: change in ankle stability, *Am J Sports Med* 23:672-677, 1995.

38. Trojian TH, McKeag DB: Ankle sprains: expedient assessment and management, *Phys Sportsmed* 26:29-40, 1998.

39. Frost HM, Hanson CA: Technique for testing the drawer sign in the ankle, *Clin Orthop* 123:49-51, 1977.

40. Birrer RB, Cartwright TJ, Denton JR: Immediate diagnosis of ankle trauma, *Phys Sportsmed* 22:95-102, 1994.

41. Birrer RB, Cartwright TJ, Denton JR: Immediate diagnosis of ankle trauma, *Phys Sportsmed* 22:95-102, 1994.

42. Aradi AJ, Wong J, Walsh M: The dimple sign of a ruptured lateral ligament of the ankle: brief report, *J Bone Joint Surg Br* 70:327-328, 1988.

43. Davis PF, Trevino SG: Ankle injuries. In Baxter DE (ed): *The foot and ankle in sport,* St Louis, 1995, Mosby.

44. Hockenbury RT, Sammarco GJ: Evaluation and treatment of ankle sprains: clinical recommendations for a positive outcome, *Phys Sportsmed* 24:57-64, 2001.

45. Kjaersgaard-Andersen P, Frich LH, Madsen F et al: Instability of the hindfoot after lesion of the lateral ankle ligaments: investigations of the anterior drawer and adduction maneuvers in autopsy specimens, *Clin Orthop* 266:170-179, 1991.

46. Colter JM: Lateral ligamentous injuries of the ankle. In Hamilton WC (ed): *Traumatic disorders of the ankle,* New York, 1984, Springer-Verlag.

47. Kelikian H, Kelikian AS: *Disorders of the ankle,* Philadelphia, 1985, Saunders.

48. Jahss MH: *Disorders of the foot,* Philadelphia, 1982, Saunders.

49. Gungor T: A test for ankle instability: brief report, *J Bone Joint Surg Br* 70:487, 1988.

50. Mennell JM: *Foot pain,* Boston, 1969, Little, Brown.

51. Reid DC: *Sports injury assessment and rehabilitation,* New York, 1992, Churchill Livingstone.

52. Alonso A, Khoury L, Adams R: Clinical tests for ankle syndesmosis injury: reliability and prediction of return to function, *J Orthop Sports Phys Ther* 27:276-284, 1998.

53. Peng JR: Solving the dilemma of the high ankle sprain in the athlete, *Sports Med Arthro Rev* 8:316-325, 2000.

54. Brosky T, Nyland J, Nitz A et al: The ankle ligaments: consideration of syndesmotic injury and implications for rehabilitation, *J Orthop Sports Phys Ther* 21:197-205, 1995.

55. Nussbaum ED, Hosea TM, Sieler SD et al: Prospective evaluation of syndesmotic ankle sprains without diastasis, *Am J Sports Med* 29:31-35, 2001.

56. Boytim MJ, Fischer DA, Neuman L: Syndesmotic ankle sprains, *Am J Sports Med* 19:294-298, 1991.

57. Wright RW, Barile RJ, Surprenant DA et al: Ankle syndesmosis sprains in national hockey league players, *Am J Sports Med* 32:1941-1945, 2004.

58. Lin C-F, Gross MT, Weinfeld P: Ankle syndesmosis injuries: anatomy, biomechanics, mechanism of injury, and clinical guidelines for diagnosis and intervention, *J Orthop Sports Phys Ther* 36:372-384, 2006.

59. Wallace LA: Limb length difference and back pain. In Grieve GP (ed): *Modern manual therapy of the vertebral column,* Edinburgh, 1986, Churchill Livingstone.

60. Thompson T, Doherty J: Spontaneous rupture of the tendon of Achilles: a new clinical diagnostic test, *Anat Res* 158:126-129, 1967.

61. Scott BW, Al-Chalabi A: How the Simmonds-Thompson test works, *J Bone Joint Surg Br* 74:314-315, 1992.

62. Simmonds FA: The diagnosis of a ruptured Achilles tendon, *Practitioner* 179:56-58, 1957.

63. Thompson TC: A test for rupture of the tendoachilles, *Acta Orthop Scand* 32:461-465, 1962.

INDEX

Note: Page numbers followed by f indicate figures; those followed by t indicate tables.